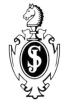

THE
SCARS
OF
VENUS

A History of Venereology

J.D. Oriel

Springer-Verlag
London Berlin Heidelberg New York
Paris Tokyo Hong Kong
Barcelona Budapest

J. David Oriel, MD

Department of Medicine, University College and Middlesex School of
Medicine, 5 University Street, London WC1E 6JJ, UK

ISBN 3–540–19844–X Springer-Verlag Berlin Heidelberg New York
ISBN 0–387–19844–X Springer-Verlag New York Berlin Heidelberg

British Library Cataloguing in Publication Data
Oriel, J. D.
  Scars of Venus: History of Venereology
  I. Title
  616.9
  ISBN 3–540–19844–X

Library of Congress Cataloging-in-Publication Data
Oriel, J. D.
  The scars of Venus : a history of venereology / J.D. Oriel.
    p. cm.
  Includes bibliographical references and index.
  ISBN 3–540–19844–X (alk. paper). — ISBN 0–387–19844–X
  (alk. paper)
  1. Sexually transmitted diseases—History. I. Title. [DNLM:
  1. Sexually Transmitted Diseases. 2. Venereology—history.
  WC 140 069s 1994]
  RC201.4.075   1994
  616.9'5'09—dc20
  DNLM/DLC
  for Library of Congress   93–34554

Typeset by Electronic Book Factory Limited, Fife, Scotland
Printed by The Alden Press Ltd, Osney Mead, Oxford
28/3830–543210 Printed on acid-free paper

Preface

Sex is a private and pleasurable activity but – the thorn on the rose – it may result in disease. If so, much of the privacy and pleasure is lost. The victim and his or her consorts will seek advice and treatment from doctors and perhaps from other medical workers, and subsequent progress will depend on their knowledge, skill and understanding. In this book I have tried to describe the development of ideas on the cause, diagnosis, treatment and prevention of venereal diseases from the ancient world until the outbreak of AIDS ten years ago. I have used the term "venereal diseases" because this, rather than "sexually transmitted diseases" was how they were described in the literature until quite recently.

Our present-day knowledge of the subject is derived from the work of doctors, laboratory scientists and dedicated laymen. Some were eminent, the subjects of full-length biographies, but others were little known even in their day and some have been completely forgotten. I have been fascinated by these people, who founded venereology and contributed so much to the welfare of the victims of venereal diseases, their sex partners and their children. Where did they work? How did their ideas develop, and how did they put them into practice? How were they regarded by their friends and colleagues? Some of them – Ricord and Fournier, for example – devoted virtually their whole careers to venereology; for others such as Bell and Hutchinson it formed only part of their professional interests and a few, such as Credé, touched and illuminated the subject only briefly.

I am not a trained historian, so cannot deploy the apparatus of scholarship. Colleagues who are expert in these matters will, I fear, be dismayed by the preponderance of secondary over primary references. I have tried to read the original papers dealing with major discoveries myself and to indicate where translations of these are available. Venereal diseases present major public health and social problems. The most important of these have been considered briefly, but I have not attempted to write a social history of venereal disease, a subject which has been undertaken by others with abler pens than my own.

I hope that this book will interest readers who are concerned in any way with patients with venereal diseases: doctors, nurses, counsellors, laboratory and public health workers. I have tried to show the debt which we owe to those who have led us here. I believe that a knowledge of the past does help to illuminate the present, although historians are notoriously bad at predicting the future.

Acknowledgements

Dr Geoffrey Ridgway most kindly read the whole manuscript, correcting errors in both grammar and microbiology. Dr Robert Morton drew on his knowledge and experience to advise me on several difficult matters, and Professor Adrian Mindel, Dr John Oates, Dr Nicol Thin and Dr Michael Waugh commented on individual chapters. I am very grateful to all these colleagues for their help; remaining errors are, of course, mine alone.

Mr William Schupbach at the Wellcome Institute Library, London, kindly provided several illustrations, and the staff of this Library, and of the Royal Society of Medicine Library, could not have been more helpful. I am indebted to them.

Every effort has been made to trace all the copyright holders of material used in this book, but if any have been inadvertently overlooked the publishers will be pleased to make the necessary arrangements at the first opportunity.

Contents

Chapter 1
Origins

─────────────

Venereal diseases are like the fine arts – it is pointless to ask
who invented them.

Voltaire, *Dictionnaire philosophique*

Thoughtful writers seeking to interpret the history of medicine have often declared that the best-known venereal diseases – syphilis, gonorrhoea, chancroid and lymphogranuloma venereum – have affected humans since the dawn of time. Seeking proof for this opinion they have pored over ancient texts and manuscripts, finding a sentence here and a few lines of verse there which convince them that they are right. To base conclusions on insufficient evidence can lead to serious errors, and the subject of the early history of venereal disease deserves reconsideration.

The evolution of disease-producing microbes is well understood. Microbiologists believe that the first bacteria appeared as free-living organisms, but as higher forms of life evolved some found a more sheltered environment by colonising the tissues and body fluids of other creatures. Many became adapted to living within the cells of their hosts, a process which was taken a stage further by other bacteria which discarded some of their metabolic equipment so that they became "energy parasites"; chlamydiae probably evolved in this way. The origin of viruses is uncertain. The dependence on the host cell which we have just noted may eventually have become absolute, the organism then consisting of no more than a molecule of nucleic acid within a protective protein coat. Alternatively, viruses may have been formed from small fragments of genetic material which had broken loose within an animal, plant or bacterial cell and become independent "footloose genes". A third view is that viruses originated very early in the evolutionary time scale as aggregates of gene-like substances which appeared in the primeval waters before the advent of cells, adopting an intracellular existence when this became possible[1].

The majority of animal parasites are harmless, living in peaceful symbiosis with their hosts, but during the slow process of evolution disease-producing mutants may appear. Pathogenicity has advantages and disadvantages for an invading organism. It may aid dissemination of the microbes to new hosts, for example by causing diarrhoea or infective discharges. On the other hand, excessive virulence may result in the host's death before there has been time for any significant spread. A balance has to be struck, and the most successful parasites are those which establish a prolonged period of infectivity, even if some may eventually inflict severe damage or death on the host. Tuberculosis, diphtheria and typhoid furnish good examples of this process. A critical point in the life cycle of a pathogen occurs when it is transferring to a new host, perhaps through a hostile environment. Sexual transmission has obvious advantages here, for the contact between infected and susceptible tissues could hardly be more direct. In some cases the infection could also be transmitted "vertically" to the host's offspring.

The identity of the primordial human sexually transmitted diseases is unknown, but some clues may come from a consideration of animal infections. As humans evolved from lower animals, their parasites probably evolved with them. As Francis Bacon (1561–1626) remarked: "Man is of kin to the beasts with his body". There is a close resemblance between some current human and animal sexually transmitted diseases – for example, trichomoniasis, genital herpes and genital warts – and these may have been the most ancient human venereal infections[2]. On the other hand, *Neisseria* are not pathogenic to animals, in whom a contagious urethritis is unknown; gonorrhoea was clearly a late arrival on the evolutionary scene. The position of syphilis is more obscure, because knowledge of the distribution of treponemes among animals is scanty. Rabbits are subject to a treponemal disease which is spread by cutaneous contact in burrows; rabbit syphilis is a dermatosis without systemic signs, resembling human pinta. An avirulent treponematosis in cynocephalus monkeys was described many years ago[3], but no disease resembling venereal syphilis affects any animal species. It is reasonable to think that while some venereal infections – genital herpes, genital warts and possibly trichomoniasis – have been inherited from mankind's remote ancestors, with relatively minor mutations in their causal organisms, others, such as syphilis and gonorrhoea, are of much more recent origin.

A study of the evolution of infectious diseases may enable us to say *how* a particular venereal infection appeared, but it will not tell us *when* or *where* this happened. To answer these questions it is necessary to peruse the old medical and non-medical literature, and many difficulties will be encountered. Primary sources are often inaccessible, translations may be inaccurate or use obsolete terminology, and the tone of much writing on medical subjects is often poetic or allegorical rather than scientific. In early times almost nothing was known about the causes of diseases, which were attributed to the effects of spirits or disorders of the Galenic humours; while several early civilisations had excellent public health facilities, the idea that contagion was a factor in the aetiology of some diseases was not acknowledged before the Renaissance. Clinical observation was often poor, and to complicate matters further some doctors regarded genital infection with distaste, as indeed they do today. According to Celsus (first century AD) both physicians and patients spoke only with reserve of the private parts: "it is not therefore an easy thing for one who wishes to observe the rules of propriety without departing from the rules of art to treat these diseases".

The first description of genital infections may have appeared in ancient China. A French naval officer, Captain Dabry, studied a compilation of Chinese medical writing which went back to 2500 BC and published his findings in 1863, but according to the French syphilologist Lancereaux[4] he did not always quote his sources or give accurate dates. He described a "corroding ulcer" of the genitals in men and women which developed a few days after coitus, followed by ulceration of the throat and anus. Some readers of his report were inclined to attribute the disorder to syphilis, but a specific diagnosis is hardly possible from the clinical information given. Other descriptions of genital lesions culled from ancient Chinese and Japanese sources have appeared, but are too remote and unreliable

2

to be considered here. In ancient Egypt the Ebers papyrus (*c.* 1550 BC) contains a reference to vulval inflammation which has, rather unconvincingly, been ascribed to gonorrhoea; in modern times, investigation of Egyptian mummies has shown no evidence of syphilitic bone disease.

In the Old Testament there are accounts of marital infidelity, prostitution, sexual orgies, phallic worship and obscene rites. Some commentators have maintained that there are references to venereal disease as well; for example, it has been suggested that the following passage refers to secondary syphilis:

> "The Lord will smite thee with the botch of Egypt, and with the emerods, and with the scab, and with the itch, whereof thou canst not be healed."
>
> Deuteronomy 28: 27

It should be remembered that this is a small part of a long list of misfortunes which, according to the author, will overtake those who do not follow Mosaic law. It is an admonition, not a clinical description of a disease. Another passage from the Old Testament reads:

> "My wounds stink and are corrupt because of my foolishness . . . for my loins are filled with a loathsome disease, and there is no soundness in my flesh."
>
> Psalms 38: 5, 7

This is part of a spiritual lamentation, and it seems very unlikely that the author intended it to be taken literally. To drag it out of context and suggest that it refers to syphilis or lymphogranuloma venereum is as absured as it would be to say that when John Keats in his *Ode to a Nightingale* wrote: "My heart aches and a drowsy numbness pains my sense" he was describing a coronary thrombosis. Some biblical characters, for example David, are said to have contracted syphilis, but the story of David and Bath-sheba, in which it is written that "she came in unto him and he lay with her, for she was purified of her uncleanness" (Samuel 2: 11, 4) could be interpreted in any way the reader chooses. Job (Figure 1.1) is another Biblical character who has been suspected of syphilis. He had many complaints, among them skin ulcers, loss of hair, foul breath, bone pains, anorexia, diarrhoea and fever, but he kept his belief in God and lived to a ripe old age. The story is far more likely to be an allegory of religious progress than a description of venereal disease.

Some commentators have been tempted to attribute some of the plagues described in the Old Testament to syphilis[5]. An example was an epidemic which followed the Israelites' worship of Baal, accompanied by wild promiscuity with prostitutes from the enemy kingdom of Moab. Moses recommended summary execution of devotees of Baal, and "the plague was stayed from the children of Israel"; however, 24000 people died (Numbers 25: 9). Syphilis seems a very unlikely cause of the plague in this context. In truth, these accounts of putative syphilis in the ancient world are simply conjectures which will not stand up to critical investigation. When syphilis *did* appear in Europe at the end of the fifteenth century it spread with alarming speed to many other localities and was uniformly regarded as a *new* disease.

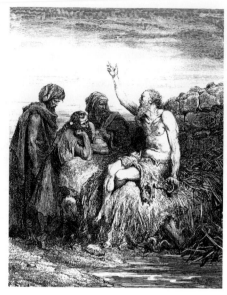

Figure 1.1. Job, suspected of having syphilis. From an engraving by Gustav Doré (mid nineteenth century).

How old is gonorrhoea? In his *Traité de la Blennorragie*, published in 1912, Georges Luys (1870–1953), a Parisian surgeon with a special interest in the subject, made a categorical statement: "Gonorrhoea is as old as mankind and urethral discharges have, no doubt, been known at all times"[6]. This *a priori* reasoning has been repeated many times. What evidence is there that gonorrhoea existed among the peoples described in the Old Testament? The medical practices of the Hebrews emphasised preventive measures, as is clear from the following well-known quotation:

> "When any man hath a running issue out of his flesh, because of his issue he is unclean. And this shall be his uncleanness in his issue: whether his flesh run with his issue, or his flesh be stopped from his issue, it is his uncleanness."
>
> Leviticus, 15: 2

In subsequent verses the contamination of persons or objects by the victim and the need for purification by washing are described at length. Clearly this passage refers to a septic discharging condition, but since the part affected is not specified there is no way of knowing whether "issue" means a contagious urethritis or a discharge from some other site. Even if "running issue" referred to a urethritis, this could just as well have been non-gonococcal as gonococcal.

The works of Hippocrates (*c.* 460–377 BC) and his pupils appeared about two centuries after Deuteronomy. Disorders of urination, menstruation and pregnancy were all described, and there is one reference to "moist ulcers, particularly of the mouth and genitals". The following fragment from *De locis affectis* has been held to refer to gonorrhoea:

4

"No disease has more varied symptoms than strangury. It is most commonly found in youths and old men. In the latter it is more rebellious, but nobody dies of it."

The proposal that the word strangury means gonorrhoea has no apparent foundation. It is derived from the Greek *stragx*, a trickle, and *ouron*, urine, and it means a squeezing out of urine in drops. Hippocrates was probably referring either to cystitis or to urinary obstruction from stricture, calculi or prostatic enlargement. It has been suggested that ancient philosophers such as Plato, Aristotle and Epicurus alluded to gonorrhoea in their works, or suffered from it themselves, but the evidence for this is meagre. The English physician and classical scholar John Davy Rolleston (1873–1946) studied the vast collection of epigrams extending over many centuries which is known as the Greek Anthology without finding anything indicative of syphilis or gonorrhoea[7]. He commented that this is all the more remarkable as two sections of the Anthology consist entirely of erotic poems and explicit references to sexual activities. In some epigrams the god Priapus threatens thieves with *pedicatio* (buggery) as a punishment; this would have been a good time to threaten gonorrhoea as well had it existed then, but there is no allusion to it.

Many of the Latin poets give a vivid picture of a world of unrestrained promiscuity. The satirists Martial (AD 40–130) and Juvenal (AD 60–127) wrote for a sophisticated public, and were quite explicit about sexual matters. In several passages they refer to anogenital warts, which were then called *fici*, figs. There is no doubt at all that the ancients regarded this disease as a result of promiscuity and homosexuality:

> In order to buy some slave boys
> Labienus sold his garden;
> But now he has only
> An orchard of figs.
>
> Martial, *Epigrams* vii, 71

> Hairy legs and forearms
> May suggest machismo,
> But the doctor smiles as he removes
> The figs from your smooth anus.
>
> Juvenal, *Satires* ii, 11

Neither of these poets referred to any disease which can be identified as syphilis or gonorrhoea. Henry St Hill Vertue (1891–1966), another English doctor familiar with the classics, having read the whole of Juvenal's *Satires* concluded that "in Juvenal's day there was no such thing as venereal disease; or to put the matter in another way the fact that Juvenal says nothing about venereal disease is alone almost proof that where he was it was not."[8] The medical historian Jean Astruc (1684–1766) pointed out that the absence of any mention of the venereal diseases by these ancient authors is in striking contrast to the outspoken comments made by French poets on the outbreak of syphilis at the end of the fifteenth century, and by Rabelais and others on gonorrhoea.

Celsus (25 BC – AD 50; Figure 1.2), the earliest Latin medical writer, devoted

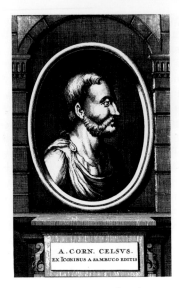

Figure 1.2. Celsus (25 BC–AD 50). From an undated portrait by J van der Spytz. (By courtesy of the Wellcome Institute Library, London.)

a whole chapter of his *De medicina* to genital diseases. He described ulceration of the glans penis complicating phimosis, retention of urine and its relief by catheterisation, and growths and gangrene of the penis. He discussed *profusio seminis* in these words:

"There is a fault in the genital region called the shedding of semen. It occurs without sexual desire or erotic dreams and in such a way that in time the patient is consumed by wasting."

Galen (AD 130–200; Figure 1.3) was the most famous Greek physician after Hippocrates and his opinions, based on the humoral tradition, dominated European medicine until the Renaissance. Like Celsus he described penile ulcers and reported anogenital excrescences which were probably warts. In *De locis affectis* he was the first to use the word *gonorrhoea* (Greek *gonos*, semen and *rhoia*, to flow) to describe a condition similar to *profusio seminis*:

"Gonorrhoea is an unwanted excretion of semen which you may also call involuntary; or to be more precise you might say a persistent excretion of semen without erection of the penis."

These descriptions do not suggest a disease resembling gonorrhoea as we know it today. Vertue comments:

"Now, is it likely that one of the most outstanding physicians that the world has known [Galen] would have passed without a word over the strongly marked features of contagious urethritis, with its unmistakable sequence of cause and event, the intense local inflammation, the

6

discharge, the stampings, gaspings, cursings of the sufferer when he is passing water, the gleet, the chordee, the relapse, the stricture, the injury to the innocent spouse, the blinded offspring? It is impossible"![8]

According to Galen's contemporary, Aretaeus of Cappadocia (second century AD), a notable Greek physician, *gonorrhoea* is a persistent flow of semen without sensation. The fluid which runs off is "thin, cold, colourless and unfruitful". Women also have the disorder, but "their semen is discharged with titillation of the parts, and with pleasure and an immodest desire for connection with men"[9]. Again, the patients became progressively more feeble. It is hard to understand what Aretaeus meant by this. What was this disease? Possible diagnoses include chronic non-gonococcal urethritis, spermatorrhoea, prostatitis and, in women, leucorrhoea; certainly it was not a gonococcal infection, unless gonorrhoea has completely changed its character since then.

Karl Sudhoff (1853–1938) held the first German chair in the history of medicine, at Leipzig; he was well known for his strict historical method, based on the use of original sources. Writing in 1917, he observed: "The literary proof that syphilis existed in Greece and Rome must, for the present at least, be considered a failure"[10]. The widely held belief that gonorrhoea existed at that time is likewise poorly supported. Balanitis, genital ulcers, gangrene and tumours, anogenital warts and retention of urine were common enough, and no doubt formed as large a part of the workload of Greek and Roman physicians as they do of today's urologists. Treatment in those far-off times was rudimentary and largely symptomatic, but catheters were used to relieve retention of urine.

Rome was sacked by barbarians in AD 410, and by AD 500 the western Empire had disappeared. Medical activity continued in the eastern Empire, centred on Constantinople; many doctors had fled there, taking their medical texts with them. The Graeco-Roman tradition established by Hippocrates, Celsus and

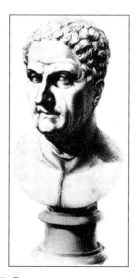

Figure 1.3. Galen (AD 130–200). From an anonymous undated marble bust. (By courtesy of the Wellcome Institute Library, London.)

Galen was maintained, but in this rigid and bureaucratic society there were no new ideas and Byzantine medicine became stagnant. Compilations of existing knowledge of genital disease were made by Oribasius (325–400) and Paul of Aegina (625–690). While some features of venereal disease were described – genital ulcers, warts and vaginal discharge – much was missing. As the medical historian Cecilia Mettler has aptly observed, "everywhere one becomes entangled in the net of humoral theory, most particularly at those points where information is most needed"[11]. According to Rolleston[7], the French dermatologist Antoine Edouard Jeanselme (1858–1935) studied the voluminous Byzantine literature for his *Histoire de la Syphilis* without finding any relevant passages, and descriptions of the pain and purulent discharge of gonorrhoea were likewise absent.

If medicine was inert in Byzantium it was flourishing in Islam. Arabic culture, centred in the huge city of Baghdad, reached its peak in the ninth and tenth centuries, with a particular emphasis on mathematics and science. The medical writings of the ancients had been translated into Arabic, and in turn Islamic physicians wrote works which were to become standard textbooks in the western world. Although again they did not describe any disease like syphilis, there seems little doubt that they were seeing patients with gonorrhoea. Rhazes (860–932) was an observant clinician. He wrote of urethral discharge and its treatment by irrigation, he was familiar with urethral stricture, and he emphasised the importance of catheterisation if there was a threat of retention of urine. Ibn Sina (Avicenna; 980–1037) was a flamboyant and highly successful physician whose *Canon of Medicine*, a compendium of medical practice, was enormously popular in the Middle Ages. He described the treatment of acute urethritis by irrigating the urethra through a silver syringe, and used catheters prepared from the skin of various animals to treat acute retention. He is said to have supplemented these measures by inserting a louse into the terminal urethra. This famous insect, sometimes transformed into a bug or flea, appears again and again in the literature[12]. A tenth-century writer, or group of writers, called pseudo-Mesue, clearly influenced by Hippocratic ideas of the benefits of suppuration, wrote:

"All inflammatory tumours formed in the passage of the urine produce at first pain accompanied by strangury; then pus is formed, and as it flows the inflammatory tumours and strangury are dispersed[13]".

Students of this literature agree that there is no evidence that syphilis existed in Europe in the early Middle Ages, and Jeanselme concluded that documents published before 1493 allegedly referring to the disease were spurious. John Freind (1675–1728) was a well-known London physician, a man of real learning and the only author mentioned in these pages to be imprisoned in the Tower of London on a charge of high treason – he became involved in a plot to restore the Stuart dynasty and was lucky to be released after only three months[14]. While immured he began his master-work, *History of Physick from the time of Galen to the beginning of the Sixteenth Century*, which was published in 1725. He placed the origin of syphilis no earlier than the fifteenth century[8]. On the other hand, Arabian physicians of the tenth and eleventh centuries were seeing patients with acute urethritis similar to the gonorrhoea we see today and unlike the "gonorrhoea" described by the ancients. The conclusion is inescapable: gonorrhoea originated in the Middle Ages, probably from a mutation of a saprophytic *Neisseria* into a virulent form. There are two possibilities. Vertue thought that in early times a precursory *Neisseria* infected the vaginal and rectal mucosae of young girls, where it caused no more than a mild vulvovaginitis. After a mutation the organism, now *N. gonorrhoeae*, became virulent and invasive and caused the disease we know today. Another possibility is that mutation to *N. gonorrhoeae* occurred in one of the non-pathogenic neisseriae which colonise the nasopharynx; the new organism could then easily reach the genital tract through oral sex.

In the ninth century a school of medicine was founded at Salerno, in southern Italy, with teaching based on Graeco-Roman and Arabian doctrines. As time went by other schools were established, and some medical texts began to appear; from these and lay writings of the period the evolution of venereology from the twelfth century onwards can be traced. Roger of Salerno (*fl.* 1170) described a disease characterised by pain, burning, redness and swelling of the penis, and difficulty in urination; this could be complicated by epididymitis, and was no doubt gonorrhoea. A Salernian aphorism of the time was *Post coitum si mingas, apte servabis urethram* (urination after intercourse protects your urethra). In England, references to *brenning* (burning), *ardor urinae* (dysuria) and, among the French speaking classes, *chaudepiss* began to appear. Perhaps because of its short incubation period its venereal nature was soon appreciated. The word *clap* replaced *chaudepiss* late in the sixteenth century. Its origin is obscure. According to the *Oxford English Dictionary*, it was first used in 1587 in the poem *King Malin* in the *Mirror for Magistrates*:

> "They give no heede before they get the clap
> And then too late they wish they had been wise."

Gonorrhoea was often treated by urethral injections, and many different agents were recommended. John of Arderne (1306–1390), who had at one time been physician to Richard II, suggested:

> "Against a burning of the male yard [penis] from heat and excoriation within, use the following soothing injection. Take the milk of a woman, a little sugar, oil of violets and barley water and administer it with a syringe."

Retention of urine was treated by introducing a wax bougie, or a small silver sound, to locate the obstruction; this was followed by dilatation, a procedure apparently introduced by Antonio Guaineri (d. 1445). Another Italian surgeon, Mariano Santo de Barletta (1490–1550) invented an instrument, the first of its kind, for the dilatation of strictures. It was long enough to reach the neck of the bladder, and was appropriately called *rostrum arcuatum*, "the beaked bow" (Figure 1.4).

Gonorrhoea was not the only genital disease described by doctors in the late Middle Ages, for there were many references to genital ulceration. The Italian surgeon Theodoric of Cervia (1205–1298) wrote a description "Of the corruptions that appear in men around the prepuce on account of coitus with an impure woman"[8]; his contemporary William of Saliceto (1210–1280) described "ulcers and pustules that arise because contact with impure women is followed by the retention of 'filth' or 'venomous material' between the glans and prepuce"[4]. Many others wrote in a similar way. The nature of this condition is unknown, but

9

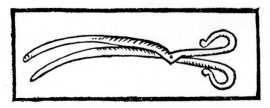

Figure 1.4. Rostrum arciatum, *the "beaked bow" (sixteenth century). Devised for the dilatation of urethral strictures.*

chancroid, genital herpes or erosive balanitis have all been suggested. Phagedenic ulceration, perhaps a related disease, was not uncommon, as it had been in the ancient world. John of Arderne described a typical case:

> "The man's yard began to swell after coit, due to the falling of his own sperm, whereof he suffered great grievousness of burning and acheing as men do when they are so hurt[15]."

Eventually John was called in, and "with a razor cut away all the dead and stinking flesh" before applying quicklime; the patient recovered. It is said that John of Gaunt, "a mighty fornicator", died of something similar. The prevention of destructive genital ulceration was regarded as an important matter. Lanfranchi (Lanfranc of Milan, d.1306), a pupil of William of Salerno, wrote that any man who wishes to preserve his member from corruption by a woman whom he suspects of uncleanliness should wash it in water mixed with vinegar, or with his own urine, after intercourse[16].

Buboes (from the Greek *boubon*, meaning groin) were often described. In earlier times the combination of abscesses in the groin and ulceration of the genitals could have been due to chancroid, or perhaps lymphogranuloma venereum. After the fifteenth century syphilis entered the diagnosis, although the indolent buboes of early syphilis seem to have been largely ignored until the end of the century. Disentangling the aetiology of inguinal adenitis, with or without genital ulceration, was not possible until the advent of microbiology.

Most of the early authors gave very little attention to the treatment of women with genital infections, perhaps because they were regarded as impure and corrupt, and they may well have received no medical attention at all. By the end of the fifteenth century the recognition of the venereal origin of some conditions often made it difficult for patients to obtain treatment. The nobility and clergy might ascribe their diseases to other causes (and hope to be believed), but the rest were regarded as victims of their own licentiousness. Many doctors, through prejudice and perhaps fear of becoming infected themselves, refused to treat them; in 1430 a regulation was enforced in London excluding patients with venereal diseases from public hospitals. And now, to add to the problems posed by gonorrhoea and genital ulceration, a new and much more terrible malady arose, the "evil pox" or "French disease", venereal syphilis.

Chapter 2
The French Disease

One sickly sheep infects the flock
And poisons all the rest.

Isaac Watts, *Against Evil Company*

The appearance of syphilis was an epoch-making event, and doctors schooled in Galenic and Arabian medicine were ill-prepared for it. The disease struck in 1493. Cases were already occurring throughout Western Europe when a major epidemic broke out in the army that the French King Charles VIII led against the Kingdom of Naples in 1494. Charles, described by the historian H.A.L. Fisher as "a young and licentious hunchback of doubtful sanity", led a cosmopolitan force of about 30 000 men, mostly mercenaries and including some from Spain; among the raggle-taggle group of civilians accompanying the army were hundreds of prostitutes. Naples was held by King Alphonso II with the help of Spanish mercenaries sent by Ferdinand and Isabella. At first Charles was successful and he captured Naples early in 1495 without difficulty, but this success was completely reversed when an Italian league was formed to eject the invaders. To make matters worse, prostitution and debauchery on both sides were followed by a widespread outbreak of the new disease. The Italian surgeon Marcellus Cumanus (*fl.* 1495), who was working in Naples, later claimed to have seen the earliest cases. Charles was forced to withdraw from Italy and discharge his soldiers, who spread the disease far and wide as they returned to their own countries. The King himself died of it in 1498.

By 1495 syphilis was raging throughout continental Europe: it was estimated that almost a twentieth of the population was infected. It appeared in France, Germany and Switzerland in 1495; in the following year the Parlement of Paris was forced to decree that no syphilitic could leave his house until cured, and infected foreigners must leave the city immediately. The homeless poor were consigned to two large barns attached to the Abbey of St Germain; these barns were the precursor of the first hospital for venereal diseases in Paris. Members of the Faculty of Medicine fled from the epidemic, leaving the field clear for the surgeons[1]. The disease reached India in 1498 and China in 1505. It was probably introduced into England by members of Charles VIII's disbanded army in 1497, and in the same year there was an outbreak in Scotland, which probably originated from Perkin Warbeck's cosmopolitan mercenaries, who had been welcomed to the country by James IV[2].

Soon after the epidemic erupted the first trickle of what was to be a flood of publications appeared. In Italy Niccolo Leoniceno (1428–1524; Figure 2.1), professor of medicine at Padua, published his *Libellus de epidemia, quam vulgo*

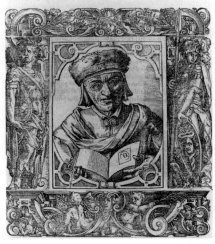

Figure 2.1. Niccolo Leoniceno (1428–1524). (By courtesy of the Royal Society of Medicine Library.)

morbum Gallicum vocent (Notes on the epidemic commonly called the French disease) in 1497[3]. He described the pustules "at first on the privates, then on the rest of the body, accompanied by great pain". His explanation of the disease was on conventional humoral lines with frequent references to Hippocrates and Galen, whose works he had translated. Nature, he wrote, relieves a corruption of the humors by "sending useless material from the internal organs to the external skin or private parts". Leonicenus said nothing about any relation between the appearance of the disease and sexual contact. He believed that it was due to the action of the noxious vapours which followed the rains and serious floods in Italy in 1494. In Spain, Francisco Lopez de Villalobos (1473–1560), a physician in Salamanca, wrote a long poem *Tratado sobre las pestiferas Bubas* (Treatise on the noxious pustules) in 1498[4]. Having searched the ancient literature he concluded that this was a new disease in Europe. He recognised its venereal origin, and was the first to describe the induration of the primary sore. He recorded the skin manifestations, including palmar and plantar syphilides, in detail, and discussed the severe bone pains. He pointed out that having affected the "shameful parts" first, the disease never left the body. This work was one of the best to be written about syphilis at the time but it did not receive much recognition, perhaps because it was written in Spanish rather than the usual Latin. Villalobos later became court physician to Charles V. For a time he was in great favour because of his knowledge and literary skill, but his caustic tongue made him enemies and his career ended unhappily. Another Spanish doctor, Gasparo Torella (*fl.* 1500) became a bishop during the pontificate of Alexander VI[5]. He saw 17 cases of the *morbus Gallicus* among the Borgias and their followers, and published his experiences in his *Tractatus cum Consiliis contra Pudendagram seu Morbum Gallicum* (Treatise and discussion of the French disease) in 1497. The book contained a series of case histories in which the author described the penile lesions, adenitis, skin rashes and osteocopic pains of the disease; he strongly suspected that it was transmitted sexually. Torella dedicated the work to the notoriously cruel and treacherous Cesare Borgia whose father, Alexander VI, apparently died of syphilis himself.

Joseph Grünpeck (1470–1532) was not a doctor, but a peripatetic priest and astrologer who was for a time amanuensis to Maximilian I, the Holy Roman Emperor[6]. He had evidently seen many cases of the new disease, perhaps during Charles VIII's Neapolitan campaign, and eventually contracted it himself. He described his experiences in his *Libellus de mentulagra alias morbo Gallico*, published in 1496. The disease was "far worse than I expected". It began with penile ulceration accompanied by gross swelling, and he then had to endure two years of recurrent skin pustules and agonising joint pains. Eventually huge ulcers, which were possibly gummatous, appeared on his shins, knees and elbows. He was treated with mercury and in the end recovered, although he said that "many others wished to die as soon as possible". His friends were unhelpful: as soon as they heard his diagnosis, they "took to their heels". The Emperor Maximilian was clearly concerned about the "bösen Blattern" (evil pocks). In an edict he described it as a disease "never seen or heard of before now" which was a punishment for blasphemy, and he sent a commission to Spain to report on the value of the drug guaiacum for treatment. Then as now, it was not at all unusual for writers on medical subjects to describe in detail diseases of which they had no personal experience, but Giovanni de Vigo (1460–1520), in his *Practica in arte Chirurgica* which was published in Genoa in 1514 said that he had treated many patients with *morbus Gallicus*[3]. He was convinced that it was a venereal disease, and described two stages. The first comprised the indurated primary sore, which was followed after some weeks by generalised skin papules and crusts, accompanied by "cruel pains" in the head, arms and legs. The second began several months later, when bony and soft tissue tumours formed and sometimes ulcerated. The disease was contagious during the first, but not the second, stage. In this work de Vigo gives a remarkably clear account of the clinical picture and time-scale of the *morbus Gallicus*, which he was careful to differentiate from gonorrhoea. His work was among the sources used by Fracastoro when he wrote his classical work in 1530.

Girolamo Fracastoro (1478–1553) was a true Renaissance man – physician, astronomer, mathematician, poet and philosopher[7]. His contemporaries described him as short, with broad shoulders and long black hair; no coeval portraits of him have survived, but many idealised pictures appeared after his death (Figure 2.2). He evidently had a gentle and retiring nature, and enjoyed nothing more than discussions about scientific matters. He kept in touch with clinical medicine through his private practice in Verona. He was in his teens when the epidemic began, so his knowledge of the first impact of *morbus Gallicus* must have come from others. The bibliographical history of his famous poem *Syphilis sive morbus Gallicus* (Syphilis or the French disease) is complicated. The first edition, in Latin, appeared in 1530 (although it may have existed in manuscript for several years before this); it subsequently went through many editions and translations. The work began with a description of the clinical features of the disease, and went on to discuss the recommended treatment, which included mercury. The discovery of guaiacum in Haiti, its introduction into Europe and its value in therapy were then recounted. Fracastoro's book ended with the well-known tale of a shepherd (or swineherd) called Syphilus who offended Apollo, the god of the sun, and was punished with a foul disease. Later, his misdeeds were forgiven, the guaiacum

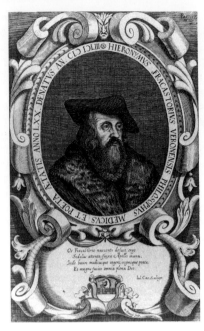

Figure 2.2. Girolamo Fracastoro (1478–1553). (By courtesy of the Royal Society of Medicine Library.)

tree appeared and a nymph advised him of the value of mercury. The poem became very well known. It was translated into English verse in 1686 by Nahum Tate, who later became poet laureate. The first time that the word syphilis was used in an English medical work was in 1717, when Daniel Turner published his book *Syphilis: a Practical Dissertation on the Venereal Disease*, and it did not come into general use until the nineteenth century. Before that the disease was variously referred to as the pox, the great pox, *lues venerea* or as the Neapolitan, Italian, French, Spanish, German or Polish disease according to the nationality and prejudices of the writer.

All contemporary accounts agree this was a very serious disease (Figure 2.3). Fracastoro said that most people become infected through intercourse, after which there was a period of three or four months before symptoms appeared. The victims felt "sad, weary and cast down", then multiple indolent recurrent genital sores developed. Next, skin eruptions appeared; the lesions were small and polymorphic to begin with, but could increase to the size of an acorn:

> "They always broke in a few days, and constantly discharged an incredible quantity of stinking matter . . . Those attacked on the upper parts of the body suffered from malignant affections which ate away sometimes the palate, sometimes the fauces, sometimes the larynx . . . Some lost their lips, some their nose, others all the genital organs. Many had gummy [gummatous] tumours on the limbs which were often the size of an egg or a small loaf[8]."

Loss of the hair and beard was common, and as if this was not enough most patients developed a characteristic symptom of persistent and unbearable pains in the limbs, particularly at night. They became "wan and emaciated, without appetite, sleepless and anxious to remain in bed". This has been called "malignant syphilis", with a short course, severe symptoms and signs and often a fatal outcome. A layman's view of syphilis in the early sixteenth century was given by the Dutch scholar Desiderius Erasmus (1466–1536) in a publication of 1520:

> "If I were asked which is the most destructive of all diseases I should unhesitatingly reply that it is that which has been raging with impunity . . . It combines in itself all the terrible features of other contagions – pain, infection, danger of death, and disagreeable and repugnant treatment which does not produce a complete cure."

Those who contracted syphilis in the early years of the epidemic were regarded with horror. The stench of the ulcers covering their bodies was such that it was rumoured that it was enough simply to smell this to become infected. Some syphilitics, with nowhere to go, roamed aimlessly until they died in the streets of the cities or in the fields beyond.

In later life Fracostoro developed the idea of contagion, and came close to expressing a modern concept of microbial infection. In 1546 he suggested that diseases could be communicated by both direct contact and fomites. The causal agents were invisible small particles, *Seminaria contagiosa* (contagious seeds), which multiplied until the entire organism was corrupted. Infection was "nothing else than the passage of a putrefaction from one body to another either contiguous with it or separated from it". In his *Syphilis sive Morbus Gallicus* he was writing 25 years after the epidemic had begun. He pointed out that although the disease was still widely prevalent it seemed to have changed. There were now fewer

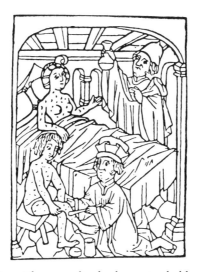

Figure 2.3. Two patients with generalised ulcers, probably syphilitic. A doctor is examining a flask of urine, and another is applying ointment with a spatula. (Woodcut from Bartholomeus Steber's Malafrantzos Morbus Gallorum, *1498.)*

15

pustules, and the osteocopic pains were less severe; on the other hand inguinal adenopathy was more conspicuous and there were more gummy tumours. Most contemporary European syphilographers recorded that by the end of the sixteenth century "malignant" syphilis had become uncommon; the disease, at least in its early manifestations, was now milder. The same sequence of events was seen when transoceanic exploration by Europeans introduced syphilis into localities such as Japan, Malaysia and Polynesia where it had been previously unknown. The resulting outbreaks of infection were severe, with widespread pustular eruptions and ulcerated mucous membranes, resembling those which had occurred in Europe in the late fifteenth century. Later the disease became less florid as it subsided into a chronic endemic state[9]. Similar phenomena have been recorded for many other infectious diseases introduced into "virgin" populations[10].

During the sixteenth and seventeenth centuries there were few dramatic advances in syphilology, but rather a steady progress towards understanding the epidemiology and clinical features of the disease. Jacques de Bethencourt (fl. 1525), a graduate of Rouen[11], wrote the first book on syphilis to be published in France, with the rather odd title *Nova penitentialis quadrigesima necnon purgatorium in morbum Gallicum sive venereum*, (A new lenten penance and purgatory in the French or venereal disease). He may have been the first to use the term "venereal disease"; he believed that it was caused by a "pestilent germ originating from a mixture of the reproductive seeds of the two sexes, or from the male seed and a menstrual discharge". Once developed, the disease spread by contagion, and could be transmitted to babies by affected parents; Bethencourt also mentioned the accidental infection of midwives and wet nurses by infants in their care. Jean Fernel (1506–1588; Figure 2.4) of Clermont, near Paris, was the greatest French physician of the Renaissance, a precise and orderly thinker and writer. According to Garrison[12] he was a man of melancholy nature and aspect, but his face lit up as he entered the sick room and no patient, however poor or humble, was turned away. He completely rejected the Galenic concept that genital lesions were secondary to humoral disorders arising in the liver. He taught that the *morbus Gallicus* was caused by a poison, a "virus". It was usually acquired through intercourse, but it was possible for a midwife to contract it through her hand, or a wet nurse through her nipple; both oral and anal lesions were potentially contagious. The virus would not pass through the intact skin – a breach in the epithelium was essential. Fernel knew that syphilis could have a long incubation period, and he recognised its prolonged latency with sudden exacerbations, the exanthemata and ulceration of the face and throat, the severe nocturnal limb pains and the alopecia. In his *De lues venereae curatione perfectissimo* (The best treatment for syphilis), published in 1556, he was among the first to use the name *lues venerea*; the word lues means simply "plague", it has no specific connotation. He regarded syphilis and gonorrhoea as separate diseases, perhaps the last author to do so for two centuries.

The Venetian surgeon Nicholas Massa (1499–1569) described the occurrence of "professional" chancres on the hands of surgeons. Torella, Fernel and others reported the transmission of syphilis by kissing and a later writer, Carlo Musitano (1635–1714) related the story of some nuns in Sorrento who contracted syphilis by kissing a little girl who had been suckled by a syphilitic woman, but he may not have been a reliable witness; the syphilologist Johann Proksch dismissed him as "an arrogant and coarse priest". The possibility that the disease could be transmitted by inanimate objects was recognised after a notorious outbreak at

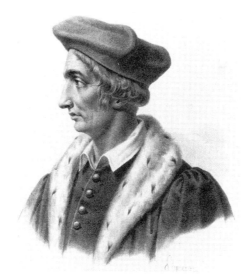

Figure 2.4. Jean Fernel (1506–1588) (By courtesy of the Royal Society of Medicine Library.)

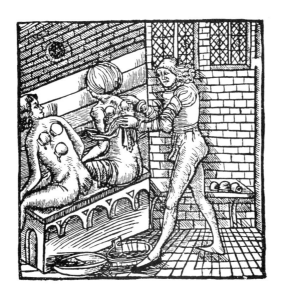

Figure 2.5. The application of cups to induce bleeding. (Woodcut from a calendar by Steffen Arends, 1519.)

Brunn (now Brno, in the Czech Republic) in 1578. According to Lancereaux[13], this was a place where the inhabitants were "much addicted to good living and the use of spirituous liquors." On certain festival days after bathing in the public baths they would have blood drawn by cupping (Figure 2.5). This practice led to an outbreak of syphilis affecting 180 people, the primary lesions being at the sites where the cupping glasses had been applied. The local Senate closed the bathing establishment – which seems to have been the sixteenth century equivalent of a leisure centre – and no further cases occurred. Several similar outbreaks from the use of cupping glasses were reported. Cases in which patients were infected by a surgeon's instruments occurred from the earliest days. The phenomenon of mediate infection as recorded in the early literature was unfortunately forgotten by later authorities such as John Hunter and Philippe Ricord, who maintained that secondary syphilis was not contagious (see Chapter 3).

The induration of the ulcer of primary syphilis had been recognised since the beginning of the epidemic. Gabriele Fallopius (1523–1562; Figure 2.6) was professor of anatomy at Padua. He described the induration as a certain sign of syphilis, and made the important observation that circumcision of men with these lesions on the foreskin did not prevent them from developing constitutional syphilis[14]. In his *Morbo Gallico* of 1560 he also distinguished syphilitic condylomata lata from other condylomatous genital lesions. The illustrious French surgeon Ambroise Paré (1510–1590) stressed not only the induration of the primary sore but the indolent inguinal bubo which often accompanied it[15]. He reintroduced the vaginal speculum (which had been used in the ancient world), and with it he could identify lesions of the vagina and cervix.

While the literature on syphilis published in continental Europe was vast, more than 80 years elapsed between the initial outbreak and its first mention by an English medical writer, William Clowes (1543–1604; Figure 2.7), who has been described as the first English venereologist[16]. He had seen service in both the army and navy (he had been fleet surgeon in the English action against the Spanish Armada) before being appointed surgeon to Queen Elizabeth's household and to

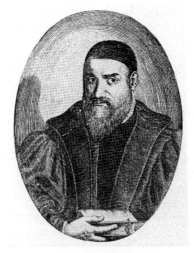

Figure 2.6. Gabriele Fallopius (1523–1562).

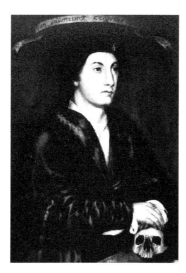

Figure 2.7. William Clowes (1544–1604) From a portrait, artist unknown, seventeenth century. (By courtesy of the Wellcome Institute Library, London.)

St Bartholomew's Hospital. His essay *A short and profitable treatise touching the cure of the disease called Morbus Gallicus by unctions* was published in 1579. He was certainly outspoken about his patients with syphilis, who evidently comprised the majority of those admitted to hospital:

> "It is wonderful to consider how huge multitudes there be of such as be infected with it and that daily increase to the great danger of the common wealth and a stain on the whole nation: the cause whereof I see none so great as the licentious and beastly disorder of a great number of rogues and vagabonds. The filthy type of many lewd and idle persons, both men and women, about the city of London and the great number of lewd alehouses which are the very nests and harbourers of such filthy creatures."

Whether he was expressing a censorious and judgemental attitude towards people with venereal diseases, or was simply writing as a bluff and rather satirical surgeon, must be a matter of opinion. The reader of Clowes' strictures may wonder whether he applied them to the many aristocrats and members of Royal houses – including Henry VIII – who contracted syphilis.

By the end of the seventeenth century early syphilis was well understood, but knowledge of late syphilis was much more scanty. Nodular and ulcerative skin disease and bone disease had been identified soon after the epidemic began; the interval between early and late syphilis was shorter then than it is today, when the onset of benign late syphilis may be delayed for many years. Knowledge of late syphilis affecting the internal organs – visceral, cardiovascular and neurosyphilis – accumulated more slowly, and this aspect of the disease was not thoroughly studied until the nineteenth century (see Chapter 4). The origin of syphilis was discussed from the time of its first appearance. The earliest writers

19

looked for sidereal influences such as the conjunction of Mars and Saturn; Bethencourt, who did not believe in astrology, suggested that Venus might be more important. Others blamed noxious effluvia from rivers and swamps. But once it became accepted that syphilis arose from coitus there were suggestions that it had come from some bizarre couplings: between menstruating prostitutes and lepers, perhaps, or between women and monkeys. Others thought that the cause might have been "cohabitation with the voluptuous Indian women of America"[17], and it was from this idea that the Columbian hypothesis arose which was to be accepted by most syphilologists until the eighteenth century. Venereologists are sometimes accused of compensating for the mundane nature of their work by developing controversies which are inherently insoluble and can therefore continue indefinitely. One such dispute concerned the use of mercury, but the origin of syphilis was far more productive of books, articles and general polemics; it lasted well into the twentieth century. There were two schools of thought. According to the first, the disease was introduced into Europe by members of Christopher Columbus's first expedition when they returned in 1493; it was conveyed by Spanish soldiers to the armies fighting in Charles VIII's Neapolitan campaign and, after this was over, to the rest of Europe. The second hypothesis was that syphilis had been present in the Eastern hemisphere under various names for centuries. It became more severe and widespread in the fifteenth century because of social factors – wars, population movement, increased promiscuity and so on – and news of the outbreak was readily communicated to literate and influential people because of the new process of printing. These proposals were subject to heated controversy. Many of the "great and good" in the medical world took sides: notable "Columbians" were Astruc, Bloch, Proksch, Jeanselme, Pusey and Harrison, while the "anti-Columbians" included Lancereaux, Sudhoff, Singer, Holcombe and Kampmeier. Some of the discussion was far from scholarly. Accusations of bad faith, alteration of dates, misunderstanding the data and misplaced patriotism filled the air, and eminent venereologists were soon calling each others' opinions prejudiced, naive or laughable.

The evidence for the Columbian hypothesis came from epidemiology and, to a lesser extent, palaeopathology. Some of the earliest colonists of Hispaniola (now Haiti) reported that the "French disease" was common among the native population. Gonzales Hernandez Oviedo y Valdes (1478–1557), who had crossed the Atlantic eight times and lived in Hispaniola for a time, was the chronicler of the Spanish colonists. In his *La general y natural historia de las Indias* he described how the disease was contracted from Indian women by the Spaniards, and through them reached the army of Charles VIII. He added:

> "The truth is that this disease was transmitted from the island of Hispaniola to Europe. It is very common among the Indians there and they know how to cure themselves, having very excellent herbs and trees appropriate for this, such as guaiac[18]."

Bartolome de Las Casas (1474–1566) was a Spanish priest who devoted much of his life to the welfare of the Indians. In old age he wrote a manuscript *Historia de las Indias*, which remained unpublished until long after his death. In it he agreed that the "French malady" originated in Hispaniola:

"I myself sometimes endeavoured to enquire of the Indians of this island whether the malady was very ancient on it, and they answered yes, before the Christians came . . . The Indians, men and women, that had it were little affected, but for the Spaniards the pains from it were an intense and continuous torment[19]."

The condition of the members of Columbus's expedition when they returned to Europe is crucial for the hypothesis. It was described by a Spanish surgeon, Ruiz Diaz de Isla (1462–1542). The first officer to arrive was Columbus's pilot, Martin Alonzo Pinzon, who had broken away and preceded his admiral to Spain, hoping to gain credit from Ferdinand and Isabella (he received a royal rebuke instead). Diaz de Isla states that on the return voyage from Hispaniola, Pinzon had been attacked by a disease which caused a severe skin eruption accompanied by much pain. Other members of the expedition developed the same condition, which he called the "serpentine disease". In his *Tractado contra el mal serpentino*, published in 1539, he claimed to have treated many such patients[20].

If the testimonies of Ruiz de Isla, Las Casas and Ovieto were correct, it became possible to trace the "French disease" to the West Indies. Since late syphilis can cause well-defined changes in the skull and long bones, there were many later attempts to find evidence of these in the skeletal remnants of people buried in the Americas in pre-Columbian times. Studies of this sort are beset with difficulties in judging the age of the bones and ensuring certainty in diagnosis; furthermore, if in any particular area the course of syphilis was mild, there might not be any such changes. Despite these problems, there have been reports of some American pre-Columbian bones which show syphilitic lesions[21]. In Europe, no authentic syphilitic bones of pre-Columbian date have ever been found, although they were common after 1493[22]. The Columbian hypothesis was generally accepted by the early syphilographers, and is undoubtedly attractive. The mild disease among the inhabitants of Hispaniola was consistent with an endemic infection whose virulence had been mitigated by the development of "herd immunity". The Spaniards, having no such immunity, developed a much more severe disease which caused the European epidemic. In recent times this hypothesis has been strenuously attacked. The evidence that venereal syphilis was prevalent in the West Indies at the time of Columbus has been dismissed as being simply hearsay, unsupported by proper medical examinations. Ruiz de Isla's observations have been viewed with profound suspicion by some workers[23], and it has even been suggested that he did not witness the events he described. The reports on ancient bones in North America have been regarded as very unreliable. The reader feels bewildered when the work of Montejo, who laboriously examined the early Spanish chronicles, receives extravagant praise from one commentator and vulgar abuse from another[23,24].

The anti-Columbian hypothesis states that syphilis was already an established disease in Europe at the time of Columbus's expeditions. In the late fifteenth century it became more common because of social disorder and accompanying promiscuity and appeared to be a "new" disease. The validity of the evidence for the existence of venereal syphilis in pre-Columbian Europe is therefore crucial. Even Sudhoff was prepared to admit that there was no literary proof that it existed in the ancient world (see Chapter 1). In the medieval literature there are descriptions of genital lesions and skin rashes, but there is not enough detail for even a tentative diagnosis to be made and no reference to the osteocopic pains which were so dominant in the later epidemic. The medical historian Victor Robinson has expressed these matters with his usual eloquence:

"There are isolated passages in the medieval writers – Saliceto, Lanfranchi, Roger, Roland, Theodoric, Guy de Chauliac, John of Gaddesden . . . suggestive of chancre. But syphilis is not a condition which can be hidden in Latin quotations. When we think of all the whoring that went on in the Middle Ages, if syphilis existed it would have manifested itself widely. In pre-Columbian Europe we cannot demonstrate syphilis; in post-Columbian Europe it strikes everywhere – in the infant's cradle and on the autopsy table, in the bordello and the monastery, in the peasant's cottage and the scholar's room, by the emperor's throne and in the papal palace. Everywhere physicians are saying, 'This is a new disease'[25]."

The same point was made by one of the early observers, Alexander Trajanus Petronius of Castile, who wrote in 1565:

"Before this disease was known in Europe, an ulcer occasioned by coition and resembling those that the French pox produces would sometimes break out on the pudenda. Buboes too and a gonorrhoea would appear, but these symptoms were easily removed[26]."

It has been argued that medieval physicians did not separate syphilis from a group of disorders collectively designated *lepra*. The term seems to have embraced true leprosy, psoriasis, impetigo and other skin diseases; among these there might conceivably have been some form of non-venereal treponematosis. Lepra was regarded as contagious, and had some ill-defined venereal connotations. John of Gaddesden (1280–1361) was court physician to Edward II, and was well enough known to be mentioned by Chaucer in the Prologue to his *Canterbury Tales*. He wrote:

"Those who cohabit with a woman who has had coitus with a leper have a stabbing between the flesh and the skin, and sometimes burning in the whole body[27]."

Bernard de Gordon (1282–1318), professor of medicine at Montpelier, was more explicit:

"A certain countess, who had lepra, came to Montpelier . . . A bachelor of medicine whom I had appointed to treat her was unfortunate enough to share her bed. She became pregnant, and he leprous[28]."

It seems unlikely that "venereal lepra" was true leprosy, which has a long incubation period and is not very contagious. Some commentators have suggested that it was venereal syphilis, but in truth it could have been almost any sexually transmissible disease.

If the Columbian hypothesis is heavily dependent on early writings of questionable validity, the pre-Columbian hypothesis has a marked tendency to collapse into a welter of unsupported hindsight and speculation. During the last few decades, however, bacteriological work has supplemented (or complicated, depending on one's point of view) the historical approach. Soon after the discovery that *Treponema pallidum* was the cause of syphilis it was found that microscopically identical organisms could be found in the lesions of pinta, yaws and endemic syphilis. All these diseases are essentially childhood infections. Pinta is a chronic skin disease of Central and South America, yaws a destructive disease of skin and bones which occurs in the tropics, and endemic syphilis (bejel) a mucocutaneous and osseous disease which is now virtually confined to the Middle East and North Africa, although it was common in some parts of Europe in the eighteenth and nineteenth centuries. All the non-venereal treponematoses give serological reactions which are identical to those of venereal syphilis, and their causal organisms cannot be distinguished in the laboratory. The apparent identity of human treponemes led to the "unitarian hypothesis"[29,30]. This postulated that all these conditions are manifestations of the same infection, the observed clinical differences being due to environmental factors, particularly temperature. The hypothesis could be made to fit the anti-Columbian theory, but a major objection is the profound clinical differences between the non-venereal treponematoses and syphilis – the latter alone showing visceral, cardiovascular, neurological and congenital infections. Some workers have rejected the "unitarian" hypothesis, and maintain that human treponemal diseases are caused by organisms which, despite their morphological identity, are subtly different from each other. If this is so, the Columbian hypothesis may be correct. The relationship between syphilis and other treponemal diseases is another of the old controversies beloved by venereologists, and has now been dragging on for half a century. Perhaps study of the molecular biology of human treponemes will resolve some of the problems, but in the mean time the relationship between the human treponemal diseases remains uncertain.

Chapter 3
"Mr Hunter's singular opinions": Early and Experimental Syphilis

Time that at last matures a clap to pox,
Whose gentle progress makes a calf an ox
Alexander Pope, *Satires of Dr Donne*

Between the sixteenth and eighteenth centuries the study of venereal diseases made only slow progress. The main clinical features of primary and secondary syphilis had been recognised, although estimates of its incubation period, and of the temporal relationship between its various stages, were very inexact. Extragenital infection, for example of the mouth, was recognised. By the beginning of the eighteenth century some of the features of late syphilis had also been described – lesions of the skin and bones, for instance – but nothing was yet known about cardiovascular or neurosyphilis, and very little about visceral involvement.

Many books about syphilis had been written, but often these were simply plagiarisms of earlier work, with very few new ideas. From time to time more important publications appeared, summarising the state of the art, with extensive bibliographies. These works were not necessarily the fruit of clinical experience, as were to be the great clinical treatises of the nineteenth century; many were products of the library rather than of the consulting room. Astruc's *De Morbis Veneris*, which was published in 1736, became the standard text on the subject for the next fifty years; an English translation appeared in 1754[1]. Jean Astruc (1684–1766; Figure 3.1) was personal physician to Louis XV. He was a scholar not only of medicine but of the Bible, and could be seen night after night working in his unheated library. He was evidently only a mediocre clinician, but he wrote more than 20 books on all aspects of medicine and surgery, including a volume devoted to the diseases of women, a branch of medicine of which he had no personal experience. In this he bears a resemblance to some of the "AIDS watchers" of the 1990s.

In the eighteenth century the cause of syphilis was unknown; indeed, the study of contagion itself was still impeded by the remains of the humoral theory. When syphilis was ascribed to "a virus", the word did not have its modern meaning; it was used to denote a poison which caused a disease. In the case of syphilis, this meant a toxic substance which was harboured in the female genital tract and transmitted to the male by intercourse; why it should have developed in the female was not discussed. A related problem which was to cause trouble for nearly a century was the connection between syphilis and gonorrhoea. The early writers, for example, de Vigo and Fernel, had regarded them as different diseases, but by the sixteenth century the distinction had been lost; there was now thought to be a single venereal poison which was responsible for both genital ulcers and genital discharges. This error cannot be blamed on any one person. The renowned Swiss physician and alchemist Paracelsus (1493–1541) was an early protagonist, calling syphilis "French gonorrhoea". Ambroise Paré (1510–1590), "the father of modern surgery", Thomas Sydenham (1624–1689), the greatest English physician of his time, the scholarly Astruc and many others were *monists*[2]. They accepted without question that syphilis and gonorrhoea were manifestations of the same disease. It is not difficult to see how this mistaken idea arose. Both diseases were contracted through intercourse, they often occurred together, and it was argued that an unsuspected intrameatal syphilitic sore could easily cause the urethral discharge of *gonorrhoea virulenta*. The relationship of syphilis to gonorrhoea was crucial, and of more than academic interest. If they were basically the same disease, patients with gonorrhoea should be treated with mercury, despite its toxicity; even though the therapy had no effect on the symptoms and signs of gonorrhoea, its timely administration should prevent the later development of syphilis.

The word *chancre* had been in use since the fifteenth century to describe a destructive genital sore. It was probably derived from the Latin *cancer*, a crab, via the old French *canker*[3]. By the middle of the sixteenth century the fact that genital ulcers had been well known in Europe before the advent of syphilis had been forgotten, and it was generally assumed that a chancre was always due to syphilis. But some workers, including Astruc, noted that not all genital ulcers were followed by constitutional syphilis. It was also observed that some men developed constitutional syphilis without any preceding genital ulcer – syphilis d'emblée – allegedly because of the direct absorption of putrid matter from the female genital tract. No integration of these disparate observations into a coherent system was possible, and none was attempted. However, there were signs of progress. In the mid eighteenth century there were moves towards the restoration of the earlier

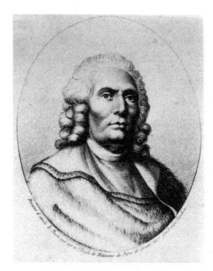

Figure 3.1. Jean Astruc (1684–1766). (By courtesy of the Wellcome Historical Library, London.)

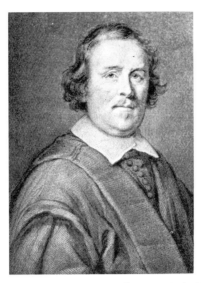

Figure 3.2. Hermann Boerhaave (1668–1738).

separation of syphilis from gonorrhoea. Hermann Boerhaave (1668–1738; Figure 3.2) was professor of medicine in Leiden, Holland, and in his day was the best known medical scientist in Europe. In 1751 he wrote a book on *lues venerea*[4] in which he differentiated the two diseases, stating that gonorrhoea was no more than a purulent catarrh, such as might occur with a head cold. Boerhaave was an influential teacher, and his ideas spread to other countries. In Scotland two Edinburgh graduates, Andrew Duncan (1744–1828) and Francis Balfour (*fl.* 1760), in England William Ellis (d. 1785), in Denmark Johann Clement Tode (1736–1805) and in Austria Gerhard van Swieten (1700–1772), who had worked with Boerhaave in Leiden, were among those who accepted the *duality of the virus*[5]. Although Ellis, and perhaps Balfour, had performed some inoculations to corroborate their views, the separation of syphilis from gonorrhoea was really no more than a hypothesis – the age of experimental medicine had not yet arrived. Nevertheless, progress in understanding venereal diseases had been made, but this was soon to receive a setback which was to last for 50 years, ironically from the hands of one of the major figures in the history of medicine, John Hunter.

John Hunter: Confusion

John Hunter (1728–1793; Figure 3.3) was born in a village a few miles from Glasgow. He did badly at school; he was a slow reader, and found writing difficult, but he showed practical ability from the beginning. He left school at the age of 13 years. In 1748 he joined his brother William in London. William was a teacher of anatomy who was later to become a well-known obstetrician. John showed remarkable skill in dissection and in investigating complex anatomical problems. Between 1749 and 1756 he also studied surgery at St Bartholomew's and St George's Hospitals. In 1760 he joined the British army and served for three years; at the time, this was recognised as an excellent way to increase surgical experience. On his return to England from service in France and Portugal he started to build up a surgical practice, augmenting his income by teaching surgical anatomy. He was still without a formal qualification, but in 1768 he obtained the diploma of the Company of Surgeons (later the Royal College of Surgeons); in the same year he was elected surgeon to St George's Hospital. From now on Hunter was an active surgeon at the hospital and in private practice, and taught surgery and surgical anatomy. He continued his meticulous dissections, and performed many experiments on animals. Although he always found writing difficult, he published books and papers on a wide range of subjects which included anatomy, physiology, surgery, venereology, zoology and geology. He had begun to collect specimens while he was working at his brother's anatomy school; this collection expanded, and eventually he set up a museum devoted to palaeontology, zoology and pathology which after his death became the Hunterian museum of the Royal College of Surgeons. His pre-eminence in surgery was generally acknowledged, and many honours and awards came his way. For the last 15 years of his life he suffered from ischaemic heart disease, from which he died suddenly at the age of 65 years after an acrimonious board meeting at St George's Hospital. Hunter was short, stocky and energetic. He could be brusque and taciturn and was reputed to be bad-tempered, but he had the gift of inspiring loyalty and affection among his associates. He spoke slowly, often correcting himself, but he could be witty and amusing[6].

There can be no doubt about Hunter's ability as a superb practical investigator, but he had never had a formal education in medicine and he was handicapped by his inability to express his thoughts clearly in either speech or writing. He

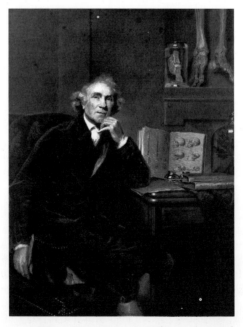

Figure 3.3. John Hunter (1728–1793) Engraving after a portrait by Sir Joshua Reynolds, 1788. (By courtesy of the Wellcome Historical Library, London.)

was not the right person to deal with the complex problems of venereal disease, and in his *Treatise on the Venereal Disease*, published in 1786[7], he propagated several serious errors, not so much of fact as of interpretation. He believed that the signs of inflammation varied according to the part affected. There was only one "venereal poison"; if this fell on a mucosal surface it would cause gonorrhoea, if on to skin it would cause a chancre, and if it was absorbed into the circulation it would cause constitutional syphilis. He put this theory to the test in his well-known experiment of 1767, in which he inoculated a recipient's glans and prepuce with material from a patient with gonorrhoea. By tradition the recipient was Hunter himself, he was portrayed as a martyr to science, and the cardiovascular disease from which he died was wrongly attributed to syphilis[8]. Since he never hesitated to experiment on humans it is more likely that the subject of the experiment was a patient. At all events, a chancre appeared 10 days after the inoculation, followed by inguinal gland enlargement, ulceration of the tonsils and a generalised skin rash, the whole illness lasting for three years. Today it seems likely that the donor had a double infection, but Hunter was convinced that he had induced syphilis by the inoculation of gonorrhoeal pus, thereby proving the identity of the two conditions. Since he believed that a patient could not have two different diseases at the same time, the frequent concurrence of syphilis and gonorrhoea lent further support to his views.

Like his contemporaries, Hunter seemed uncertain about the incubation period of primary syphilis, saying that this could be between one day and several weeks. His powers of observation are shown in his accurate clinical descriptions of many syphilitic conditions, although the indurated "Hunterian chancre" of primary syphilis had been depicted by de Vigo in 1514 and by many others since then[9]. Hunter believed that there were other causes of genital ulceration besides syphilis and that their distinction was important, although this could often be made only by observing the response to mercury, which was active against syphilis alone. Hunter made repeated attempts to induce chancres by inoculating patients with secondary syphilis with material from their own lesions or blood. These were invariably unsuccessful, and he concluded that constitutional syphilis was not contagious. As Lancereaux has remarked "It never struck him that to ascertain whether syphilitic blood is contagious it is necessary to inoculate a healthy person and not one already syphilised"[10]. In due course this was done, but not by Hunter. His conviction that the blood of a person with syphilis was not contagious led him into a further error, that congenital syphilis could not be contracted in utero but only during delivery. Forgetting the history of the past, he also denied that an infant could contract syphilis by suckling a wet nurse with lesions on the breasts.

Hunter did not clearly differentiate the lesions of secondary and tertiary syphilis, and his descriptions of the latter are disappointing. The great German syphilographer Johann Karl Proksch (1840–1923) lamented:

"Hunter dealt the most terrible blow to the doctrine of the involvement of the internal organs by syphilis. With a few calmly written lines he annihilated a doctrine which for three centuries had been proved upon countless bodies and accepted by all the physicians of the world ... Hunter merely said superficially: 'I have not seen that the brain, heart, stomach, liver, kidneys and other viscera have been attacked by syphilis, although such cases have been described', but this amply sufficed to cause visceral syphilis almost completely to disappear for more than half a century from textbooks upon venereal diseases[11]."

Hunter left venereology in a thoroughly confused state. His well-known remark to Edward Jenner ". . . but why think? Why not try the experiment?"[12] exemplified an approach which had hitherto worked very well, but of course the experiment should be the right one, properly conducted and controlled, and the result interpreted correctly. Hunter's failure in these respects led him to perpetrate serious errors, but his prestige ensured that his opinions were accepted almost without question. Any disagreements with his views on venereal disease were dismissed by his supporters as expressions of envy and malice. Although Hunter's teaching was partly erroneous, it did embody traditional doctrines which were defended by many celebrated practitioners. But there were those who did not accept these; in particular, Boerhaave's ideas had not been forgotten in Scotland, and were to come to fruition in the work of one of the greatest figures in the history of venereology, Benjamin Bell.

Benjamin Bell: Clarification

Bell (1749–1805; Figure 3.4) was another Scot, born in Dumfries to a family of landowners, and he received a classical education at a local grammar school. He had always been interested in surgery, and after leaving school he was apprenticed to a local surgeon before, at the age of 17, he joined the Medical School at Edinburgh. The school was prestigious, having men of the calibre of the Monros and Cullen on the staff. Bell did well as a student, and in 1771 he became a Fellow of the Royal College of Surgeons of Edinburgh. He then spent several months in postgraduate study in Paris and in London, where he met the Hunter

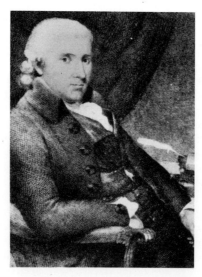

Figure 3.4. Benjamin Bell (1749–1805).

30

brothers. He was impressed by John; he wrote in a letter to Cullen: "I have had the pleasure of a most agreeable, and at the same time most useful acquaintance I ever met with, for there is scarce an article, either in physic or surgery, that Mr Hunter has not got something new upon, and there is none more ready of communication than he is"[13]. He returned to Edinburgh in 1772; he was appointed surgeon to the Royal Infirmary, and started a private practice. But just as things were beginning to go well for him he sustained a serious injury through falling off a horse and was incapacitated for two years. He eventually recovered and resumed his surgical practice. This prospered, and in time he became widely known as a careful and skilful surgeon; it was said that nobody should think of dying before Mr Bell had seen him. Demands for his opinion necessitated many journeys, and he had an oil lamp fitted inside his carriage so that he could read and write as he travelled. He had a lifelong interest in agriculture, and he was an able businessman. He wrote a series of essays on political economy which led to a correspondence with William Pitt, the British Prime Minister. He "respectfully declined" the offer of a baronetcy[14].

During his enforced retirement Bell had planned some major works on surgery which were published between 1777 and 1788 and were well received. But his greatest work was his *Treatise on Gonorrhoea Virulenta and Lues Venerea* which appeared in 1793[15]. He had evidently devoted much thought to the monist – dualist controversy, and in his opening chapter he presents his conclusions:

(1) The symptoms and signs of gonorrhoea and syphilis are quite different.

(2) Gonorrhoea does not progress to syphilis. Cases in which they have occurred together can be explained either by their having been contracted at the same time, or by one having been contracted before the other had resolved.

(3) The diseases in sex partners match the diseases in index cases.

(4) Experimental proof of the unity of syphilis and gonorrhoea would require many inoculations of infected material. Bell expressed doubts about the ethics of this, and in an obvious reference to Hunter added that a single experiment performed by an already biased investigator proves nothing. Despite these misgivings, he seems to have organised an experiment himself: "Two young gentlemen of this place [presumably his students] failed to induced gonorrhoea in themselves by inoculating material from a chancre, or syphilis by inoculating gonorrhoeal pus".

(5) In Scotland *Lues venerea* had been prevalent for many years under the name *sibbens*. He had never seen a patient with sibbens develop gonorrhoea: "These are poor country people whose manners do not expose them to the hazards of being infected with gonorrhoea".

(6) Medication which cures syphilis, particularly mercury, is ineffective against gonorrhoea.

These arguments, set out at length with many illustrative case histories, made Bell's case. The contrast with Hunter's approach is obvious, and indeed the two men were very different. Bell was better educated, and he was a fluent writer. He was not an experimental surgeon but he kept careful notes and, like Ricord and Hutchinson, could always support his opinions from his own large clinical experience. It is hard to resist the conclusion that, despite his earlier admiration,

Bell had a poor opinion of Hunter as a venereologist. He criticised his opinions several times in his book, and at one point referred to "Mr John Hunter, whose ingenuity and abilities are only to be equalled by his singular opinions". Bell was not infallible. He probably confused syphilitic chancres with other types of genital ulceration, particularly chancroid. Although he saw syphilis as progressive, he did not suggest the orderly temporal arrangement of symptoms and signs delineated by Ricord in the next century. Nevertheless, his contribution to venereology was crucial, for as long as it was believed that there was only one venereal disease progress was impossible. We do not know how his *Treatise* was received, and it was to be his last work. His health failed comparatively early, and he died in 1805 at the age of 57 years. His best epitaph was given by his grandson: "With great store of information on most subjects, he had the art of always appearing to derive instruction rather than give it . . . He never seemed to be in a hurry, but bestowed as much attention upon each of his patients as if he had no other to occupy his thoughts"[16].

Bell's Successors

Although Bell never attained Hunter's prestige, his work was influential. Jean Francois Hernandez (1769–1835), working at the School of Naval Medicine at Toulon, was stimulated by his *Treatise* to inoculate gonorrhoeal pus into the skin of a group of convicts under his care; he failed to produce syphilis in any of them, and these experiments further weakened the unitary hypothesis[17]. Among the many other physicians who were interested in the relation between syphilis and gonorrhoea was Francois-Xavier Swediaur (1748–1824; Figure 3.5), a contemporary of Hunter and Bell. Of Swedish descent, Swediaur was born near Linz, in Austria, and received his medical education at Vienna[18]. After graduating he moved to London, where he made friends among the more

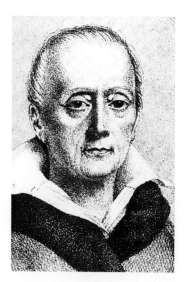

Figure 3.5. Francois-Xavier Swediaur (1748–1824).

influential physicians and soon built up a large practice. In 1783 he visited Cullen – one of Bell's former teachers – in Edinburgh:

"A pale youth, made thin by long vigils passed in study, presented himself ... He held under his arm a manuscript [of his work on venereal diseases]. Cullen read it, and was so impressed that he told his students 'My old age is suffused with the most pleasing consolation of being the first to announce the appearance of a mind destined to give a great stimulus to medical science'[18]."

Although he was was interested in the scientific aspects of medicine, Swediaur is best remembered through his two books. *Practical Observations on the More Obstinate and Inveterate Venereal Complaints* was published in London and Edinburgh in 1784, and a revised edition of the book, now called *Traité Complet sur les Symptomes, les Effets, la Nature et le Traitement des Maladies Syphilitiques* in Paris in 1798. Both were very successful, and ran through many editions and translations. The books did not contain much in the way of original work or new ideas; they were textbooks of venereology, flavoured with quotations and criticisms. At some point in his career Swediaur had fallen foul of Hunter, or maybe he was jealous of him. He referred to him in terms which these days would bring libel lawyers buzzing round his head: "[Hunter] is a low and vain man, ignorant of the different writings and discoveries made by his contemporaries, and can attribute to himself what should have been attributed to others". Hunter's *Treatise on the Venereal Disease* was "full of errors, founded on vague empiricism, with a wealth of false advice. It is almost forgotten in England"[19].

Swediaur wrote particularly well on the clinical picture of secondary syphilis – the fever, weakness, lassitude and joint pains – which have deceived so many clinicians over the years. But when he came to discuss the relation of syphilis to gonorrhoea he equivocated:

"Some persons [he was referring to Bell] maintain that the virus of gonorrhoea never produces chancres and that the virus of chancres never produces gonorrhoea ... I do not deny that this is frequently the case; but frequent observations have equally well proved to me that this assertion is very far from being generally correct. I know of many cases in which patients with gonorrhoea with no ulcer communicated chancres and vice versa."

Swediaur died at the age of 76 years from uraemia due to enlargement of the prostate and bladder stones. Like Unna (see, pp. 151–152) he gained an international reputation without having any official appointment in a hospital or university. He did not make any major contribution to venereology, but he was a keen observer and an excellent writer. We will meet him again when we come to consider gonorrhoea.

The problem of the "duality of the virus" was not the only one to perplex syphilologists at the end of the eighteenth century. The temporal relationship of the signs of syphilis, the contagiousness of its lesions, the ease with which these could be inoculated, and the natural history of congenital infections were

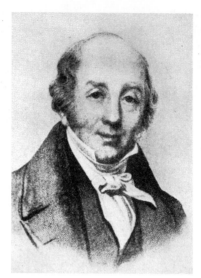

Figure 3.6. Abraham Colles (1773–1843).

all questions requiring answers. In addition, there was a seemingly endless controversy over the treatment of syphilis, particularly with mercury. Some of these difficulties were taken up by Abraham Colles (1773–1843; Figure 3.6), a Dublin surgeon who also described a well-known wrist fracture. He published *Practical Observations on the Venereal Disease and the Use of Mercury* in 1837[20]. He did not agree with the opinion held by many of his contemporaries that the different rashes of secondary syphilis indicated different forms of the disease and, without giving details, he reported observations which indicated that the lesions of both primary and secondary syphilis were contagious. He pointed out that even very early excision of a primary chancre would not arrest the development of constitutional signs. Colles' well-reasoned and informative work was subjected to a withering review in *The Lancet*, possibly by Wallace, who disliked him:

> "even the ancient author himself has no suspicion that he is really adding nothing to our stock of knowledge . . . the whole volume is a crude jumble of facts with which, and with many more, all intelligent practitioners are already acquainted . . . Dr Colles has taken care to keep from his pages the names of Carmichael and Wallace, brethren residing in the same city, highly appreciated there, well known as distinguished contributors to our knowledge of venereal diseases, and received as authorities where the name of the superannuated Professor of Surgery to the Dublin College [Colles] has hardly yet been heard[21]."

William Wallace (1791–1837) was born at Downpatrick, in Ulster, and studied medicine in Dublin, where he qualified in 1813. He spent the next five years in postgraduate study in London, and on his return to Dublin was appointed surgeon to the Jarvis Street Hospital. He was already interested in dermatovenereology; during his apprenticeship he had worked at the Dublin Lock Hospital, a large institution for the treatment of venereal diseases, and he had studied dermatology during his stay in London. In 1818 he founded the Dublin Hospital for Diseases of the Skin, the first such hospital in Europe. Like Hunter, Wallace was at heart a scientist. He soon began to study the contagiousness of secondary syphilis by the experimental inoculation of syphilitic secretions, some into patients already infected with syphilis but others into healthy subjects who happened to be in hospital for other reasons[22]. Material from ulcers or condylomas thought to be syphilitic was used. It seems uncertain whether all these lesions were due to secondary syphilis – some of the ulcers may have been primary chancres, or even due to chancroid – but a few of the inoculations were valid, and were followed after four weeks by first primary then secondary syphilis. The ethical aspects of these experiments do not seem to have concerned him. Although his results made little impact at the time, he was one of the first workers to show that the lesions of secondary syphilis were contagious. His other major contribution to venereology was his introduction of potassium iodide for the treatment of syphilis (see Chapter 5). Wallace was a lone wolf, and he could be outspoken and argumentative. His scientific interests led him into frequent acrimonious disputes with his colleagues, and when he died of typhus at the early age of 46 there were few to mourn him[23]. Nevertheless, he made significant contributions to syphilology.

Philippe Ricord's "Steadying Influence"

During the first decades of the nineteenth century it was becoming increasingly clear that the current fragmented and contentious opinions about syphilis needed what Mettler has called "some comprehensive, steadying influence", and this came from the work of Philippe Ricord (1800–1889) and his school.

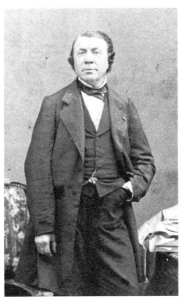

Figure 3.7. Philippe Ricord (1800–1889). (By courtesy of the Royal Society of Medicine Library.)

Ricord (Figure 3.7) was one of the most charismatic figures in the history of venereology[24]. He was born in Baltimore, USA, where his parents had emigrated from Marseille to escape the Terror which followed the French Revolution. Owing to shortage of money he had to leave school early, and he worked in a series of clerical jobs, but he studied natural history and medicine in the evenings. At the age of 20 years he was able to return to France, and his medical education continued in Paris, first at Val de Grace Hopital, then at Hôtel Dieu under Dupuytren and finally at l 'Hôpital de la Pitié under Lisfranc. He graduated in 1826, and as no hospital appointments were available he spent the next few years in rural general practice. In 1831 he was offered a post as surgeon to l 'Hôpital du Midi, one of the great Parisian hospitals for venereal diseases. Although he had no experience of the subject he accepted the offer, and remained at the Midi for the next thirty years.

Ricord was a skilful clinician with great personal charm, and it was not long before he became one of the most popular doctors in Paris. He was an excellent teacher. In the summer his lectures were held out of doors; according to a contemporary they were "like a chat, with language clear and full of imagery, brightened by recollections of incidents in the hospital and out of town." His *bons mots* were legendary. Ricord considered himself a surgeon, and wrote many articles on surgical topics, but his main interest was venereology, which he took very seriously. He deplored the inadequate methods of examination then in use, particularly for women; inspection of the vulva and palpation of the vagina were regarded as enough for a doctor to declare a woman to be "infected" or "not infected." He reintroduced the vaginal speculum, which had fallen into disuse, and designed a trivalve instrument himself (Figure 3.8) with which he was able to demonstrate unsuspected vaginal and cervical lesions, including chancres.

Ricord's second diagnostic aid was autoinoculation. He was firmly convinced that it was wrong to inoculate healthy people with diseases whose results were unpredictable. Instead, he inoculated pus from a urethral discharge, genital ulcer or draining bubo into the patient's own thigh, covered it with a watch glass and examined the site daily for the development of lesions. Between 1831 and 1837 he performed more than 2500 of these inoculations. He came to believe that the technique could be used not only for research but to also to aid diagnosis;

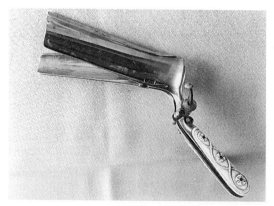

Figure 3.8. Ricord's uterine speculum, c. 1865. This trivalve instrument is made of brass, with an ivory handle. (By courtesy of Musée des Hôpitaux de Paris.)

he called it the "sole rigorous method available," although future events were to show him wrong about this. He published the results of his experiments in his *Traité Pratique des Maladies Vénériennes*[25]. This appeared in 1838, and was a great success. His conclusions were: (1) an ulcerated chancre, or its resultant bubo, will always reproduce a chancre when reinoculated; so will the pustule caused by the autoinoculation; (2) reinoculation of material from the ulcers of secondary syphilis will not produce a chancre; and (3) reinoculation of the pus of blennorrhagia [gonorrhoea] will not induce a chancre. He concluded that syphilis had one specific cause, that gonorrhoea was not caused by syphilis, and that secondary syphilis was not contagious. Of course, his interpretation of these results was faulty. We now know that although autoinoculation from a primary syphilitic sore of short duration is sometimes successful, developing immune responses prevent inoculations from the sores of late primary and secondary syphilis from "taking". While some of the chancres which he successfully reinoculated may have been syphilitic, many must have been due not to syphilis but to chancroid; this was very common at the time, and can be easily reinoculated. These experiments also led Ricord to define an incubation period for syphilis of only a few days; again, this is much more consistent with chancroid than with syphilis. He recognised the existence of hard and soft chancres, but taught that both were forms of syphilis. Thus the failure to separate the three major venereal diseases, gonorrhoea, syphilis and chancroid, was only partly resolved by Ricord's work. A few years after the publication of the *Traité* his former pupil Bassereau showed that there were three veneral "poisons" involved: one associated with gonorrhoea, the second with hard chancres and constitutional syphilis and the third with soft chancre (chancroid) and its local complications. The story of this discovery is told in Chapter 8. It helped to explain the discrepancies among Ricord's cases, and eventually he had to abandon his unitary view of genital ulceration.

Ricord's conclusion that the lesions of secondary syphilis were not contagious was a serious mistake which was to cause a great deal of trouble. Proksch commented:

"This assertion tempted 19 medical men in all countries to infect and ruin for life 77 persons on whom they made experiments. Before that very year 1838, 50 monographs had been written on the same subject – all of them positive in their proof of the dangerous nature of secondary syphilis. As early as 1496 a heavy fine was imposed in Switzerland on those who used for a second time a knife or instrument which had been used on a syphilitic patient. Epidemics of cupping-transferred syphilis were observed in Brunn in 1577 and afterwards in many other places. Extragenital infection had been treated in all textbooks for hundreds of years and in more than one thousand monographs. And still these facts were not known to Ricord[26]."

Ricord clung on to the results of his inoculation experiments and would not give way, but others would not allow the matter to rest there. Vidal de Cassis (1803–1856), a junior colleague at the Midi, believed that clinical observation supported the idea of secondary contagion, and this belief was strengthened by reports of apparently successful inoculations of normal "volunteers" with material from patients with secondary syphilis which had been performed by

Wallace and other investigators. Blood had also been inoculated. Lancereaux wrote:

> "What Hunter did not do, Waller of Prague had the boldness to do. On 27 July 1850, in the presence of a great number of physicians and pupils, he inoculated a boy age 15 years with the blood of a woman affected with secondary syphilis. On the 31st of the following month tubercles were observed at the point of insertion which were followed soon after by secondary symptoms. Gibert performed a similar operation with equal success. In 1856 the Secretary of the Medical Society of the Palatinate announced that a physician who wished to remain incognito had inoculated nine healthy individuals with the blood of a person with secondary syphilis; of this number three, in whom a large absorbing surface had been rubbed, developed syphilis[27]."

Ricord categorically refused to consider experiments of this sort, saying that they were unethical. Indeed they were, but it is hard to understand how he could have ignored the results, and the historical evidence mentioned by Proksch, unless he was unaware of them. At all events, Vidal de Cassis did not share Ricord's scruples and in 1851 inoculated a pharmacy student with pus from a lesion on the breast of a patient with secondary syphilis, inducing a primary chancre after six weeks and secondary manifestations three months later. Ricord was still unconvinced, suggesting that the source lesion was a primary chancre; by now he was a powerful figure in European venereology, and he managed to silence opposition for the time being. However, by 1858 the position had become so unsatisfactory that a committee of the Academy of Medicine was convened to study the whole question; it was chaired by Camille Gibert (1797–1866), a miserable and grumpy individual but an able venereologist, on the staff of St Louis Hospital in Paris, who had performed some successful inoculation experiments himself. He presented the committee's report the following year. The evidence – historical, epidemiological, clinical and experimental – was overwhelming and Ricord, now aged 60, was obliged to make a humiliating public pronouncement that for all these years he had been wrong[28].

The vogue for experimental inoculations reached its apogee in the controversy over "syphilisation"[29]. A young Parisian graduate, Joseph-Alexandre Auzias-Turenne (1812–1870), inoculated pus from human chancres into animals and described the development of lesions which he thought might be syphilitic. Repeated autoinoculation, reinoculation and further autoinoculation eventually produced a state where no lesion could be induced by inoculating material from any source. He performed a small number of experiments on prostitutes with similar results, but he noticed that if syphilitic lesions were already present they seemed to improve. He thought that "syphilisation" might induce immunity to syphilis, and perhaps be of value in therapy. Ricord was implacably opposed to the whole idea, and succeeded in having Auzias' experiments on prostitutes banned. However, he continued other experiments. Trouble was inevitable, and it came in 1851 when a young German doctor called Lindemann, who had performed repeated self-inoculations, finally gave himself syphilis. Auzias treated him by syphilisation, but he died. The "Lindemann case" caused a major scandal and effectively ended syphilisation in France, although it lingered for a few years in some other countries. Auzias himself died a forgotten man, and it is sad to report that his body was found to be covered with scars from his own attempts at syphilisation.

Ricord gave careful thought to the natural history of syphilis. This subject had been tackled many times by earlier investigators, and various systems based on pathological anatomy, dermatological signs and so on had been suggested. Ricord proposed a simple scheme which was to become generally accepted[30]:

(1) *Primary lesion*, a chancre, the immediate result of contagion.
(2) *Secondary lesions*, constitutional poisoning, resulting from that infection.
(3) *Tertiary lesions* [gummas], which rarely appeared before the end of the sixth month, and whose development could be delayed for many years.

Another French venereologist, Joseph Rollet of Lyons, was also studying syphilis. In 1859 careful clinical studies enabled him to define its incubation period as approximately three weeks. This was in accordance with the results of the inoculation experiments of Wallace and others, which had shown incubation periods of 18–35 days. Rollet also confirmed the contagiousness of secondary syphilis in an ingenious way. He had noted that the disease was occurring in glass workers who were passing the blowpipe back and forth from mouth to mouth. A worker with mucous patches in his mouth could thereby infect his colleagues, and Rollet collected many cases where this had happened[31].

Despite several setbacks Ricord remained the best known venereologist of his time. He retired from the Midi in 1860, but remained active for another 25 years. In old age he was "full of wit, brimming over with kindness, eager to hear all the news of his old friends and thoroughly au fait with the doings, scientific and personal, of the leading men in the profession"[32]. He died at the age of 89 from pneumonia shortly after climbing the new Eiffel Tower. It is said that a successful general requires luck as well as skill. Ricord had both. His autoinoculation technique was basically flawed, but it enabled him to confirm that gonorrhoea and syphilis were separate diseases – and to get the credit for the discovery. He failed to recognise the "duality of the chancre" and the contagiousness of secondary syphilis and, as we will see in a later chapter, he did not understand gonorrhoea. In some ways the complexity of the venereal diseases were too much for him. On the other hand, he greatly improved the standards of clinical diagnosis in women and he introduced a valid grading of the stages of syphilis which has stood the test of time. Above all, he founded a school and a tradition; his pupils, who included Bassereau, Diday and Fournier, were to make important discoveries. Ricord transformed venereology, and through his personal magnetism he made it respectable.

By the middle of the nineteenth century early syphilis in men had been described so well that only a few points of detail needed to be added. The incubation period had been defined. The classical indurated penile chancre was well known, and it was realised that atypical forms, and multiple chancres, could occur. In men, the urethral chancre (*larvated chancre*) had been described by Ricord. Astruc had referred to anal chancres in a roundabout way as "the contamination which may follow from the abominable and unnatural intercourse of persons of the same sex". Ricord's knowledge of these enabled him to explain some cases of *syphilis d'emblée*, a concept which he had found difficult to understand.

"In England they seldom search for chancres at the anus; their medical customs reflect the innate modesty characteristic of the nation. I was shown [at St Bartholomew's Hospital, London] a group of men and women with secondary syphilis supposedly due to immediate contagion [syphilis d'emblée]. I still have to laugh at the startled expression of the house officer and his assistants when, carrying a bold finger and scrutinising gaze into certain mucous folds I succeeded in discovering a rear entrance to perfidious Albion[33]."

It was reported that primary chancres could not be seen in some women with undoubted early syphilis. This may have been because of failure to diagnose cervical chancres. These had been described as early as 1843 by Gousselin, who commented that their identification was one of the advantages of speculum examination[34]. They were thought to be uncommon; Fournier stated that only five percent of chancres in women were on the cervix, and this view was echoed by many subsequent authors. The subject was resurrected by the British venereologist Anwyl Davis in the 1930s. He had a quite different opinion, claiming that in women the cervix was the commonest site to be infected by T. pallidum, over 40% of chancres being on this site[35].

Extragenital chancres had been recorded since the earliest times, particularly in the mouth – described by Rollet as "the great laboratory of secondary syphilis". Infection of a suckling's mouth from syphilitic lesions on the breast of a wet nurse had been described since the fifteenth century, although both Hunter and Ricord, whose inoculation experiments had led them to believe that secondary syphilis was not contagious, refused to accept the idea that babies could be infected in this way. Everyone agreed that a wet nurse could develop a primary chancre on the breast by suckling an infected infant. Another source of extragenital infection in babies was vaccination against smallpox, which had been introduced by Edward Jenner in 1796. The usual practice was to use lymph from a recently vaccinated child to vaccinate others. Although the possibility that syphilis might be transmitted in this way was pointed out early in the nineteenth century major epidemics of vaccination syphilis had occurred. Lancereaux relates that in 1841 a child born of syphilitic parents furnished lymph for 64 children; most of them developed syphilis, and eight died[36]; in the USA in the 1860s there were mass infections from this cause among Confederate troops[37]. Although the risk of transmitting syphilis by arm-to-arm vaccination was acknowledged in Europe, in Britain it had been dismissed as negligible until in 1877 Jonathan Hutchinson, one of the great figures of Victorian medicine, published an illustrated account of a series of cases where primary chancres had developed at the site of vaccination (Figure 3.9)[38]. This needed courage, because at the time there was a violent controversy between supporters and opponents of compulsory vaccination. Hutchinson himself favoured it, but said that "concealment in such a matter appears to me the very worst policy". Eventually measures to prevent these infections by the careful examination of the vaccinifer were adopted, and after the use of calf lymph became compulsory in the 1880s vaccination syphilis disappeared.

Most of the clinical features of secondary syphilis were well known in the mid nineteenth century. Skin eruptions were classified as erythematous, papular, pustular and squamous, as they are today. Alopecia, mucous patches, condylomata lata, generalised lymphadenopathy and systemic symptoms such as

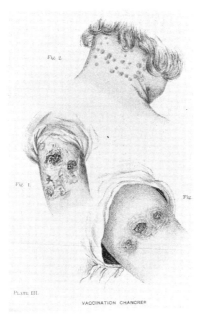

Figure 3.9. Vaccination chancres, with a secondary syphilitic rash on the neck of one patient. From Hutchinson's Syphilis, *1887.*

malaise, fever and loss of weight were all recognised. The pioneer syphilographers had described many neurological disorders in patients with early syphilis, and after the introduction of lumbar puncture by Quinche in 1891 it it was found that abnormalities of the cerebrospinal fluid were not uncommon, even in those with no symptoms[39]; evidently, infection of the meninges by *T. pallidum* was a more frequent event than had been supposed (see Chapter 4). Iritis in secondary syphilis was described in 1830 by Sir William Lawrence (1783–1867), a surgeon at St Bartholomew's Hospital, London[40], and subsequently examined in detail by many ophthalmologists and physicians (including Ricord). After the invention of the ophthalmoscope in 1851 by Hermann von Helmholtz (1821–1894) the ocular changes in early syphilis could be studied in detail and choroidoretinitis was identified as a cause of loss of vision in the secondary stage, occurring later than iritis. In 1896 Hutchinson described deafness in some patients with secondary syphilis[41]; the cause of this was shown, many years later, to be a syphilitic pachymeningitis[42]. Thus for more than three centuries fresh discoveries were made about early syphilis, which revealed it to be a disease of the most fascinating interest.

Experimental Syphilis

The eighteenth and nineteenth-century masters were unrivalled clinical observers, but they undoubtedly found some aspects of syphilis hard to understand. For example, what was its minimum and maximum incubation period? How long did patients remain infectious? Was it possible for an untreated syphilitic to be reinfected, and did a patient who had been treated for syphilis have any immunity against further attacks? Questions of this sort were difficult to answer from clinical observations alone, and many workers looked for explanations by performing experiments on either human volunteers – sometimes including the experimenter himself – or unsuspecting hospital patients. The practice was widespread. Although some physicians – Ricord was one – strongly disapproved, the majority seem to have had no qualms. As the nineteenth century progressed, however, public opinion hardened against the experimenters, so that by the end of the century few studies with dangerous pathogens were being undertaken. One of the last seems to have been performed on an unfortunate medical student called Paul Maisonneuve. In 1905 Metchnikoff and Roux had shown that calomel ointment was an effective prophylactic against experimental syphilis in monkeys, and Maisonneuve was persuaded to participate in a human venture. Although the prophylaxis was successful there were persistent rumours that he had developed syphilis and could therefore not be trusted to look after patients; he spent years trying to convince his colleagues that he had not been infected[2].

It was obvious that it would be much easier to study the natural history of syphilis if a suitable animal could be found. No animal is naturally subject to a disease like human syphilis, so a search was made for a species which could be infected with the disease. From the mid nineteenth century attempts were made to inoculate the syphilis "virus" into dogs, cats, pigs, rabbits and other animals, all without success. It is possible that some of the early experimenters succeeded in inoculating apes, but priority is usually given to Metchnikoff and Roux, who addressed the problem in 1903. Elie Metchnikoff (1845–1913; Figure 3.10) grew up in Tsarist Russia. He began his career as a zoologist but in 1882, after a nervous breakdown, he resigned his appointments and left Russia. While living in Messina, Sicily, he discovered the phenomenon of phagocytosis and in 1888 he took his discoveries to the Pasteur Institute in Paris. Here the weary

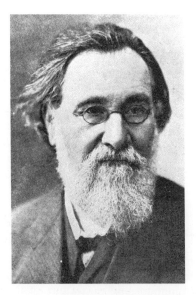

Figure 3.10. Elie Metchnikoff (1845–1916).

exile at last felt at home, and he never returned to Russia. Pasteur provided him with laboratory space to continue his studies of immunology. In 1895 he succeeded Pasteur as director of the institute, and in 1908 he shared the Nobel Prize for Medicine with Paul Ehrlich. Metchnikoff was brilliant, excitable and flamboyant, in complete contrast to his collaborator in the study of experimental syphilis, Pierre-Paul-Émile Roux (1853–1933) who was quiet and methodical. Roux had previously discovered the exotoxin of diphtheria, and had worked with Pasteur on rabies.

After several failures with lower animals Metchnikoff and Roux thought they might be more successful with primates, and they inoculated the clitoris of a chimpanzee with syphilitic material. Three weeks later a classical primary chancre appeared, followed by inguinal adenopathy. The animal was shown at a meeting of the Academy of Medicine in Paris, and the lesion was closely inspected by many eminent venereologists, including Fournier. One month after the chancre appeared the chimpanzee developed undoubted secondary syphilis; the search for a susceptible animal was over. The work was published between 1903 and 1905[43], amid mounting excitement. Among the many researchers who wanted to pursue the subject was Albert Neisser, who had discovered the gonococcus in 1879. At one time he had a colony of 200 monkeys in the grounds of his own house at Breslau but the animals, besides being expensive, failed to thrive in the cold winters of north Germany. He therefore decided to move his laboratories and staff to Batavia (now Jakarta) in Java, where monkeys were plentiful. In February 1905, accompanied by his wife, he set out. The work continued for two years (Figure 3.11); at first it was funded from Neisser's own resources, but later he received some outside help. When he returned to Breslau he brought with him the material for his *Beiträge*[44], perhaps the most comprehensive account of experimental syphilis ever published. Its incubation period was established, and

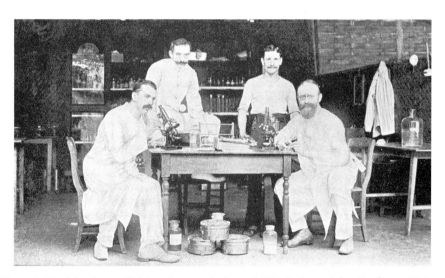

Figure 3.11. Members of Neisser's team in Java, 1906. Left to right: Professor Neisser, Dr Bruck, Dr Kaiser, Karl Leschner (a technician) (From Neisser: Beiträge zur Pathologie und Therapie der Syphilis, *1911.)*

it was shown that the "virus" was present in the blood within a few hours of inoculation, from which it followed that the destruction or excision of a primary chancre, which was often performed at the time, was useless. The contagiousness of secondary syphilis was confirmed, and an old controversy was settled when it was shown that while an animal with active syphilis could not be reinfected, an animal cured of the infection had no immunity. Neisser's group was unable to immunise monkeys against syphilis, and since no tertiary lesions appeared in the experimental animals the pathogenesis of late syphilis could not be studied.

Between 1906 and 1914 a voluminous literature on experimental syphilis appeared, and in time some other susceptible animals were found which were cheaper and more manageable than monkeys. An American scientist left this account of a visit to Europe in 1908:

> "Professor Hoffmann has under his charge quite a menagerie of monkeys, sheep, goats and rabbits that he has infected with syphilis. While standing in the pen watching him examine some infected monkeys I felt a slight tugging at my coat, and turned to find a syphilitic almond-eyed goat nibbling at the hem. After this I confess to having a very creepy feeling in Dr Hoffmann's barnyard[45]."

Much was learned from these experiments, but large animals are expensive; suitable small animals proved very difficult to find, although rabbits could be infected with human syphilis, developing primary and secondary lesions. Unfortunately neither rabbits, monkeys or any other animal develop any disease resembling late syphilis.

Chapter 4
"He sees syphilis everywhere":
Late Syphilis

their worm dieth not, and the fire is not quenched

Mark 9:44

Since the time of Ricord it has been customary to divide the "syphilis drama" into three stages. Nowadays the signs of tertiary syphilis rarely appear less than two years from the original infection, but in earlier times some of these seem to have appeared well before this; indeed, a "galloping syphilis" was described in which tertiary lesions followed the secondary stage after only a few months. This makes it more than usually difficult to interpret many of the early clinical descriptions, in particular to decide whether the authors were describing late syphilis or merely a prolonged secondary stage.

The characteristic lesion of late benign syphilis is the gumma: Lancereaux's "gummy product". Deep-seated lesions of the skin and subcutaneous tissue were described by the earliest syphilographers; for example, Fracastor wrote of their "eroding the flesh and eating down to the bone"[1]. Chronic cutaneous syphilides, in their bewildering complexity, were among the commonest signs of late syphilis; they gave rise to a massive literature, and helped to unite the disciplines of dermatology and venereology. Late syphilis affected the bones almost as often as the skin, and bony swellings were described by Jean de Vigo, Fallopio and other masters. According to Virchow, Jean-Louis Petit, a Parisian surgeon, gave the first good account of syphilitic exostoses in 1735. Twenty years later a Polish physician, Jan Frederyk Knolle, wrote his doctoral thesis on bone syphilis[2]. Like many other eighteenth-century clinicians he divided the course of untreated syphilis into "liquid" and "solid" stages; it was held that the venereal poison was first absorbed into the body fluids, causing the manifestations of early syphilis, and later affected "solids" such as the bones.

Gummatous affection of the nasal bones and cartilages was formerly quite common, and many surgeons found fame and fortune in their ability to repair the deformities. In a more robust age than our own these misfortunes brought ribald comments. The essayist Richard Steele wrote in *The Tatler* in 1710:

> "I shall close this paper with an admonition to the young men of the town ... The general precept I will leave with them is to regard every town woman as a particular kind of syren that has a design upon their noses, and that amidst her flatteries and allurements they will fancy she

speaks to them in the humorous phrase of old Plautus, "Keep your face out of my way or I will bite off your nose."

Lord Chesterfield warned his son of this danger in one of his letters[3]. Syphilitic disease of the testicle was recognised by many surgeons, Bell, Astley Cooper and Dupuytren among them. Bell contrasted the painless swelling of syphilis, in which the testis alone was affected, with the painful swelling of the epididymis which occurs in gonorrhoea[4]. It was noted that syphilitic disease of the testis could occur within a year of the primary infection, earlier than most of the classical manifestations of late syphilis; this led Hutchinson, writing in the nineteenth century, to include it in an "intermediate" group of disorders which included some skin eruptions, choroiditis and cerebrovascular disease, which he regarded as relapses of secondary syphilis rather than signs of true late syphilis – he called them "reminders".

Visceral Syphilis

Giovanni Battista Morgagni (1682–1771) was a pioneer in the study of morbid anatomy. When he dissected the bodies of syphilitics he noted lesions of the heart, aorta and cerebral arteries, but the possibility of visceral syphilis – affecting the internal organs – attracted little interest until the nineteenth century. Hunter roundly declared that it did not exist. He wrote that the skin, throat and nose were readily affected by the *lues venerea*, then the bones and periosteum, but the "vital parts" were probably not susceptible to the disease[5].

Hunter's great authority, combined with his poor understanding of syphilis, held back studies in this area for many years. Ricord and his contemporaries were familiar with at least some forms of visceral syphilis: of the liver, for example, although they recognised the difficulty of distinguishing it from other diseases[6]. This became easier when the pathology of late syphilis was studied by Rudolf Virchow (1821–1902). Virchow (Figure 4.1) was one of the founders of scientific medicine. Born in Pomerania, he graduated at Berlin in 1843, and was then appointed morbid anatomist at the Charité Hospital. In 1848 he was sent to investigate an epidemic of typhus in Silesia; unfortunately his report, which recommended political as well as sanitary reforms, gravely offended the authorities and he was dismissed. He was soon appointed to the chair in pathological anatomy at Wurzburg, and seven years later, in 1856, he returned to Berlin as professor of pathology. He now embarked on a study of late syphilis, investigating not only its morbid anatomy but its cellular pathology[7]. By this time microscopes were well developed, and Virchow cut sections by hand and stained them by the simple methods available at the time. He undertook a detailed study of the bony and cutaneous effects of late syphilis, and described gummas at various sites. He discussed syphilitic cirrhosis and its differentiation from other forms of liver disease. He had seen two cases of cardiac gumma, and he raised the possibility of a syphilitic myocarditis, a thorny subject which was debated for many years. Virchow was uncertain about the effects of syphilis on the central nervous system, and questioned whether syphilitic disease of the lungs was a real entity. He described the classical histological picture of perivascular cuffing with lymphocytes, epithelioid and giant cells as specific to syphilis; the

46

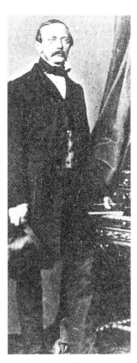

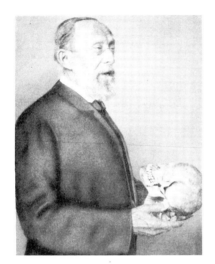

Figure 4.1. (left) Rudolf Virchow (1821–1902). (Courtesy of Dr M.A. Waugh.)

Figure 4.2. (right) Felix von Baerensprung (1822–1864).

plasma cell, another important component of the cellular reaction to syphilis, was discovered by Unna (see p. 151–2) in 1891. Virchow's work had a profound effect on the way in which syphilis was regarded, and he made it possible for clinicians aided by pathologists to determine the full extent of the involvement of organs and tissues in late syphilis[8].

Virchow had wide scientific, cultural and political interests. He became a member of the Reichstag in 1880. His republican views brought him into conflict with Bismarck, who is said to have challenged him to a duel (he declined the offer). His political views unfortunately coloured his relationship with Felix von Baerensprung (1822–1864; Figure 4.2), who was director of the syphilis clinic at the Charité Hospital and had supported Ricord's opinion on the separate identity of syphilis and gonorrhoea. Although relations were harmonious to begin with, in later life they fell out over the pathology of syphilis; moreover, von Baerensprung was staunchly conservative and a supporter of Bismarck. Disagreements led to vicious personal attacks on Virchow by von Baerensprung which became so paranoid and intemperate that it was realised that he had serious mental disease. In fact, like many venereologists of his period he had developed general paresis, from which he died at the early age of 42 years[9]. Virchow went on to become famous throughout Europe as a pathologist, epidemiologist and public health physician. Physically he was short and active, with dark eyes, and he revelled in polemics and controversy. Some of his opinions were certainly unconventional: he rejected Darwin's theory of evolution through natural selection, and was unconvinced of the importance of bacteriology. But in believing that disease should be studied by clinical observation supported by pathology, particularly at the cellular level, with animal experimentation if possible, he was very much a modern man and he had enormous influence. He died at the age of 81.

Samuel Wilks (1824–1911; Figure 4.3) was another pioneer in the study of visceral syphilis. He spent most of his professional life at Guy's Hospital; kindly and genial, he was described by Osler as one of the handsomest men in London. He began his report with these words:

> "The syphilitic affections of the internal organs of the body constitute a subject which is comparatively novel and one, therefore, which is still open to further investigation. Although it is but a few years since specimens illustrating it were received with more than incredulity by the medical profession, yet so strong has been the evidence in favour of modern observations that few pathologists now retain any doubts about their general truth[10]."

He went on to describe examples of syphilitic disease of the liver, spleen, lungs and other organs. Some of his cases, for example, a prostitute with an abdominal aneurysm, may not have been syphilitic.

Cardiovascular Syphilis

From the mid nineteenth century onwards clinical and pathological observations gradually clarified the extraordinary diversity of the lesions of late benign syphilis; it seemed that no organ or tissue could escape. However, although some of these

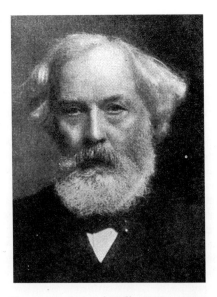

Figure 4.3. Samuel Wilks (1824–1911).

conditions had effects that were anything but benign most people who died of syphilis did not die of these, but of either cardiovascular or neurosyphilis. It is strange that for many years these serious diseases were unrecognised. Some of the early masters groped after a connection between syphilis and aortic aneurysm, although they were inclined to attribute it to the effects of mercury. In 1634 Ambroise Paré mentioned this in the following dramatic description of a fatality:

> "The aneurysmals which happen in the internal parts are incurable. Such as frequently happens to those who have often had the unction and sweat for the cure of the French disease, because the blood being so attenuated and heated therewith that it cannot be contained in the receptacles of the artery, it distends it to the largeness as to hold a man's fist. Which I have observed in the dead body of certain Taylor, who by an aneurysma of the arterious vein suddenly, while he was playing at tennis, fell down dead, the vessel being broken. His body being opened, I found a great quantity of blood poured forth into the capacity of the chest, but the body of the artery was dilated to that largeness I formerly mentioned, and the inner coat thereof was bony ... whilst he lived he said he felt a beating and a great heat over all his body by the force of the pulsation of all the arteries, by occasion whereof he often swooned[11]."

Giovanni Lancisi (1654–1720), the greatest Italian clinician of his time and physician to several popes, saw a link between cardiac disease and syphilis. In a posthumous work published in 1728 he noted chronic dilatation of the heart as a sequel of syphilis. He called the condition "aneurysma gallicum" (aneurysm due to the French disease) but whether he was describing aortic aneurysm or cardiac enlargement secondary to aortic incompetence is uncertain[12]. Morgagni, in his account of more than 600 autopsies published in 1761, reported that he had found lesions in the heart and aorta of syphilitic subjects, but after this no more was heard about cardiovascular syphilis for over a century. Aneurysms were common, and were attributed to physical exertion and arteriosclerosis. Virchow did not discuss aneurysm, although he did describe a syphilitic myocarditis, and Lancereaux referred to "gummy tumours of the heart". But little was added to the understanding of cardiovascular syphilis, and the seminal observations of Lancisi and Morgagni were forgotten.

In the later part of the nineteenth century medical officers of the British army expressed concern over the high incidence of deaths from aortic aneurysms in soldiers, and it was recognised that these often appeared to be free from the ordinary atheromatous changes. The connection with syphilis was established by Francis Henry Welch (1839–1910). He studied medicine at the London Hospital, and soon after qualifying joined the Army Medical Service. Between 1871 and 1876 he was assistant professor of pathology at the Army School at Netley, Hampshire. Later, he saw active service in Egypt and Afghanistan; he rose to the rank of surgeon colonel before retiring in 1895. He died in England at the age of 71 years. It was during his time at Netley that he presented a paper "On aortic aneurysm in the Army and the conditions associated with it" to a meeting of the Royal Medical and Chirurgical Society of London. He had studied 34 fatal cases, whose average age was 32 years. In half there was a history of syphilis, and in two-thirds there were characteristic changes in the wall of the aorta which impaired its elasticity and contractability and resulted in its dilatation. These changes could also damage the aortic valves and lead to cardiac hypertrophy. Welch described the macroscopic and histological features of these lesions, and emphasised the difference between these and atheromatous changes. He concluded that the most important cause of aortic aneurysm and its associated lesions was syphilis[13]. Outside the army this work had a chilly reception. It was argued that the real cause of aortic aneurysm was atheroma, to whose contributory causes – alcoholism and the "rheumatic diathesis" – soldiers were especially liable. The connection with syphilis was dismissed as fortuitous. A year before his death Welch wrote to Osler:

> "The only individual who gave me the slightest support in 1876 was Sir James Paget, and since then one or two others have written giving me their experience, but for long after, as could be seen in the narration of annual cases in the professional journals, there was a dead set against my deductions[11]."

Despite his rough handling, Welch was not alone in his opinions. Many Scandinavian physicians believed that syphilis and aneurysm of the aorta were closely associated, and in Stockholm Mamsten described a "sclero-gummatous aortitis" which he believed to be specific. However, the first clear definition of syphilitic aortitis as a precursor of aneurysm was made in 1895 by Dohle, a pupil of Arnold Heller at the Pathological Institute at Kiel; he described round and plasma cell infiltration of the vasa vasorum, scarring of the intima and fibrous thickening of the media and adventitia. This work was not generally accepted, and in the end Heller spoke himself on the subject at a meeting of the German Pathological Society in 1899. There was a long discussion, in the course of which most of the well-known pathologists of Germany ridiculed the work of the Kiel team, who had no supporters. One of the long-running disputes so common in the history of syphilis ensued until in 1903, at another meeting of the same Society, there was a reluctant admission that Heller, Dohle and their colleagues were correct[14]. Since then, a vast amount of work has confirmed the importance of obliterative changes in the vasa vasorum in the pathogenesis of syphilitic disease of the aorta and aortic valves. In 1906 Reuter was the first to demonstrate spirochaetes in an aortic lesion, and from 1908 onwards the Wassermann reaction was used to provide further proof that Francis Welch had been right all along[15].

Neurosyphilis

The idea that syphilis could affect the nervous system came early in the epidemic. Such masters as Niccolo Leonicino (1497) and Niccolo Massa (1556) described patients with headache or paralysis which they thought might have been due to the *morbus Gallicus*. In the seventeenth century there were references to epilepsy, loss of vision, vertigo and paralysis supposedly due to syphilis, but the early observers were handicapped by a poor understanding of the structure and function of the nervous system, and of the pathological processes involved in the infection. A notable advance came when in 1761 Morgagni described some features of the morbid anatomy of cerebral syphilis; he discussed cerebral arteritis, and pointed out that gummas could involve the brain as well as the skull.   There was a setback for many years after John Hunter in 1790 stated that in his view the brain was not affected by syphilis, although during this time the understanding of neurology was steadily improving. In 1834 the French pathologist Claude Francois Lallemand (1790–1853) presented a collection of brain disorders which he believed were caused by syphilis, and from 1847 onwards Virchow contributed a detailed description of the morbid anatomy and histopathology of cerebral gummas and arterial lesions. This paved the way for many clinical and pathological studies of neurosyphilis which appeared in the second half of the nineteenth century. For example, the French master Lancereaux, in his *Traité historique et pratique de la syphilis*, published in 1862, was able to devote 82 pages to the subject. In many ways the work has a modern flavour. The conditions he described now included headache, fits, cranial nerve palsies and hemiplegia.

Von Helmholtz had invented the ophthalmoscope in 1851, so Lancereaux was able to discuss papilloedema, and blindness due to optic atrophy. He attributed most of these disorders to either meningitis or gummas, and gave many examples of a good response to treatment with iodides and/or mercury. In 1870 Clifford Allbut (1836–1925), regius professor of physic at the University of Cambridge, described the histology of syphilis of the cerebral arteries, and in 1874 Otto Heubner (1843–1926) published a classical monograph on syphilis of the cerebral arteries and its clinical effects: predominantly headache followed by a stroke of some kind[16]. The reader scans this literature in vain for any reference to tabes dorsalis or general paresis. The attribution of these devastating diseases to syphilis was a late development which was the subject of much controversy until the truth was established. At the centre of these disputes was one of the giants of syphilology, Jean Alfred Fournier (1832–1914; Figure 4.4).

Fournier was born in Paris and, like Benjamin Bell, had a classical education. He began his medical studies in 1854, and was soon allotted an internship under Ricord at l'Hôpital du Midi. Ricord liked Fournier and had a great influence

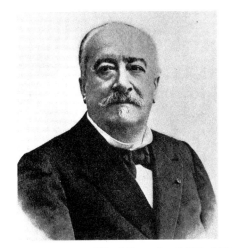

Figure 4.4. Jean Alfred Fournier (1832–1914).

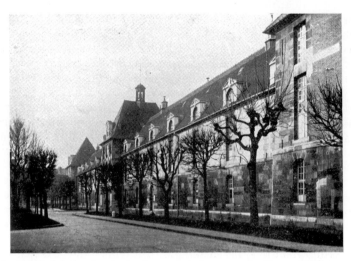

Figure 4.5. Hôpital Saint Louis (early twentieth century). (From Shelley and Crissey, Classics in clinical dermatology, 1953. Courtesy of Charles C. Thomas, Publisher, Springfield, Illinois.)

on his later career; no doubt this was the reason why the younger man chose "syphilitic contagion" as the subject of his doctoral thesis. After various junior appointments, in 1876 Fournier became chief of service at l'Hôpital St Louis, the renowned skin and venereal disease centre (Figure 4.5), and he remained there until 1902. In 1879 he was admitted to the Academy of Medicine, and in the following year became the first occupant of a chair of dermatology and syphilology in the faculty of medicine[17]. Although in his younger days Fournier published work on skin diseases, gonorrhoea and chancroid, he soon devoted himself almost exclusively to the study of syphilis. He was an outstanding clinician, and his skill in history taking combined with his meticulous technique of clinical examination enabled him to resolve many complex problems. He was a brilliant teacher, and his Friday morning lectures at St Louis became legendary; like his master Ricord he used anecdotes and reminiscences to lighten case presentations and serious analysis and keep his audience's attention. In his heyday he was an impressive figure, tall and broad-shouldered and with close-cropped hair, looking (as Garrison said) like a retired artillery officer. He had a clear, harmonious voice, impeccable manners and was always immaculately dressed. Not surprisingly, he had a huge private practice. It is said that he had four waiting rooms, one for men, one for women, one for doctors and one for prostitutes; it is reassuring to know that doctors were always seen first. Although he always denied that he was obsessed with syphilis, his devotion to the subject brought him some (presumably good-natured) jibes; the Hungarian dermatologist Louis Nekam maintained that Fournier classified skin diseases as syphilitic, parasyphilitic, syphiloid and asyphilitic[18].

Fournier in France and Hutchinson in England were the two outstanding syphilogists of their time. Fournier's most important contributions to medical science concerned congenital syphilis and neurosyphilis, but he illuminated all clinical aspects of the disease. In later life he became involved in the social and preventive aspects of venereal disease, and in health education. He founded the Society of Sanitary and Moral Prophylaxis in 1901, and wrote essays and pamphlets on syphilis and marriage, and tracts for young people and soldiers. A play called *Les Avaries* (Damaged Goods) about the disastrous effects of syphilis within a family was dedicated to Fournier, who had given the author technical advice. The contrast between Fournier's zealotry and his master Ricord's tolerant attitude towards these matters could hardly have been greater. Fournier's closing years were clouded by his wife's prolonged illness and his own struggle against arteriosclerosis, and he died at the age of 82 at Neuilly, a suburb of Paris.

Fournier's involvement with tabes dorsalis began in the 1870s. The early history of this disease, and its nomenclature, are somewhat confusing. The word *tabes* had been used since the time of Hippocrates to describe a combination of spinal weakness and spermatorrhoea whose nature is now unknown, and it was not used in its modern sense until after the fifteenth century. The earlier physicians had found it difficult to classify the various types of ataxia and paralysis. Some features of a disorder which may have been tabes dorsalis were mentioned by eighteenth-century authors, but it was not until 1844 that Martin Steinthal in Berlin gave the first good description of the characteristic gait, the paraesthesiae, the lightning pains and the visceral "crises." Soon after this, Jean Cruveilhier, who held the first chair of pathology at the Paris faculty, recognised the degeneration in the posterior columns of the spinal cord. In 1846 Moritz Romberg, of Meiningen, who was the first physician to write a formal treatise on neurology, gave a detailed description of tabes and described its association with the eponymous sign that ataxics cannot stand still with their eyes shut[19]. In 1869 a Scottish eye surgeon, Argyll Robertson, described a case of tabes (although he did not name it as this) in which he noted the abnormalities of the pupillary reactions which have born his name ever since[20]. In 1859 Guillaume Duchenne differentiated tabes dorsalis from other diseases of the spinal cord. Duchenne was one of medicine's eccentrics. He roamed around Parisian hospitals without invitation, examining interesting cases and holding informal discussions with the medical staff. In the end his honesty and enthusiasm overcame opposition, and he became one of the great French neurologists, welcome everywhere[21]. Duchenne was astute. He was the first physician to notice that tabetics gave a history of syphilis more often than would be expected from chance; he also introduced the term "locomotor ataxia" which held the field for many years, until in 1881 the British neurologist Hughlings Jackson suggested that the older name was reinstated because many patients with the disease were not ataxic.

Duchenne's contemporary, Jean Charcot had created at the Salpetrière the greatest neurological clinic of his time. Besides elaborating the list of symptoms and signs of tabes he described the associated joint affections which bear his name, but he ignored the association with syphilis which Duchenne had described. Study of the pathological changes in tabes began with Virchow, and later investigators included Cruveilhier, Charcot and the British neurologist William Gull (1816–1890). They established the degeneration of the posterior nerve roots and posterior columns of the spinal cord which lie at the heart of the disease; this was thought to be of inflammatory origin, although there are now some doubts about this.

In 1876 Fournier reported a definite history of syphilis in 24 of 30 patients with tabes; while he was confident that it was the cause of the disease in some cases, he thought that in others it might be only a "predisposing factor." Three years later the association of syphilis with tabes was confirmed by two neurologists, Edme-Félix Alfred Vulpian in France and William Gowers in England. The possibility of a syphilitic aetiology was received at first with some scepticism. It was only to be expected that in Fournier's practice there would be a large number of patients with syphilis, and it was hinted that "he sees syphilis everywhere". However, in 1881 Wilhelm Heinrich Erb, an influential German neurologist, published a large series of 1100 tabetics and no less than 10 000 controls and reported results very similar to those of Fournier. Fournier himself returned to the subject in a long book published in 1882 in which every aspect of the problem was discussed and his conclusions re-stated[22]. After this his ideas on the aetiology of tabes were generally accepted, although Charcot still maintained that syphilis had nothing to do with it. Fournier was never sure that syphilis was the *sole* cause of every case of tabes, and he was to have the same difficulty when he came to study general paresis.

For many centuries there had been a poorly defined relationship between "venery" and insanity. Some of the features of "dementia paralytica", later to be called "general paralysis of the insane" and in modern times "general paresis", had been described by the end of the sixteenth century, but the first full acount was given in 1798 by John Haslam, a physician at the Bethlehem Hospital, an institution for the insane just outside London. He described four cases of paralytic insanity with disturbances of speech. All of them died; post-mortem examination showed "thickening of the arachnoid membrane and an increased consistency of the brain", but Haslam was not sure whether these appearances were the result or the cause of the insanity[23]. In 1822 a Parisian internist, Antoine-Laurent-Jessé Bayle, described the clinical and pathological features of six similar cases, and became the first physician to separate this disease from other forms of insanity. Six years later the French physician François Broussais gave this description of a patient with unmistakable dementia paralytica:

> "There is an embarrassment of speech as well as memory . . . by degrees the face loses its expression, they become indifferent to what passes around them and they seldom speak. We see them immovable, silent and sitting or laying down for days together. If paralysis proceeds at an equal pace with dementia the patients are at last deprived of the power of executing any voluntary movement, their food must be put in their mouths and they must be kept constantly clean[24]."

The first observers to suggest a link between general paresis and syphilis were Johann Friedrich von Esmarch, a German military surgeon, and his colleague Peter Willen Jessen. In a paper "Syphilis and mental disturbance" published in 1857 they reported a history of syphilis in several of their patients; this was also mentioned by Kjelberg in Uppsala in 1863.

Fournier had observed concurrent tabes and general paresis in some patients, and in the early 1880s he started to collect data on a possible connection between general paresis and syphilis. It was obviously much more difficult to obtain reliable retrospective information about patients with general paresis, many of whom were demented, than about patients with tabes. Nevertheless, Fournier persisted, and after several interim reports set out his final conclusions in a famous paper read before the Academy of Medicine in 1890. He began by stating that some patients with late syphilis showed features suggestive of general paresis, but post-mortem examination revealed only meningovascular or gummatous changes. He called this entity "general syphilitic pseudo-paralysis", and regarded it as "an *ensemble* of cerebral syphilis and nothing else". He then proceeded to establish the relationship between "true general paralysis" and syphilis. First, there was a past history of syphilis in 50 to 90 per cent of patients, second, long-term surveillance of people with early syphilis showed that some went on to develop general paresis, third, although the disease was uncommon in women most of those who did develop it were prostitutes, at high risk of syphilis, and fourth, there was no doubt that juvenile general paresis could follow congenital syphilis. At this point in his argument the author felt obliged to hedge:

> "Some observers, much more courageous than I, regard general paralysis as a direct consequence – a direct effect of syphilis. According to this idea, general paralysis occurring in the syphilitic would be the equivalent of any other entirely specific symptom as, for example, a mucous patch or a gumma. So far as I am concerned, it is impossible for me to agree with this theory[25]."

Fournier's problem lay in the failure of general paresis to respond to anti-syphilitic treatment with mercury and iodides; this led him to conclude that post-syphilitic general paresis is syphilitic in its *origin* but not in its *nature*. He called it (together with tabes dorsalis and primary optic atrophy) *parasyphilis*; in modern terminology, syphilis was *necessary* but not *sufficient* for the development of general paresis. Like others, Fournier thought that general paresis could be produced "independently of any syphilitic taint." He honestly admitted that he could not explain the relationship between the two "as long as the microbe of syphilis remains undiscovered and its various possible reactions upon the organic tissues are unrecognised".

Fournier's proposal that syphilis was involved in the pathogenesis of general paresis was not well received. Clinicians simply could not imagine that diseases as different from each other as early syphilis and general paresis could have a common cause, or be separated by many years of apparently perfect health. They preferred the older explanations: paresis was due to alcoholism, business worries, bereavement and other types of stress. Nevertheless, it was hard to escape the syphilis connection. Richard von Krafft-Ebing, a neuropsychiatrist from Mannheim, inoculated nine paretics with material from lesions of early syphilis, with negative results in every case, which suggested that the patients had been exposed to the infection and become immune to it. He made the well-known comment that general paresis is "a product of civilisation and syphilisation". Another psychiatrist, Emil Kraeplin, wrote in 1904: "We can today declare with the greatest certainty that syphilitic infection is essential for the later appearance of paresis", and Max Nonne in Berlin, a well-regarded and experienced neurologist, found evidence of previous syphilis in 90 per cent of his cases.

In Britain the idea that general paresis was a syphilitic disease was accepted by only a minority of psychiatrists, but opinions changed after the work of Frederick Mott (1853–1926; Figure 4.6), an outstanding figure in neurology and scientific psychiatry. He received his undergraduate education at University College Hospital and qualified in 1881. After postgraduate study in Vienna he

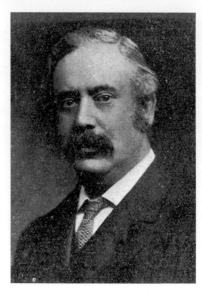

Figure 4.6. Frederick Mott (1853–1924).

was appointed to the consulting staff of Charing Cross Hospital, where he soon developed a special interest in neurology. His studies on the neuropathology of the psychoses led to his appointment as pathologist to the Central Laboratory of London County Asylums. Almost immediately he became involved with general paresis, and collected a vast amount of clinical and pathological data. He found that 80 per cent of his series of patients either gave a history of syphilis or showed clinical evidence of it, and he was struck by the development of juvenile paresis in some patients with congenital syphilis. In the laboratory he demonstrated characteristic perivascular cuffing in the cerebral cortex and meninges of paretics. These studies convinced him of the syphilitic origin of the disease. He published his results in the first edition of *Archives of Neurology* (a journal which he founded) in 1899[26]. After this, the opinions of the French and German workers were gradually accepted in Britain. Mott continued with his work on scientific psychiatry. He participated in the foundation of the Maudsley Hospital, where he directed the pathology laboratory until his death. He was knighted in 1919, and received many academic honours. Withal, his personality was quiet and unassuming, "a kindly friend and a generous host"[27]. He died at the age of 73.

General paresis was a very important disease in the nineteenth century and claimed many eminent victims, but the long struggle to understand it was coming to an end. In 1906 Wassermann and Plaut reported positive serological reactions for syphilis in the cerebrospinal fluid in 90 per cent of paretics, and in 1913 Noguchi and Moore, working at the Rockefeller Institute in New York, clinched the matter by demonstrating spirochaetes in the brains of a series of paretics[28]. This was the end of the long argument, and it was soon generally accepted that syphilis was the only cause of general paresis, and that tabes was – as Fournier had believed – a closely related condition.

Hutchinson

The systemic effects of syphilis had been plain from the earliest days of the epidemic, and as time went by clinical and pathological studies showed that virtually no organ or tissue was spared. Moreover, syphilis was common and difficult to treat. Throughout the nineteenth and early twentieth centuries the need for expert skill, knowledge and judgement was met by a series of outstanding syphilologists: we may think of Barensprung and Lesser in Germany, Sigmund and Neumann in Austria, Lancereaux and Fournier in France and Bumstead and Morrow in the United States. In Britain the acknowledged master was Jonathan Hutchinson (1828–1913). Hutchinson (Figure 4.7) was born in Yorkshire in 1828 and was taught medicine first at York, then at St Bartholomew's Hospital in London. After a few years in junior hospital posts he obtained a remarkable series of appointments, becoming surgeon to the London, Metropolitan Free and Moorfields Eye Hospitals and physician to Blackfriars Skin Hospital.

Osler said that Hutchinson was "the greatest generalised specialist of his generation, the last of the polymaths". Certainly his wide experience formed an ideal background for his study of syphilis, a disease which fascinated him throughout his long life[29]. His major contribution to syphilology concerned congenital infections, which will be discussed in the next chapter, but he cared for many adults in both hospital and private practice; it was said that he had seen a million syphilitics. He used to say that he was able to learn about the disease because many of his patients belonged to the "educated classes" – they could give clear histories of their illnesses, and could be kept under surveillance for many years after treatment. His clinical experience enabled him to see the many resemblances between syphilis and other conditions. He embodied his ideas in a famous paper on "syphilis as an imitator"[30], and generations of

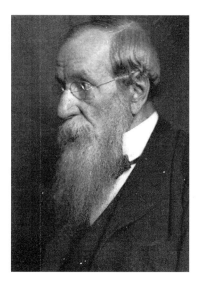

Figure 4.7. Jonathan Hutchinson (1828–1913). (Photograph by courtesy of Miss M. Hutchinson.)

medical students learned never to forget syphilis in differential diagnosis. With the decline of syphilis this advice has, alas, been forgotten but it may have to be re-learned one day. Like his close friend Fournier, Hutchinson was not very interested in bacteriology. His reception of the discovery of *Treponema pallidum* in 1906 was rather cool, but it underlines the fact that nearly all the discoveries about the manifestations of syphilis had been made by clinicians who had no idea of its cause:

> "To those minds incapable of accepting as practically proven anything not actually demonstrated, the discovery is invaluable; and at the same time it furnishes an important weapon of defence to those who for themselves had long ago accepted its conclusion[31]."

Hutchinson was a serious man, a workaholic who never took a holiday. He was a natural teacher, with a remarkable memory; his students thought him infallible, and would pack the lecture theatre to "hear what Jonathan would say". A contemporary described him as: "A tallish dark figure . . . dark eyes that seemed to look past you through his spectacles, black hair and beard lengthening and becoming grey with age"[32]. His knowledge of syphilis was phenomenal. No clinical aspect of the disease escaped him, and he communicated his ideas in masterly lectures, books and articles. He was essentially a naturalist, and in later life he established at his home at Haslemere, in Surrey, an educational museum; at first it was devoted to local natural history, but it was gradually enlarged to include fossils, specimens and illustrations of evolution, an aviary and a vivarium. Hutchinson liked nothing better than to show visitors round the museum and explain the exhibits. It is there to this day. He spent the closing years of his life in Surrey, where he died in 1913 at the age of 85 years. He was one of the great figures of Victorian medicine, and an outstanding syphilologist.

Syphilis had become a crucial component of medical practice. It was a major cause of disability and death, and its protean effects demanded from those attending its victims a broad knowledge not only of medicine but of many of the major specialities. It is no wonder that at the turn of the century William Osler, the greatest physician of his time, wrote: "Know syphilis and all its manifestations and all things clinical will be added unto you".

Chapter 5
"The sins of the fathers": Congenital Syphilis

I never asked you for life. And what sort of life have you given me?

Henrik Ibsen, *Ghosts*

Within a few years of the first outbreak of syphilis in Europe Gabriele Torella (*fl.* 1500) noted signs of syphilis in neonates, and in 1529 the German alchemist and physician Paracelsus (1493–1541) was the first to state "it is a hereditary illness, and passes from father to son". After this came a period which was short on facts but long on unsupported assertions. To be sure, the natural history of syphilis in adults had not been defined, but in congenital syphilis there was an additional and confusing factor – the role of the wet nurse. There were case reports of infection of healthy nurses by syphilitic babies and of normal babies by syphilitic nurses, and there were descriptions of families in which successive children had developed the disease. For two centuries the origin of congenital syphilis was endlessly discussed, but the number of possible permutations and combinations of father, mother, infant and wet nurse meant that almost any conclusion could be drawn. One can sympathise with Diday (1812–1894) who, having waded through this literature, came across a remark by Guillaume Rondelet (1507–1566): "I have seen children born entirely marked with the pustules of the morbus gallicus". Diday's comment was: "A fact! Something precious for that period!". Even such eminent syphilographers as Boerhaave, van Swieten and Jean Astruc, while they admitted the hereditary transmission of syphilis, had little of interest to say about it.

In the eighteenth century good clinical descriptions of early congenital syphilis began to appear, although the mechanism of transmission remained mysterious. John Hunter[1] believed that the only syphilitic lesion which was infectious was the primary chancre, and he therefore taught that infection of the baby could occur only during delivery. Benjamin Bell[2] on the other hand, while accepting that this was possible if the mother had primary syphilis, was convinced that infection of the foetus in utero was possible: "Children may receive, and frequently do receive, the venereal disease from their parents labouring under it in a constitutional form". In insisting that infection occurred only from a maternal primary chancre, Hunter had "unguardedly fallen into error". Bell went on to advocate breast feeding of an infected infant by its mother but not by a wet nurse, and said that both mother and baby should be treated with mercury; he would not hesitate to treat a woman with syphilis during pregnancy. Bell's enlightened opinions on congenital infections were well in advance of his time.

In 1780 interest in the subject was reawakened by the opening of a hospital in Paris for the care of pregnant women with syphilis and their babies. Among the physicians to the hospital was René-Joseph Bertin (1767–1828). In 1810 he published a monograph, *Traité de la maladie vénérienne*, in which he described the mucocutaneous lesions of congenital syphilis and mentioned some bony abnormalities. He put a particular emphasis on ophthalmia neonatorum, which he regarded as a serious and potentially blinding disease. At the time when he was writing many people still believed that syphilis and gonorrhoea were the same disease, and the ophthalmia which he ascribed to congenital syphilis was almost certainly gonococcal.

Paul Diday

Paul Diday (1812–1894; Figure 5.1) was the first of the great French venereologists to make a major study of congenital syphilis. He received his medical education in Paris under Dupuytren, and after graduating was appointed *chirurgeon en chef* at l'Hospice de l'Antiquaille at Lyons. He returned to Paris for a period of postgraduate study, and began to attend Ricord's clinics. He found venereology fascinating; he was a regular participant in the legendary conferences under the lime trees at l'Hôpital du Midi and became one of the master's favourite pupils, and a personal friend. When he returned to Lyons he set to work to establish a school of venereology along Ricordian lines. In this he was successful, and in time l'Antiquille became a major centre. Diday himself was a tireless enthusiast, interested in all aspects of the speciality, even to the point of self-experimentation. Like many others, he tried to inoculate animals with the "virus" of syphilis with the idea of eventually developing a vaccine. The result of one of these experiments was alarming. Having raised a pustule on a cat's ear, he inoculated the material into his own penis. The result was a severe phagedenic ulcer which took many months to heal[3].

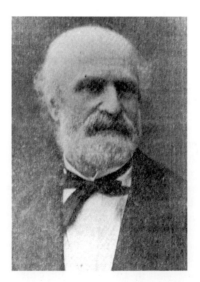

Figure 5.1. Paul Diday (1812–1894).

will have received an impress which is seldom effaced in later life". In 1858 he read a paper *On the means of recognising the subjects of inherited syphilis in adult life* at a meeting of the British Medical Association[12]:

> "First among the peculiarities by which these patients may be identified is the *tout ensemble* of the physiognomy. A bad pale earthy complexion, a thick and pitted skin, a sunk and flattened nose, and scars of old fissures about the angles of the mouth often give the countenance so much of peculiarity that the condition may be recognised at a glance. The opinion is usually borne out by observing further that the subject is of short stature, has a large protruberant forehead and a heavy aspect."

He went on to describe the state of the teeth and the frequent destruction of the soft palate. Acute iritis could occur in syphilitic infants, but as the subject became older interstitial keratitis or choroidoretinitis were more likely. He concluded that: "It is not by any one symptom that the diagnosis of hereditary syphilis can ever be supported but by the careful estimation of the entire group".

In a previous chapter we have discussed Étienne Lancereaux's fine *Treatise on Syphilis*[13]. Lancereaux was a contemporary of Hutchinson and knew about his work. He drew a clear distinction between "hative" and "tardive" types. In his description of the former he included the features detailed by Diday, but splenomegaly was now added to the list; bony and periosteal lesions were still considered to be rare. Lancereaux thought that the "tardive" signs bore resemblances to the tertiary manifestations of acquired syphilis, but he also included the stigmata and the dental and ocular conditions described by Hutchinson. He gave a pathetic example of the havoc congenital syphilis could cause in those days:

> "This woman, who believed that her husband had had syphilis, did not pretend that she herself had been quite free from symptoms of that disease. She had had four children, of whom one died at the age of seven, another at three and a third at two years of age. She had had four miscarriages, three at seven months and the fourth at two months. The only child left was twelve years old, but did not look more than six or eight years. His head was extremely small and the bones of the cranium appeared united. The child walked when led, and was almost completely devoid of intelligence and memory ... The nose was flattened. The two first incisors were notched and studded with small depressions – there was a true arrest of dental development. On the upper part of the tibia there was a fistulous opening and necrosis of several months standing."

Alfred Fournier was junior to Diday. He was as interested in congenital syphilis as his friend Hutchinson and in 1886 he published in Paris a monumental work, *La Syphilis Héréditaire Tardive*. He described the retarded development, facial deformities, stigmata, eye and ear abnormalities and bony malformations in detail, besides discussing the many associated marital, social and medicolegal problems. It is one of the landmarks of French venereological literature.

The "Laws"

Although in the nineteenth century there were misconceptions about the natural history of congenital syphilis, enough was known for some empirical observations to be made which, although partly flawed, reached the status of "laws". The first of these came from the Irishman, Abraham Colles. In his book on syphilis published in 1837[14] he made this statement:

> "I have never seen or heard of a single instance in which a syphilitic infant (although its mouth be ulcerated), suckled by its own mother, had produced ulceration of her breasts; whereas very few instances have occurred when a syphilitic infant had not infected a strange hired wet nurse who had previously been in good health."

Colles added that he knew of cases where the father of a child had been treated with mercury for early syphilis and declared cured, yet subsequently had syphilitic children, even though both he and his wife showed no clinical signs of the disease. He did not attempt to explain these phenomena, he simply recorded them. The other eponymous "laws" were by Profeta and Kassowitz. Guiseppe Profeta (1840–1910), the Italian author of several large books on the venereal diseases, stated that a healthy child of a syphilitic mother could be suckled with impunity by her or by a syphilitic wet nurse[15], and the Viennese dermatologist Max Kassowitz (1843–1913) said that the effect of maternal syphilis on the baby diminished in successive pregnancies[16]. These "laws" are really statements about the immunology of syphilis, which was poorly understood at the time. They were often quoted in discussions on the thorny subject of the transmission of congenital syphilis.

Bony Abnormalities

The clinical studies of Diday, Hutchinson and Fournier, excellent though they were, could not embrace every aspect of the subject, and of course the masters were not infallible. For a long time bony lesions were a controversial subject. Some of the first observers referred to their occurrence in syphilitic infants, but they were thought to be very rare, even by such eminent syphilogists as Diday, von Baerensprung and Lancereaux. In 1863[10] Hutchinson had written: "Nodes are not common in young infants, but do every now and then occur". In 1870 George Wegner (1843–1917), then assistant to Virchow in Berlin, published a classical paper, largely based on the study of autopsy material, in which he gave a detailed description of the histopathology of the bone lesions of 12 cases of foetal or neonatal syphilis; he pointed out that far from being rare these osteochondritic lesions were actually quite common[17]. Wegner was closely followed by the French paediatrician Marie Jules Parrot (1829–1883, Figure 5.5); he had studied the bones of syphilitic foetuses and infants, and concluded that nearly all the bones were involved in almost every case of congenital infection[18]. He had noticed that infants rarely moved affected limbs – "Parrot's pseudoparalysis" – and he described changes in the bones of the skull: cranial nodules and areas of periostitis leading to frontal "bossing". He disagreed with Wegner, who thought

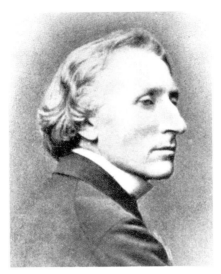

Figure 5.5. Marie-Jules Parrot (1829–1883).

that the syphilitic process was inflammatory, an osteochondritis; Parrot regarded it as a dystrophy, and the debate on the relative importance of inflammatory and trophic influences has persisted to this day. Unfortunately, Parrot also came to believe that syphilis might cause rickets. At a meeting in London in 1879 (chaired by Hutchinson) he went so far as to say "without hereditary syphilis there is no rickets"[19]. The ensuing controversy, which was further confused by statements that rickets was a congenital disease, occupied the decade between 1880 and 1890; eventually it became clear that cases of so-called congenital rickets were really syphilitic and that rickets and congenital syphilis were two common but different diseases which could easily occur in the same child. A subdivision of the same controversy concerned the widespread belief that softening of the vault of the skull (craniotabes) was a sign of syphilis, whereas it is now known to be due to rickets. Parrot did not live to see the end of these disputes, as he died in 1883.

In 1875 the New York venereologist Robert William Taylor (1842–1906) wrote a monograph on the bony lesions in congenital syphilis[20] which included the first description of syphilitic dactylitis. Taylor strongly disagreed with Parrot over the *post hoc ergo propter hoc* argument which he had used to link syphilis with rickets, which he regarded as fallacious. A further development came in 1886 when Clutton, a surgeon at St Thomas' Hospital London, described bilateral painless chronic synovitis of the knees in 11 patients aged 8–21 years. All showed evidence of either interstitial keratitis or Hutchinson's teeth, and Clutton suggested that this synovitis was a late manifestation of congenital syphilis[21]. Another late sign, bowing of the tibia (sabre shin), due to recurrent attacks of periostitis, was well known[22].

In venereology as in other branches of medicine there is a limit to the discoveries which can be made by clinical observation, even when supported by histopathology, and by the end of the nineteenth century this limit had been reached. However, Roentgen had discovered X-rays in 1895, and it was not long before the new science of radiology was applied to congenital syphilis. At the German Congress of Natural Sciences held at Aachen in 1900 Hochsinger presented the first radiographs of bone lesions in the disease and four years later he published a two-volume work in which he described every aspect of the subject in detail, incidentally confirming Parrot's observation that there was evidence of osteochondritis in almost all syphilitic foetuses[23]. Oluf Thomsen, working in Denmark[24], was the first to show that congenital syphilis can be diagnosed radiologically in neonates with no abnormal clinical signs. Events were now moving fast. In 1906 Levaditi and Sauvage demonstrated *Treponema pallidum* in the bone marrow of an infant with congenital syphilis and in the same year the Wassermann reaction was introduced. With the availability of radiology and serology the study of bone involvement entered the modern era.

Systemic Diseases

A systemic reaction in which haemoglobinuria follows chilling was first described by Dressler in 1854 as "intermittent albuminuria and chromaturia". His patient was a 10-year-old child with congenital syphilis, but he did not seem to appreciate the aetiological importance of the infection[26]. Other cases were described in the following years, and it was suspected on anamnestic and clinical grounds that the disease in a child might be related to parental syphilis; this was confirmed when serological tests for syphilis became available. At one time late congenital and acquired syphilis were the leading causes of the condition, whose underlying mechanism was elucidated by Donath and Landsteiner in 1904[27].

Neurological disorders in children – convulsions, paralysis, mental subnormality and so on – were poorly understood in the early part of the nineteenth century, so it is not surprising that the syphilologists of the day were unaware of the frequent involvement of the central nervous system in congenital syphilis. Hutchinson[11] gave one of the first descriptions: "Chronic arachnitis as evinced in a tendency to hydrocephalus is very common in syphilitic infants, and occurs in almost all who suffer severely from the taint in question." Although this observation does not seem to have made much impact at the time, later in the century it was realised that meningovascular syphilis in infancy is not unusual. While all the varieties of neurosyphilis which occur in adults can affect children, general paresis was probably the commonest. It was first described by Clouston, an Edinburgh physician, in 1877[28]. He had seen a 16-year-old boy who showed typical signs of the disease; there were no stigmata, and Clouston does not say whether he thought it was due to syphilis. However, it soon became clear that there was a definite link between juvenile paresis and congenital syphilis; for example the British neurologist Frederick Mott, writing in 1899, said that he had personally seen 22 such cases in three years in London County asylums, and was satisfied that in the majority there was evidence of a syphilitic origin either from the presence of stigmata in the patients or from a history of syphilis in the parents or other siblings[29]. The clinical picture of juvenile paresis is so unlike the adult form that it was probably often overlooked in the nineteenth century, and many victims dismissed as having epilepsy or mental disease.

Whether congenital syphilis could cause mental subnormality alone was the subject of much discussion. Hutchinson[30] thought that it could: "As a matter of clinical observation I would suggest that it is not at all uncommon to note a slight deficiency in vigour of intellect in the subjects of infantile syphilis, but that anything amounting to dementia is certainly rare". A parallel problem concerned convulsions. These are not uncommon in children, and it was often difficult in an individual case to decide whether or not they were due to syphilis. After the introduction of lumbar puncture for patients with syphilis in 1901, and examination of the cerebrospinal fluid by the Wassermann reaction in 1906, the diagnosis became easier, but the relationship between congenital syphilis, mental subnormality and convulsions remained controversial until well into the twentieth century. The prognosis for all forms of neurosyphilis in children was poor, and unless the diagnosis had been made early treatment was largely ineffectual. Fortunately it is uncommon today, for it was one of the saddest manifestations of the infection.

Myocardial lesions, variously described as myxoma, gumma and myocarditis, had been noted at autopsy of babies with congenital syphilis since the 1860s; soon after the discovery of *T. pallidum* in 1907 a type of interstitial myocarditis in which the organisms were present in large numbers was described[31]. Many workers observed histological changes in the aorta in early congenital infections, but aortic valve disease from this cause was not recorded until 1915[32]. Syphilitic aortitis resulting in aortic dilatation and aneurysm was commoner in acquired than in congenital syphilis, but even in the 1930s it was said that in people under the age of 30 years syphilitic cardiovascular disease was usually due to a congenital infection[33].

The Origin of Congenital Syphilis

Almost without exception nineteenth-century venereologists believed in the paternal origin of congenital syphilis; it was thought that a father's "tainted" semen infected an infant at the time of conception, the mother remaining uninfected. This doctrine was accepted by Diday, who regarded paternal transmission as "settled". Nevertheless, he also thought it possible for a foetus to be infected by the mother if she already had syphilis, or if she contracted it during pregnancy, as Bell had suggested. Both Ricord and Diday stated that Hunter's idea of infection of the baby from a maternal primary chancre during delivery was possible, but unlikely. Ricord believed that a foetus, having been infected by its father, could transmit syphilis to its mother across the placenta: he called it "choc en retour". This provided an explanation for the common observation of a mother, having been perfectly well during pregnancy, showing signs of syphilis after delivery. Diday and others were doubtful about "choc en retour," but the doctrine of "sperm inheritance" held good. It was endorsed by Hutchinson, who regarded the evidence in support as "overwhelming". After the discovery of *T. pallidum* it was remarked that this organism was too large to be conveyed by spermatozoa, but even then Hutchinson was reluctant to abandon something which he regarded as a clinical fact: "We listen with much respect to the arguments which those who propound these views [against sperm transmission] urge in their support, but decline to accord them the infallibility which they seem desirous to claim"[34]. Some diehards never abandoned "sperm transmission", which was promulgated as "at least possible, and even probable" as late as 1947[35]. It was admitted that if the mother was "tainted" before conception, or contracted syphilis during her pregnancy, the infection could pass from her to the foetus via the placental circulation. Hutchinson and his contemporaries were quite willing to accept this, although they regarded it as much rarer than paternal transmission.

Soon after the introduction of serological tests for syphilis in 1906 it became clear that with very rare exceptions the mother of a child with congenital syphilis was seropositive, and a few years later it was shown that congenital syphilis could be prevented if cases of maternal syphilis were identified by the Wassermann test and treated with arsenicals. These discoveries, although they established the overwhelming importance of maternal transmission, by no means solved all the problems of the natural history of congenital syphilis. Venereologists struggled without success to explain why so many mothers of babies with congenital syphilis were symptomless during pregnancy, and despite much effort and innumerable theories this problem has not been solved to this day. It was difficult to explain why in contradiction to Kassowitz's "law" congenital syphilis was sometimes much more severe in a later than in an earlier child, and that in twin pregnancies one child sometimes developed congenital syphilis while the other remained well. "Third generation syphilis" was much discussed. For example, was it possible for a woman with untreated congenital syphilis married to a healthy man to bear a syphilitic infant? Most nineteenth-century observers, including Fournier, thought that this could occur, but the English authorities, headed by Hutchinson, rejected the idea. The main difficulty was to exclude acquired syphilis in the second generation, but enough cases were reported to indicate that third generation syphilis was at least possible. A related problem concerned the development of acquired syphilis in individuals with untreated congenital infections; here, the consensus was that this too was possible. Although these arcane matters generated a large literature, the truth will probably never be known. Nevertheless, the elucidation of the pathogenesis of congenital syphilis and the abandonment of the concept of paternal transmission were of great importance; they led the way to the effective control programmes which have made this horrible disease rare.

Chapter 6
Spirochaeta pallida: The Microbiology of Syphilis

If circumstances lead me, I will find where truth is hid
William Shakespeare, *Hamlet*

The idea that some human diseases might be caused by the transmission of minute living creatures originated among the myths and legends of the ancient world, and had been seriously suggested by Fracastoro in his *On contagion* in 1546. Proof that such agents existed had to await the construction of microscopes. The first instruments of good quality were built by the Dutch naturalist Anton von Leeuwenhoek (1632–1723); some of these could magnify objects more than 250 times. The examination of various body fluids revealed many "animalcules" and "infusoria", but nobody knew what these were or what they meant. A major step was taken by the French microscopist Alexandre Donné (1801–1878), who later became Inspector General of the University of Paris. The design and performance of microscopes was by now much improved, and Donné made some important discoveries, which included blood platelets and the leucocytosis of leukaemia. In 1836 he published his studies "as to the nature of various genito-urinary discharges in both sexes"[1]. In specimens from women with vaginitis he had seen many flagellated protozoa:

> "The animalcule is of a size double that of a human erythrocyte, or about the size of a pus cell, namely 1/40 mm in diameter. The body is round, but may elongate and assume diverse forms. At the anterior end is a long flagellum-like appendage, very thin, which may wave back and forth with great rapidity. On the under part are a number of very fine cilia [later found to be an undulating membrane] that cause a rotating movement. At the posterior end are a number of appendages of uncertain structure."

Donné concluded that this was a new genus and proposed the name *Trico-monas vaginale*, later changed to *Trichomonas vaginalis*. For the next 80 years little interest was taken in this organism, which was thought to be a harmless commensal. In 1894 *T. vaginalis* was found in the male urinary tract, and it was suggested that it might be sexually transmissible[2]. It was not until 1916 that Hoehne proposed that it was a cause of vaginitis[3], and not until the 1930s that the concept of trichomoniasis as a sexually transmitted disease was firmly established.

Trichomonads were not the only organisms identified by Donné. He described microbes resembling vibrios which he had seen in syphilitic chancres. At first he wondered whether these might play any part in causing syphilis, but by 1844 when he published his "Course of microscopy" he had abandoned this idea; he thought the vibrios were present merely by chance. In Donné's time there was no science of microbiology. This developed after Louis Pasteur had proved that fermentation and putrefaction were initiated by airborn micro-organisms. He believed that some microbes could cause human disease, and his German contemporary Robert Koch developed the experimental methods which proved this to be true. Once bacteria had been shown to cause many infectious diseases it was natural that attention would be paid to syphilis, and for 20 years many investigators applied themselves to this disease. Many candidate organisms were proposed, and as many rejected; eventually it was reluctantly concluded that the search for a "syphilis bacterium" had failed[4].

The Discovery of *Spirochaeta pallida*

Some scientists conjectured that syphilis might be caused by a protozoon; in some ways it resembled the equine disease dourine, which was known to be caused by a trypanosome. One worker went further than this. In 1905 Siegel, an assistant at the Institute of Zoology at the University of Berlin, claimed to have found a flagellated protozoon in syphilitic lesions which he thought was their cause. Most workers greeted this claim with scepticism, but in Berlin it was taken very seriously. Kohler, director of the Imperial Health Institute, asked Lesser, the head of the Clinic of Dermatology and Syphilis in Berlin, to participate in a joint clinical and microbiological study. The work was entrusted to Schaudinn, an expert protozoologist, and Hoffmann, Lesser's first assistant; Neufeld, an assistant at the Institute, was co-opted as bacteriologist. Fritz Schaudinn (1871–1906; Figure 6.1) was born in Roeseningken, a village in East Prussia[5]. Having received his basic education locally, in 1890 he was admitted to the University of Berlin, where he obtained a degree in zoology. He soon became interested in protozoa, and after becoming Privatdozent (a recognised teacher not a member of the salaried staff) he undertook research on amoebiasis, malaria and hookworm disease. In 1904 he was appointed director of the new division of protozoology in the Imperial Health Institute. Eric Hoffmann (1868–1959; Figure 6.2) was born in Witnitz in Pomerania and educated at a grammar school in Berlin before studying medicine at the Military Medical Academy. After a short tour of military duty Hoffmann asked if he could study under Lesser at the Skin and Syphilis Clinic, and this was agreed[6].

The team started work at the beginning of 1905. They soon found that Siegel's protozoon did not exist; he had mistaken organic debris for a micro-organism. But on March 3 Schaudinn, using a Zeiss microscope with an apochromatic objective, examined a fresh preparation which Hoffmann had prepared from an eroded vulval papule in a woman aged 25 with secondary syphilis. He saw several pale spiral organisms which he had never seen before; they rotated about their long axis, glided forwards and backwards, and underwent movements of flexion (Figure 6.3). He called in Hoffmann and Norfeld, and they all looked at them – perhaps "with a wild surmise" – for after 400 years the cause of syphilis had been found. The following month Schaudinn and Hoffmann found *Spirochaeta*

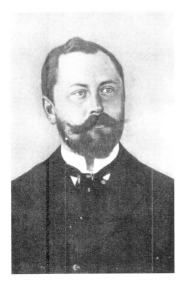 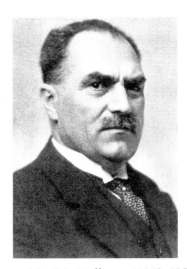

Figure 6.1. Fritz Schaudinn (1871–1906).   *Figure 6.2. Eric Hoffmann (1868–1959).*

pallida, as it was now called, in both fresh and Giemsa stained preparations from 11 patients with early syphilis; Hoffmann provided fluid from ulcerated and non-ulcerated lesions, and he also used a technique of lymph node puncture and aspiration which Koch had used for trypanosomiasis. Spiral organisms had previously been reported in both syphilitic and non-syphilitic genital lesions, and from the beginning Schaudinn and Hoffmann differentiated pale finely coiled *Spirochaeta pallida* and the dark, coarser *Spirochaeta refringens* which was present in many non-syphilitic specimens.

These results were discussed informally at the Imperial Health Institute and early publication was agreed; Neufeld withdrew, and Schaudinn and Hoffmann wrote a paper *Preliminary report on the presence of Spirochaetes in syphilitic*

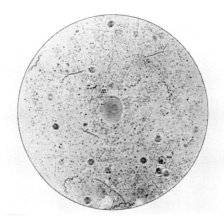

Figure 6.3. Photograph by Schaudinn showing seven spirochaetes in a Giemsa-stained smear. (From Schaudinn and Hoffmann's first paper, 1905.)

73

lesions and in Papillomas[7], which appeared on 10 April 1905 (Figure 6.4); a second paper on the findings with lymph node aspirates followed soon afterwards. At a meeting of the Berlin Medical Society on 17 May they presented their results, together with some further exciting news: Metchnikoff had found *S. pallida* in several chancres in apes inoculated with syphilis, and other investigators had found the organisms in specimens from infants with congenital infections. The findings were discussed at a further meeting of the Society the following week, but their reception was cool. To be fair, we must remember that there had been many claims that the cause of syphilis had been discovered, since Donné saw "vibrios" in a vulval chancre in 1836. The dermatologist Oskar Lassar said that in the last 25 years there had been 25 organisms supposed to be the cause of syphilis, and the President concluded by saying: "I am hereby closing the meeting until the next organism of syphilis claims our attention". Many other venereologists were also doubtful. Neisser, in a letter from Java, wrote: "We are still toiling with the syphilis spirilla. Here and there we find something positive, but we are more convinced than ever that these spirilla are not really the cause of syphilis". But by the following year, after confirmatory reports by many workers, including some members of his own team, he had changed his mind. In 1906 Karl Landsteiner introduced dark field microscopy, which made it easier to see the organisms, which were soon to be placed in a new genus and called *Treponema pallidum*. By the end of 1906, 750 papers on the subject had appeared.

Vorläufiger Bericht über das Vorkommen von
Spirochaeten in syphilitischen Krankheitsprodukten und bei Papillomen.

Von

Dr. Fritz Schaudinn,   und   **Dr. Erich Hoffmann,**
Regierungsrat   Privatdozent.

(Aus dem Protozoen-Laboratorium des Kaiserlichen Gesundheitsamtes und aus der Königlichen
Universitätsklinik für Haut- und Geschlechtskrankheiten zu Berlin.)

Auf Veranlassung des Herrn Präsidenten des Kaiserlichen Gesundheitsamtes Dr. Köhler und unter Mitwirkung des Herrn Professor Dr. E. Lesser wurden von uns in Gemeinschaft mit den Herren Dr. Neufeld und Dr. Gonder Untersuchungen über das Vorkommen von Mikroorganismen in syphilitischen Krankheitsprodukten begonnen. Hierbei fand Schaudinn am lebenden Objekt sowie in gefärbten Präparaten Organismen, die zur Gattung Spirochaete gestellt werden müssen, einer Gattung, deren systematische Zugehörigkeit zum Stamm der Protozoen Schaudinn auf Grund seiner Untersuchungen an der Spirochaete ziemanni des Steinkauzes behauptet hat. Die Spirochaeten konnten bisher sowohl an der Oberfläche sezernierender syphilitischer Effloreszenzen als auch in der Tiefe des Gewebes und in den spezifisch erkrankten Leistendrüsen nachgewiesen werden.

Um die baldige Nachprüfung dieser Befunde zu ermöglichen, sollen sie schon jetzt unter Beifügung von zwei Mikrophotogrammen kurz mitgeteilt werden.

Neben Fällen von reiner Syphilis wurden auch solche untersucht, die durch andere Erkrankungen kompliziert waren, und schließlich auch bei nicht an Syphilis leidenden Patienten nach dem Vorkommen von ähnlichen Organismen in der Genitalgegend des Körpers gefahndet.

In den folgenden Zeilen sollen zunächst die angewandten Untersuchungsmethoden und die Eigenschaften der aufgefundenen Parasiten in Kürze geschildert, dann die wichtigsten der untersuchten Krankheitsfälle unter Zufügung der parasitologischen Befunde skizziert werden[1]).

Für das Auffinden der außerordentlich zarten, schwach lichtbrechenden, dabei aber sehr lebhaft beweglichen Spirochaeten in den syphilitischen Geweben eignet sich am besten das lebensfrische Material, das sofort nach der Entnahme vom Körper des

[1]) Die parasitologischen Angaben dieser Arbeit stammen von Schaudinn, die klinischen und literarischen von Hoffmann. Herrn Dr. Gonder sind wir für die eifrige Mitarbeit bei der Herstellung, Färbung und Durchsicht der Präparate zu großem Dank verpflichtet.

Figure 6.4. Title page of Schaudinn and Hoffmann's first paper in Arbeiten aus dem Kaiserlichen Gesundheitsamt *reporting the discovery of* Spirochaeta pallida, *1905.*

Schaudinn and Hoffmann succeeded because one was a microbiologist with superb technical proficiency and the other a venereologist able to provide specimens of high quality from accurately diagnosed patients. Their work was to have a profound influence on future research into syphilis, but the partnership ended sadly. In January 1906 Schaudinn was appointed Director of the Institute for Ship and Tropical Hygiene in Hamburg, where he hoped to continue his studies in an environment where there would be unlimited opportunities for research. He travelled to the International Medical Congress in Lisbon, and he described his reception in a letter to his wife:

"The dermatologists paid me a tribute today which I will probably never experience again. The old French Professor Hallopeau asked those present to stand, and led me to the chairman's seat. I was then greeted with such a storm of applause that I could not get a word in edgeways. Every time I opened my mouth they clapped like madmen[8]."

But Schaudinn was not well. He had a chronic rectal infection, and had developed an abscess. An emergency operation was performed in Hamburg, but it was unsuccessful and soon afterwards he died at the age of 34 years. He was sincerely mourned. He was a large man, outspoken and robustly humorous, but his friends also spoke of his sensitivity and tenderness. His relaxation came from his young family and from his skill as a pianist. Von Prowazek arranged for the publication of his remaining papers, but who knows what he might have achieved had he lived? Hoffmann survived him for many years. In 1910 he became professor of dermatology at Bonn. Like Crick and Watson, he had made his greatest discovery early in his career. His later life was spent in clinical work, teaching and writing – he was the author of a standard textbook on dermatovenereology which went through many editions. Hoffmann always spoke his mind, and he was rash enough to criticise Hitler and the Nazis not only to his friends but in public. This led to his premature retirement in 1934. Fortunately he was still able to travel, and he gave many lectures during his visits to friends overseas, besides writing two volumes of memoirs. He died in 1959, at the great age of 91.

Improvements in Technique

Soon after the discovery of T. pallidum it was found that although the organism could be stained with various dyes they were exceedingly difficult to see against a background of tissue or debris. Constantin Levaditi (1874–1953), a Roumanian bacteriologist working in Metchnikoff's laboratory in Paris, devised a silver nitrate impregnation method to demonstrate T. pallidum in tissue sections, which made the organisms much clearer[9]. This technique was used by Hideyo Noguchi (1876–1928; Figure 6.5), a Japanese pathologist working in New York, to demonstrate treponemes in the brain in cases of general paresis and tabes dorsalis[10], and they were occasionally found in gummas and cardiovascular lesions. Clinical resemblances between syphilis and yaws had been noted for many years, and in 1905 Aldo Castellani (1877–1971),

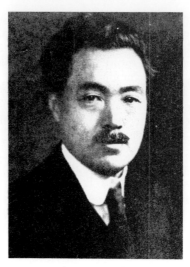

Figure 6.5. Hideyo Noguchi (1876–1928).

working in Ceylon (now Sri Lanka), found a spirochaete, *Treponema pertenue*, by microscopy of wet and stained specimens from patients with yaws; he had been in touch with Schaudinn, who examined some of his specimens and confirmed his findings[11]. *T. pertenue* was later proved to be the cause of the disease.

It was inevitable that attempts would be made to culture *T. pallidum*. Noguchi was the first to claim, "beyond all doubt" as he put it, that he had obtained a pure culture of the organism in fluid media; he stated that with some of these cultured strains he had produced syphilis in rabbits[12]. However, virulence was not maintained on passage, and both Roux and Levaditi thought that the Noguchi strain, although a treponeme, was probably a contaminant of the original inoculation. Since then, despite countless attempts, there has been a general failure to culture and maintain virulent *T. pallidum* in vitro[13]. There are, however, several non-virulent strains which can be passaged indefinitely in the laboratory. The so-called Reiter treponeme originated from a patient with early syphilis who was seen at the Kaiser Wilhelm Institute in Berlin in 1924. It received its name from Hans Reiter, who was well-known for having described a patient with the eponymous syndrome in 1916. After being passed through rabbits it was established in non-living fluid media. Its subsequent chequered career – the strain was actually lost on one occasion – has been described by Reiter himself[14], who insisted that it had remained pathogenic, although few workers agreed with him. Because it could be kept viable in relatively simple media it was used for some years as antigen in a serological test for syphilis. The only way by which *T. pallidum* can be kept both alive and virulent was found to be serial passage in living animals, of which the rabbit was the most convenient. The best known rabbit-adapted strain of *T. pallidum* is the virulent Nichols strain, which was established in 1912 by Henry James Nichols (1877–1927), then a captain in the United States army working in the Rockefeller Institute in New York; this has remained pathogenic to humans ever since.

Serological Tests for Syphilis

The development of syphilis serology is firmly linked to the name of August Paul von Wassermann (1866–1925; Figure 6.6). He was born in Bamberg in Bavaria and studied medicine in Erlangen, Vienna, Munich and finally Strasbourg, where he graduated MD in 1888. In 1891 he became assistant in the scientific and clinical division of Koch's Institute for Infectious Diseases in Berlin. For the next few years he conducted many studies in the expanding field of immunology. He became Privatdozent in internal medicine in 1901, was named professor in 1902, and in 1906 was appointed director of the division of experimental therapy and serum research in the institute.

Wassermann and Neisser were old friends, and when Neisser returned from Java in 1906 he went to see him in Berlin. In the course of their discussion Neisser complained that there was still no satisfactory serological test for syphilis, and either he or Wassermann (accounts differ) suggested that it might be possible to apply a complement fixation reaction to this disease. The reaction had been devised in 1901 by Jules Bordet and Octave Gengou, working in the Pasteur Institute, and Wassermann had used it to try to demonstrate tuberculin in tuberculous organs. It was agreed that the study with syphilis would be worth doing. Neisser was to supply extracts of syphilitic organs from apes and humans to use as antigens, and test and control sera from his apes; Wassermann would provide the laboratory expertise. Wassermann's and Neisser's assistants, Schucht and Bruck, were to prepare the material and perform the tests.

The team had immediate success[15], and the first results were published in 1906 (Figure 6.7). Laszlo Detre (1875–1939), a Hungarian physician, had the misfortune to publish his own results with a similar test a few weeks later, but Wassermann's team had priority. They reported that immune sera from apes

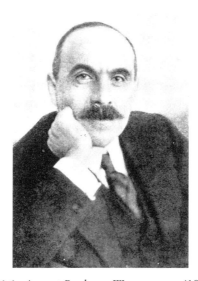

Figure 6.6. August Paul von Wassermann (1866–1925).

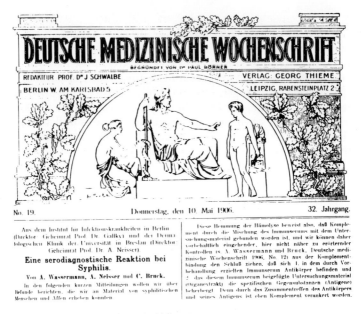

Figure 6.7. The announcement of the first serological test for syphilis by Wassermann, Neisser and Bruck. From Deutsche Medizinische Wochenschrift *(1905).*

contained complement fixing antibodies against "specific syphilitic substances", while control sera gave no reactions, and concluded:

> "The practical importance of these findings is obvious. We are in a position to determine in vitro whether a human or animal serum contains antibodies specific for substances of the syphilitic agent, and we should be able to quantify these antibodies ... It would be of the greatest diagnostic and therapeutic value if one could regularly demonstrate syphilitic material or antibodies in the circulating blood of syphilitics."

This hope was realised when the group examined human sera, although they obtained positive results in only 49 of 257 "certain" syphilitics. In collaboration with Felix Plaut, Wassermann tested the spinal fluid from 41 paretics, with positive reactions in 32[16].

Bruck appeared as co-author in one of the papers, although he later complained that he had done most of the work for which Wassermann received the credit; Schucht was not listed at all. Neisser's role in these studies seems to have been peripheral, but in later years he often paid tribute to Metchnikoff, Roux, Schaudinn, Wassermann and Bruck. Wassermann and Neisser presented their results at a Congress for Internal Medicine in Vienna 1908, a meeting which one would like to have attended. Osler was there, and he wrote in a letter:

> "On Tuesday morning Professor Neisser of Breslau opened the discussion on 'The present position of the pathology and therapy of syphilis'. This was a splendid address, given without notes, in a good clear voice, the

subject matter arranged in a most orderly manner ... Neisser was followed by Professor Wassermann, who also gave a model address."

From now on, Neisser's interest in syphilis was centred on therapy, but in 1911 he gave some advice on the performance of laboratory tests which no doubt would be echoed by microbiologists working today:

"The [Wassermann] reaction is so complicated that in my experience it should be performed in a large laboratory in which many specimens are examined every day by a fully trained staff. This seems to me to be quite essential, since even an experienced person can make mistakes if he examines only a few sera at a time ... For this reason it is out of the question for the test to be performed satisfactorily in a practitioner's office, and it seems inadvisable to provide the reagents for a doctor to do the test himself[17]."

A vast literature on the "Wassermann reaction" and its successors now developed. Wassermann had thought that the test detected specific antibodies to T. *pallidum*, but this was not so. It was soon found that the antigen in the test was not specific to syphilis, as it could be found in some normal human and animal tissues. This led to a long debate on the nature of the "antibody" in syphilitics, now called "reagin", which to this day has not been completely decided. But to clinicians working in the first decades of the twentieth century this was academic. The test appeared to be for the most part *clinically* specific, and made it possible to confirm a provisional diagnosis, to detect the presence of syphilitic infections in patients with no symptoms or signs of the disease, and to assess responses to treatment. Two generations of venereologists worked with the "WR", they understood its behaviour in the various stages of syphilis, and its occasional "false positive" reactions. The test transformed medical practice, and added a new dimension to the mass of clinical observations which had been made in the nineteenth century.

As experience with the Wassermann reaction increased, it was used to confirm that some constitutional diseases which had long been thought to be due to late syphilis were indeed so caused. This was of particular value in neurosyphilis. Lymphocytosis in the cerebrospinal fluid of patients with tabes and general paresis had been reported in 1901[18], and in 1906 the Wassermann reaction was found to be positive as well[16]. A further important discovery was made in 1913; studies of the spinal fluid from patients in the various stages of syphilis showed that the Wassermann reaction was positive in some individuals with no clinical evidence of neurosyphilis. This important discovery led to recommendations which were followed for many years:

"A negative Wassermann reaction in the blood is no evidence that the nervous system is not affected, and every patient with increased cells, globulin, or a positive reaction in the spinal fluid needs active antisyphilitic treatment. No patient who has been infected with syphilis can conscientiously be discharged as cured until the spinal fluid has been examined and found to be normal, even though he remains free from signs and symptoms and has a persistently negative Wassermann reaction in the blood[19]."

Carl Bruck (1879–1944) went on to become senior physician in Neisser's Department of Dermatology in Breslau, and was eventually appointed professor of dermatology at Hamburg-Altona. He published many articles and books on the serology of syphilis. Wassermann himself did little further work on the subject after 1906. His main interest now was the chemotherapy of malignant disease, but this was abandoned during the First World War, when he was responsible for the control of infectious diseases in the Prussian army. After the war he became director of an expanded Institute for Experimental Therapy and Biochemistry in Berlin, but in 1924 he developed glomerulonephritis, from which he died in the following year. Wassermann was a short man, with bright blue eyes. Impulsive and highly intelligent, he had the gift of explaining complicated matters clearly and simply, and he was evidently a brilliant speaker[20]. His work on syphilis made him famous; and he received many honours and decorations, but he described himself simply as "a laboratory worker".

The complement fixation procedure was time-consuming, and a simpler serological test was needed. It had been discovered in 1907 that mixing a syphilitic serum with antigen and complement caused a visible precipitate[21], but this was not put to practical use until 1921, when Reuben Kahn at the University of Michigan introduced a precipitation test along these lines. The Kahn test proved very popular and was soon followed by a multitude of similar tests named after their discoverers: Kline, Eagle, Price, Mazzini, Hinton, and so on.

In 1941 the serologically reactive substances cardiolipin and lecithin were isolated from the crude alcoholic extract of beef heart which had previously been used as antigen, and a "cardiolipin Wassermann reaction" was developed and used in many laboratories. From the mid 1940s onwards cardiolipin gradually became accepted as the best antigen for flocculation tests, and it was used in the Venereal Disease Research Laboratory (VDRL) test which gradually replaced the others and came into general use in the early 1950s.

Since the early days it had been known that the Wassermann test could give positive results in some people without syphilis, and as experience with reagin tests accumulated it became clear that a truly specific serological test was needed. This was provided by the *Treponema pallidum* immobilisation (TPI) test, which was introduced by Robert Nelson and Manfred Mayer, working in the Johns Hopkins School of Hygiene and Public Health in 1949[22]. For 25 years the TPI test dominated syphilis serology. It was highly specific but technically demanding and, since live virulent treponemes were used, not without risk to laboratory staff. It never became a routine screening test, but was used to categorise sera which had given discordant results with reagin tests. Many workers tried to devise a simpler verification test, and at least 20 of these were developed[23]. The Reiter Protein Complement Fixation test, which used an antigen extracted from Reiter treponemes, was introduced in the early 1960s and was perhaps the best known of these. Although it was not entirely specific, it was used for a time in conjunction with reagin tests in many venereal disease clinics. The only one of the multitude of tests devised for the serological diagnosis of syphilis to survive into the modern era is the VDRL test; the remainder, including the original Wassermann reaction which achieved so much, are now obsolete.

Chapter 7
"For one pleasure, a thousand pains":
The Treatment of Syphilis

Physicians of the utmost fame
Were called at once; but when they came
They answered, as they took their fees,
'There is no cure for this disease'

Hilaire Belloc, *Cautionary Tales*

At the beginning of the syphilis epidemic doctors had no idea how they should treat its victims. Measures such as diet, bleeding, purging and sweating were used while the pharmacopoeias were hurriedly consulted. External applications of mercury compounds had been used on a small scale by the ancient Greeks, and in the early Middle Ages were studied more thoroughly by Arabian physicians. In the twelfth century applications of mercury (*Unguentum Saracenicum*) were advocated by Roger of Salerno for the treatment of some chronic skin diseases. Toxic symptoms such as salivation, which had been noted by the Arabs, were now regarded as beneficial, and "salivation cures" were initiated, chiefly for gouty conditions[1]. Mercury was prescribed for syphilis because Celsus had advised doctors confronted with a new disease to try remedies which had been found to be effective against similar conditions; syphilitic skin eruptions often resembled other skin diseases, so mercury was used by many of the early syphilologists, including Torella, Cataneus and de Vigo. Ointments of various strength were applied, sometimes just to the lesions but often more widely.

Ulrich von Hutten (1488–1523) was a German knight, a humanist and defender of Luther[2]. Cantankerous by nature, he passed his life in a series of literary and philosophical squabbles. He had no medical training, but he wrote a treatise about the French disease which was a combination of his personal experience – he had contracted syphilis early in life (Figure 7.1) – and his gleanings from ancient and contemporary literature. He received no less than 11 courses of mercury, and he described the technique of inunction:

> "They anointed the joints of the arms and legs, some the spine and neck and others again the whole body, some once a day, some twice and some three or four times . . . they anointed him and placed him on a bed laid in the hot room, and with many covers laid over him forced him to sweat[2]."

Treatment was continued for three for four weeks. Various agents were added to the mercury rubs to improve their action: aloes, myrrh, sulphur, camphor, and

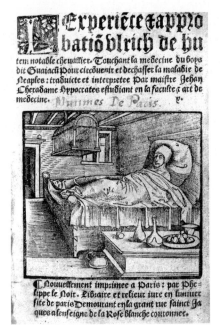

Figure 7.1. Ulrich von Hutten suffering from syphilis. Woodcut by P. le Noir (1520?). (By courtesy of the Wellcome Institute Library, London.)

sometimes more exotic ingredients such as viper's fat, earthworms fried in oil, frogs ground up alive and human fat. Mercurial fumigation was also used:

> "The patient was first bled and purged and then put into a kind of well-warmed tent. At his feet was placed a pan of charcoal, and the substances intended for the fumigation were thrown in at intervals so that the patient remained exposed from head to foot to the smoke which was thrown off, and perspired freely. If by chance he was observed to be near fainting he was allowed to apply his mouth to a hole made for the purpose, or breathe fresh air through a tube[3]."

Overdosage must have been common, with frequent toxic effects such as hair loss, abdominal pain, diarrhoea, mouth ulcers and copious salivation. Von Hutten had endured these himself:

> "The ointment caused such profuse salivation that the patients were in danger of losing their teeth unless care was taken. The throat, palate and tongue became ulcerated, the gums swelled, the teeth became loose and there flowed incessantly from the mouth a very stinking secretion."

Mercury was administered not only by doctors but by charlatans and quacks, who asserted that they alone understood the secrets of successful therapy;

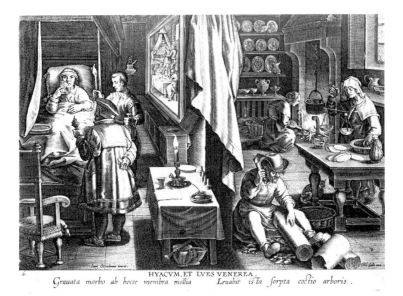

HYACVM, ET LVES VENEREA.
Gruuata morbo ab hocce membra mollia   Leuabit ista forpta coctio arboris.

Figure 7.2. A sixteenth-century patient with syphilis taking a guaiac preparation, which is being prepared from wood shavings in the next room. Engraving after Jan van der Straet, 1570. (By courtesy of the Wellcome Institute Library, London.)

sometimes healthy people were persuaded that they had syphilis and required a course. The treatment was responsible for many deaths. Patients dreaded it, and many doctors regarded it as harmful and ineffective. At one time medical students at Heidelberg University were obliged to take an oath that they would never prescribe mercury for syphilis[4]. Some workers believed that once absorbed it accumulated in syphilitic lesions, especially in bones; Fernel, an antimercurialist, wrote that "the more compact bones become carious. Upon opening such decayed bones with a knife I have often discovered quivering droplets of mercury"[5].

Guaiacum

Alternative and gentler remedies were needed, and many medicaments from the ancient pharmacopoeias were tried. Sarsaparilla, the dried root of the briar vine, had no significant activity, but guaiacum, the "holy wood", which was introduced in 1508, was thought to be effective and soon became very popular (Figure 7.2). The plant grew in the West Indies, and those who believed that syphilis had come from the New World thought it appropriate that its cure should come from the same place. It was given by mouth, and had no major side effects. Von Hutten said that he had been cured by guaiacum while mercury had failed, and he enthusiastically recommended it[2]. His optimism was ill-founded, for he died of late syphilis some years later. Guaiacum seems to have been no more than a sudorific, and it was eventually abandoned. Doctors were forced to accept that despite its side effects mercury was the drug of choice for syphilis.

Oral Mercury

The use of mercury for the treatment of syphilis was strongly supported by one of the most remarkable men of the age. Philip Aureolus Bombastos von Hohenheim (1493–1541; Figure 7.3) – Paracelsus was a nickname – was born near Zurich. A physician's son, he studied medicine, mineralogy, chemistry, alchemy and philosophy, and wandered through Europe acquiring knowledge of these various subjects[6]. He obtained a degree in medicine under Leoniceno at Ferrara, and in due course was appointed professor of medicine at Basel University; his nonconformity was expressed at once, as he publicly burned the works of Galen and Avicenna and insisted on giving his lectures in German rather than Latin. He maintained that clinical experience and original thinking were far more important than slavish adherence to ancient doctrines; the physician should direct treatment specifically at the cause of a disease rather than resorting to sweating, bleeding and purging. Paracelsus himself used his knowledge of chemistry to devise many new remedies. Not surprisingly, he antagonised the authorities at Basel; he was forced to leave and resumed his wanderings, practising medicine and surgery all over Germany with considerable success. He died in Salzburg at the age of 48 years, perhaps from a wound received in a tavern brawl, although others said that he had been thrown over a cliff by thugs hired by a group of physicians and apothecaries whom he had offended – a lesson to those who are inclined to upset the medical establishment.

Paracelsus was a heavy drinker, obese, truculent and argumentative, but he achieved real advances in both chemistry and medicine and his influence lasted until well into the eighteenth century. He was also important in the history of venereology, a subject on which he wrote several tracts. Although he failed to distinguish gonorrhoea from syphilis he was the first physician to recognise congenital syphilis. He defended the'use of mercury, advocated oral therapy and warned against overdosage. The first mercurial preparation given by mouth seems

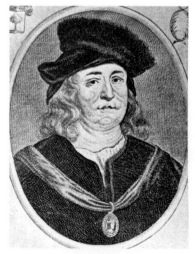

Figure 7.3. Paracelsus (1493–1541).

to have been mercuric oxide, called "red precipitate" or "angelical powder". Later, metallic mercury was preferred. It was contained in some famous pills which originated in the Middle East, and it was rumoured that the first Christian who dared to take one dropped down dead on the spot. Paracelsus himself introduced "blue mass", a preparation of metallic mercury, and "sweet mercury" (calomel) and "white precipitate" (mercuric nitrate) were also prescribed.

Treatment with mercury could provoke profuse salivation, but this was regarded as beneficial because it washed away the venereal poison; some doctors insisted that the dose was increased until at least three pints of saliva a day were produced. The removal of the poison was, it was thought, aided by inducing copious sweating in a sweat room or bagnio, the patient lying on a couch in a room heated by dry air or steam (Figure 7.4). A plan has survived of a bagnio at St Thomas' Hospital, London, one of a group of rooms in which the treatment of syphilis was undertaken[7].

By the eighteenth century mercury was the linchpin of the treatment of syphilis for all but a few venereologists. Oral therapy was now preferred, the choice lying between metallic mercury or one of its salts. Paracelsus's "blue mass" was bulky and inconvenient to take, and was replaced by the famous "blue pill", a mixture of mercury, confection of roses and powdered liquorice, and in the nineteenth century mercury with chalk (*Hydrargyrum cum creta*). Mercuric chloride (corrosive sublimate) was advocated by Hermann Boerhaave early in the eighteenth century. A pupil of his, Gerhard van Swieten (1700–1772) was "head-hunted" by the Austrian Empress Maria Theresa to take the chair of medicine at the University of Vienna. He experimented with various preparations of mercuric chloride until, in 1750, he heard that a Russian surgeon called

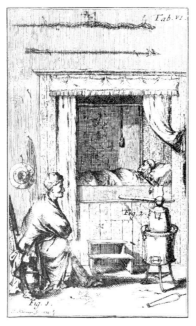

Figure 7.4. A patient undergoing a "sweat treatment" for syphilis. Stephen Blankaart, 1685. (By courtesy of the Wellcome Institute Library, London.)

85

Sanchez had successfully used a solution of the salt in brandy. He adopted this preparation, which became known as *liquor Swietenii* and was used for many years.

However it is administered mercury is toxic, and side effects with all these preparations were common. The need for salivation was controversial. The eminent English physician Thomas Sydenham (1624–1689) taught that syphilis could not be cured by mercury without salivation and Benjamin Bell advocated a dose (by inunction) sufficient to "render the mouth gently sore", but Francois-Xavier Swediaur declared: "I have not found one patient [with syphilis] who required salivation but I have, on the contrary, observed that the greater the salivation the less certain and effective was the cure"[8]. Salivation was not the only side effect of mercury; gastroenteritis, skin rashes, liver and kidney damage were all common. Some authors suggested that many of the so-called signs of secondary syphilis were really due to mercury. There were even some extreme "avirulists" who doubted whether syphilis existed at all except as a mild superficial disorder, its alleged major effects being iatrogenic.

At the end of the eighteenth century an earlier controversy erupted again: was treatment with mercury effective, and in view of its side effects was it justifiable? During the Peninsular campaign of 1808–1814 British army surgeons were puzzled by the good results that their Portuguese colleagues seemed to obtain without specific treatment. Some experiments were performed in the hospital of the Coldstream Guards, and were published in 1817[9]. Soldiers with primary syphilis were treated simply with rest and soothing local applications; the chancres healed, and only a few developed systemic disease, but these patients were not followed for long enough to establish the value of this non-specific treatment.

Nineteenth Century Treatment Regimens

By the nineteenth century the majority of venereologists accepted that, as Bell had said, "under proper management mercury may be considered as a certain remedy for syphilis," but looked for improvements in its administration. Inunctions had never been completely abandoned and were revived in Vienna by Karl von Sigmund (1810–1883). He has been described as an Austrian Ricord, charming and elegant, and he was fluent in seven languages. He wrote many well-regarded books on infectious diseases and syphilology. A convinced mercurialist, he believed that inunction was the best method of administration. His obituarist Doyon saw groups of patients sitting in the middle of Sigmund's clinic, all industriously performing their "frictions" under the vigilant eye of a male nurse[10]. "Grey ointment", a trituration of metallic mercury in animal fat, was widely used. The inunction was usually performed once a day for at least twenty minutes; those who could afford them employed professional "rubbers". There were side effects, of course; salivation was not sought but could occur, and gastrointestinal symptoms, if less common than with oral therapy, still troubled some patients. There was also a risk of contact dermatitis. Inunctions may have been dirty and disagreeable but many people preferred them to oral therapy, with its inevitable diarrhoea. Mercurial injections were introduced by the Viennese dermatologist Ferdinand von Hebra (1816–1880) in 1861. He used mercuric chloride, but others preferred calomel. A later preparation was the infamous "grey oil", *oleum cinereum*, which was a mixture of oil, fat and metallic mercury. This was devised by Edward Lang in Vienna in 1887[11], and later modified by Neisser. Mercury injections were at first given subcutaneously, but these were very painful and often caused sloughing of the skin. Later workers gave the injections by deep intramuscular injection, claiming that these were less damaging and gave better absorption[12].

How mercury should be used – the timing, route, dosage and duration of therapy – was endlessly discussed. In the early days, treatment was deferred until the appearance of signs of secondary syphilis confirmed the diagnosis and was then continued until all lesions had healed, but as time went by treatment began earlier; Ricord, for example, taught that a patient with an indurated primary sore should receive mercury straight away[13]. Another problem was treatment of the chancre itself. In 1793 Bell stated that "chancres at first are always local, and are the source of whatever matter enters the system". However, uncertainty over the speed with which the virus of syphilis spread after inoculation made it difficult to decide whether excision of a chancre was desirable. In 1837 the Irish venereologist Colles stated that this was futile: "I have known a chancre completely cut out on the first or second day of its appearance, yet the occurrence of secondary symptoms was not prevented"[14]. Ricord compromised, recommending excision only within the first five days. Eventually, with the early use of mercurials, aggressive treatment of primary chancres was abandoned.

Iodides

During most of the nineteenth century the importance of iodides for the treatment of syphilis was second only to that of mercury. Iodine was discovered in 1811 by a French chemist, Bernard Courtois. Crude iodine-containing preparations such as seaweed and burned sponge had been used medicinally for many years and in 1821 Johann Christian Martini of Lübeck used iodine successfully for the treatment of syphilitic ulcers of the throat. In the same year Laurent Theodor Biett, a dermatologist working at l'Hôpital St Louis, used iodine combined with mercury for the treatment of gummas. Potassium iodide was introduced by Charles Coindet of Geneva in 1820 and in 1831 Jean Lugol, a French physician, used a mixture of iodine and potassium iodide for the treatment of late syphilis. The way was thus prepared for the studies of William Wallace in Dublin. He first investigated the kinetics of iodine and iodides in dogs; then, in a series of experiments which began in 1832, he showed that after oral administration iodides were present in many body fluids, including the milk of nursing mothers. In 1836 he described the successful treatment of 139 cases of post-primary syphilis[15], and his results were soon confirmed by others. Ricord observed that iodides were more effective in late than in early syphilis; the drug was particularly valuable for the treatment of deep-seated gummas and syphilitic disease of bones, neither of which responded well to mercury. In 1866 Lancereaux declared that "the two substances, iodine and mercury, are incontestably the chief agents which we are now able to oppose to the ravages of syphilis"[3]. Despite their side effects, mostly coryza and skin rashes, iodides retained their place in the treatment of late syphilis, and in combination with mercury, arsenicals or penicillin were used well into the twentieth century.

Fournier's "Chronic Intermittent Therapy"

In the second half of the nineteenth century the duration of therapy was still contentious. Ricord had broken with tradition by advocating prolonged treatment: "Six months of mercury followed by three of iodide, such is the medication, gentlemen, which gives the most sustained cures in the enormous majority of cases"[13]. His pupil Fournier developed a different approach. In his *Traitement de la Syphilis* (1893) he stated that "a maladie chronique il faut traitement chronique", and believed that a patient gradually became accustomed to mercury, so that it slowly lost its effect; furthermore, prolonged courses of treatment increased the risk of toxicity. He therefore proposed that instead of a period of intense treatment with mercury as advocated by Ricord, several courses, separated by courses of iodides, should be given over three or four years, followed by a further course twice a year until 10 years had elapsed. This was Fournier's "traitement chronique intermittent", which was widely used in Europe at the end of the nineteenth century and endorsed by such eminent physicians as Neisser and Hutchinson. There were many variations in the strength, length and duration of the mercurial "cures" and in the intervals between them. A fashionable version was the so-called "Aachen treatment", named after the spa town in Germany. This was based on mercurial inunctions "by the bare hands of a skilled rubber", with sulphur water internally and externally[16]. Some venereologists supplemented systemic therapy with the application of mercurial ointment or iodoform to syphilitic rashes and lesions; Hutchinson favoured a preparation of calomel with the ominous name "black wash". The treatment of late syphilis began with a course of sodium or potassium iodide, followed by a course of mercury; recurrences were so frequent that these courses were repeated indefinitely.

Most venereologists were very cautious in their management of men with early syphilis who were married or intending to marry. All too often they had seen infected wives, wrecked marriages and diseased children follow unwise medical advice. Hutchinson, for example, insisted on an interval of two full years between the date of contracting syphilis and marriage or the resumption of marital intercourse[17]. Cutting corners in this regard undoubtedly led to many disasters; a notorious case which occurred in the 1880s may serve as an example. Lord Colin Campbell, a young Scottish aristocrat, contracted syphilis for which he was still receiving treatment from Sir Henry Thompson, a well-known London surgeon, when he became engaged. He told his fiancée that because of his illness – he did not disclose its nature – they would have to occupy separate bedrooms for some time after they married, and she raised no objection. On their honeymoon the bridal couple were accompanied by a nursing sister who administered mercurial inunctions to Lord Campbell, who was by this time a virtual invalid. The marriage was consummated three months later, and inevitably his wife contracted syphilis; she was granted a divorce because of this, and soon afterwards Lord Campbell died of his infection[18].

Did the "two specifics" cure syphilis? It is impossible to say. Mercury, and to a lesser extent iodine, are treponemacidal, and suppressed many of its clinical signs. For four centuries most clinicians believed mercury to be effective, and it would be rash to assume that they were all mistaken. But a drug can be effective without being curative. Relapses after treatment were common, and the very long regimens recommended by experienced clinicians like Fournier and Hutchinson suggest a lack of confidence in their efficacy. Although the prevention of neurosyphilis by the energetic treatment of early syphilis was often discussed and evidently regarded as important, it is doubtful whether it was achieved. It seems likely that mercury was suppressive rather than curative. The effectiveness of mercury/iodine regimens could have been determined by long-term clinical and serological surveillance, but this was not practicable until early in the twentieth century, and by this time made no appeal to investigators excited by new discoveries.

Organic Arsenicals: The Work of Paul Ehrlich

The modern era of syphilis therapy began with the introduction of organic arsenicals by Ehrlich and Hata in 1910. Paul Ehrlich (1854–1915; Figure 7.5), one of the great figures in the history of medicine, was born in Strehlen, in Prussian Silesia (now Strzelin, Poland), the son of a Jewish distiller. After attending a local elementary school he went to St Maria Magdalen Grammar School at Breslau, where he was a classmate of Albert Neisser. He studied natural science, then medicine, at Breslau, Strasbourg and Freiburg. While still a student he became interested in aniline dyes, which had been introduced into microscope technique by the German pathologist Karl Weigert (1845–1904), Ehrlich's cousin. Ehrlich studied their use in haematology and histology, and was struck by their selective action on different cells and tissues. This led him to the concept that chemical affinities govern all biological processes, which was to underly much of his future work.

Ehrlich graduated at Leipzig in 1878, and was appointed physician in Friedrich von Frerich's medical clinic at the Charité Hospital in Berlin. It was a fortunate appointment for him because von Frerich, a clinician with a major interest in

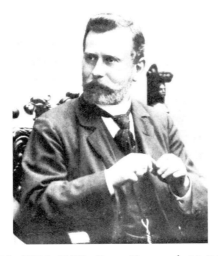

Figure 7.5. Paul Ehrlich (1854–1915). From Marquardt M (1949) Paul Ehrlich. (By courtesy of Butterworth-Heinemann Ltd.)

experimental pathology himself, encouraged Ehrlich's histological and biochemical research, and from this period came his definition of eosinophils, a method for staining the acid-fast tubercle bacillus (which had defeated its discoverer, Robert Koch), and a diazo reaction for detecting bilirubin in the urine. He also found that malaria parasites stained with methylene blue, and administered the dye to two patients with malaria, apparently successfully – an experiment with future significance. He became Privatdozent in 1886. Two years later, suffering from what seemed to be persistent catarrh, Ehrlich detected tubercle bacilli in his own sputum. Accompanied by his young wife, whom he had married in 1883, he went to Egypt for a year and underwent tuberculin therapy. He returned to Berlin in 1889. He now had no job, so he set up a small private laboratory and began a series of studies on the immune reactions of mice to various plant proteins which led him to develop the doctrine of active and passive immunity. In 1891 Koch gave him a small laboratory in his new Institute for Infectious Diseases in Berlin, where he worked unpaid for the next three years. At first he studied tuberculosis with Koch, then turned to the problem of diphtheria. Emil von Behring (1854–1917), who was also working in Koch's Institute, discovered the principle of antitoxic immunity to tetanus and diphtheria in 1890. He had difficulties over the production of diphtheria antitoxin, and Ehrlich set out to produce potent sera by the active immunisation of large animals, and used his chemical skill to devise methods by which the potency of toxins and antitoxins could be measured. In 1894 he reported the successful treatment with antitoxic sera of 220 children suffering from diphtheria.

In 1896 Ehrlich was appointed director of a new Institute for Serum Research and Testing at Steglitz, a suburb of Berlin. Those who knew him have described his joy in at last having a laboratory of his own[19]. Here he established standards for the assay of toxins and antitoxins and developed his "side-chain" theory, which proposed that a toxin is bound to a cell because of an affinity to a "receptor" in the cell, and that antitoxins are "receptors" thrown off into the circulation. These studies made him famous, and in 1899 he moved to Frankfurt to become director of the purpose-built Royal Prussian Institute for Experimental Therapy. Here he concluded his work on diphtheria and studied the mechanism of haemolysis; Wassermann later said that he could not have developed his complement fixation test for syphilis without Ehrlich's work on this subject. In 1906 a Research Institute for Chemotherapy, called the Georg-Speyer-Haus, was endowed and erected alongside Ehrlich's institute and placed at his disposal. He was now able to embark on a systematic investigation of the action of synthetic chemicals against pathogenic microbes, a subject which had occupied his mind since early in his career. In an address at the ceremonial opening of the Georg-Speyer-Haus in 1906 Ehrlich had prophesied the creation of substances "in the chemist's retort" which would

"be able to exert their full action exclusively on the parasite harboured within the organism and would represent, so to speak, magic bullets which seek their target of their own accord[20]."

At a later date he spoke of *therapia sterilans magna* – one-shot cure, it would be called today – but this dream was never to come true in his lifetime. In 1904 he had discovered that trypan red cured mice experimentally infected with *Trypanosoma equinum*, which caused a disease of horses and mules

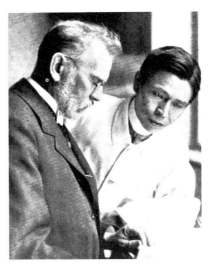

Figure 7.6. Paul Ehrlich and Sahachiro Hatta. From Marquardt M (1949) Paul Ehrlich. *(By courtesy of Butterworth-Heinemann Ltd.)*

in South America. Some trypanosomes became resistant to trypan red, and these strains responded to a pentavalent arsenical compound, atoxyl. At this time it was thought that there were resemblances between trypanosomal and spirochaetal infections, and atoxyl was tested against fowl spirillosis and syphilis in rabbits, apes and a small number of humans. It had some activity, but was unacceptably toxic. Ehrlich set out to find a derivative of atoxyl which was safe and effective, assisted by chemists at a dyestuffs factory in Frankfurt who synthesised compounds to his specification. In 1908 he reported that a trivalent arsenobenzene compound, number 418 in his series, was very active against trypanosomal disease, although it gave poor results in rabbit syphilis.

At this point, in 1909, Sahachiro Hata arrived (Figure 7.6). A Japanese, he had been working on experimental syphilis in rabbits and had come to Europe to study under Ehrlich. He was a patient, tireless and meticulous worker and Ehrlich thought highly of him. Hata tested hundreds of chemical compounds against infected rabbits. After one of these trials he showed his results to Ehrlich with the famous words "Believe 606 very efficacious"[21]. At first Ehrlich did not believe him (the compound had been reported as ineffective by a previous worker) but Hata repeated the experiments many times with the same results, and Ehrlich was convinced. He released small amounts of "606" for clinical trials against human syphilis. The first results were spectacular. After a single injection the lesions of early syphilis melted away, and treponemes disappeared with a rapidity which contrasted sharply with their sluggish response to mercury and iodides. Many patients were cured who had been labouring under ineffective treatment for months. Among the clinicians who performed a clinical trial on "606" was Ehrlich's old friend Albert Neisser, "Albertus Maximus" as he called him. Neisser was enthusiastic. "We must advise everyone with syphilis . . . to seek the new medicine"[22]. Prophetically, he thought that the currently recommended dosage, two or three injections, might be too small, and he suggested that additional treatment with mercury might also be advisable. But for the most part the verdict

91

was unanimous: "606" was highly effective against syphilis (Figure 7.7), and there seemed to be no serious side effects. The possibility of a quick and complete cure for a disease which had plagued mankind for 500 years caused a furore among clinicians greater, according to the veteran United States venereologist Rudolph Kampeier (1898–1990), than greeted the advent of penicillin in the early 1940s[23]. Leader writers in the medical press excelled themselves; an article in the *New York Medical Journal* stated:

> "No matter what qualifications the present statements may have to undergo, this great fact is well assured – a single injection of a synthetically made compound is capable of completely sterilizing the diseased animal body in a very short time . . . If reports continue to hold what they promise, syphilis could be eradicated from civilized humanity in two or three decades. What a hope, what a dream!"[24]

Ehrlich himself advised caution, and tried to restrict supplies of "606" to investigators whom he knew personally, but in vain. By the end of 1910, "606", now called arsphenamine, had been patented under the name of Salvarsan and large-scale manufacture begun.

The early hopes of a complete cure from a single injection of arsphenamine were not fulfilled. Many patients treated in this way for early syphilis developed recurrences, and even several injections could not be relied on to eradicate the infection in all cases. Some patients with late syphilis died shortly after receiving the drug, presumably because of Jarisch – Herxheimer reactions (see below). Side effects, which included dermatitis, jaundice and blood dyscrasias, were not uncommon. It was inevitable that the pendulum should swing the other way, and some physicians began to suggest that arsphenamine was too

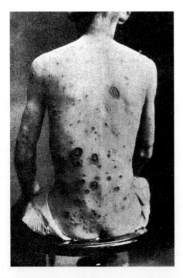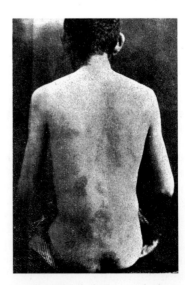

Figure 7.7. A youth suffering from syphilitic sores on his back, before and after treatment with "606". Erkenne deine Krankheit 1910. (By courtesy of the Wellcome Institute Library, London.)

toxic for general use. However, "If hopes were dupes fears may be liars", and many of these problems were due simply to lack of experience with a new and potent medicament and were eventually overcome. Nevertheless, for several years after its release Ehrlich had a hard time. He was bombarded by doctors and patients with requests for supplies of the drug and advice on its use, and he felt obliged to investigate personally each complaint of adverse reactions. The result of all this was that his institute was full of people all day long, and the pressure on him was enormous. Despite this he managed to bring out his 914th compound, called Neosalvarsan, which could be administered by intramuscular rather than intravenous injection[25]. Many venereologists, however, preferred the parent compound.

Ehrlich was subjected to a great deal of personal criticism, compounded of malice, envy and perhaps antisemitism. He was accused of charlatanism, profiteering and ruthless human experimentation. In March 1914 the Reichstag was forced to debate the merits of arsphenamine; although it concluded that it was "a valuable enrichment of the remedies against syphilis", Ehrlich found the experience humiliating. Worse was to come, for three months later he was a defence witness for Frankfurt Hospital, which had been accused by a journalist of forcibly submitting prostitutes to treatment with this "dangerous" drug; the hospital was acquitted and the journalist jailed for a year, but Ehrlich was distressed by the whole affair. He became even more dispirited after the outbreak of the First World War in August 1914; members of his staff left to join the army, some of his laboratories were given over to the preparation of vaccines for military use, and he felt deeply his isolation from colleagues in other countries. He was worn out by years of overwork, aggravated by heavy smoking and diabetes. In December 1914 he had a slight stroke, and in August of the following year a further stroke ended his life at the age of 61. His old friend von Behring delivered the oration at his funeral, and he was buried in the Jewish Cemetery at Frankfurt.

Ehrlich's capacity for original thought and his technical ingenuity had a lasting effect on medicine. His idea of therapeutics based on specific chemical affinities permeated much of his work and eventually led not only to arsphenamine but to the sulphonamides, antibiotics and many other agents. His life was centred in his laboratory. He undertook only a few lecture tours: to England in 1900, the USA in 1904 and Sweden in 1908. He would not speak at lay organisations, as he did not want to be accused of self-advertisement. A German gynaecologist left this account of his lectures:

"His discourses were all received with enthusiasm, although many among his audience were unable to follow his ideas. He would ask 'Is everything perfectly clear?' and everyone shouted 'Yes, yes!' Who would admit to the kind professor that his theories were actually quite difficult to grasp?[26]"

He received many honours, culminating in a Nobel prize for medicine in 1908, which he shared with Metchnikoff, for his contributions to immunology. He was nominated for a further prize in 1912 and 1913 for his work on arsphenamine, but because of the war and his death in 1915 this was never implemented.

Ehrlich had the ability to direct several lines of research at the same time and the will-power to abandon those which were unproductive. He was always genial and friendly to his colleagues and assistants, judging them solely by their knowledge and achievements, never by their personal weaknesses. He was angered only by meanness, unfair criticism or false claims of priority. His working methods have been vividly described by his secretary and biographer Martha Marquard[27] and by Johan Almqvist, a Swedish dermatovenereologist who visited him in 1911 and got to know him well[28]. Being untidy and rather absent-minded he depended on his staff, particularly the porter of the laboratory, Kadereit, who had followed him from Steglitz and become a discreet and reliable factotum. Countless times during the day the call was heard, "KA-DE-REIT!" as Ehrlich asked for mineral water, more cigars or missing documents. He was devoted to his wife and two daughters, and enjoyed jokes and banter with his friends. He had little interest in literature or the arts; he read only detective stories, and liked his wife to play him waltzes and operetta music rather than the classics. Even at home his work predominated. After his guests had gone he would retire to his study, where he remained in a pall of cigar smoke until after midnight. Ehrlich was a modest and lovable man, and he transformed the treatment and prognosis of syphilis.

Continuous Therapy

During the decade which followed the discovery of arsphenamine treatment was gradually rationalised. It was clear that infectious relapses and persistently positive Wassermann reactions often followed too small a number of injections. Courses of treatment became progressively longer, and eventually it was proposed that they should continue for at least a year; furthermore, in order to prevent drug resistance courses of arsenic should alternate with courses of mercury. Fournier's "chronic intermittent therapy" was abandoned in favour of a single continuous course of treatment[29]. These ideas were consolidated by the work of Albert Keitel, who had opened the Johns Hopkins Department of Syphilis in 1914, and his successor Joseph Earle Moore, who was to become the doyen of American syphilologists. In 1926 they stated:

> "Treatment [of early syphilis] shall be continuous, consisting of courses of arsphenamine alternating with mercury by inunction (or of insoluble bismuth salts intramuscularly [see below]) plus potassium iodide, treatment shall be carried out under full serological control, and treatment shall be prolonged without intermission for one year after the blood and spinal fluid have become and remained completely negative[30]."

This view was accepted by many venereologists, but as so often before in the history of the subject there were disagreements and arguments not only about details but about some basic concepts so, for example, in England Harrison still favoured intermittent therapy. Continued investigation of the arsenicals had led to the introduction of silver arsphenamine in 1918, stovarsol in 1921 and mapharsen in 1934; none of these had major advantages over the earlier compounds. Moore wryly commented: "As late as 1943 there was still disagreement among doctors as to the best method of treating even the simplest form of syphilitic infection"[31].

Bismuth

Bismuth became an important drug in syphilotherapy. Some early work with this agent had been interrupted by the First World War, and after it was over two Parisian physicians, Sazerac and Levaditi, resumed the study. First, they used injections of sodium and potassium bismuth tartrate to treat experimental syphilis in rabbits, and when these experiments were successful they used the same preparation to treat a group of human patients. Their results were published in 1921[32], and showed a good response in both early and late (gummatous) infections. Subsequent work indicated that bismuth had a treponemacidal action intermediate between that of arsenic and mercury; moreover, side effects were minimal – no more than a blue discoloration of the gums – and Jarisch – Herxheimer reactions very mild. Bismuth was immediately accepted, and within a short time had replaced mercury. Numerous compounds were marketed, at one time there was a choice of 113, but eventually intramuscular injections of metallic bismuth or one of its insoluble salts were favoured.

Fever Therapy

Syphilis was treated with combinations of arsenicals, mercury, bismuth and iodides for over 30 years. How effective was this therapy? The prognosis of early and latent infections was good. If patients were treated expertly and co-operated in a full course of treatment which was not disrupted by side effects 85–95 per cent were permanently cured[33]. This was a big "if", of course – late syphilis could still develop in one third of those inadequately treated – but the outlook for those who completed therapy was good. Similarly, less than 10 per cent of infected mothers treated before the fifth month of pregnancy had babies with congenital syphilis. The results of the treatment of late syphilis were less satisfactory. Gummatous disease responded well, although there might be a residual disability from its destructive effects before treatment. Cardiovascular syphilis reacted less favourably, because structural disease was often well established by the time the diagnosis was made. Treatment also gave poor results with neurosyphilis, unless it was very early.

General paresis, with its inexorable slide towards dementia and death, was particularly dreaded. The most effective therapy was devised by Julius Wagner von Jauregg (1857–1940; Figure 7.8), an Austrian neurologist and psychiatrist who for many years occupied the chair in psychiatry at the University of Vienna. It had been observed that some psychotic patients improved after a febrile illness, and Wagner von Jauregg had the idea that they might be victims of a pathological process which responded to fever. From 1888 onwards he used a variety of agents, including tuberculin and typhoid vaccine, to induce fever in patients with general paresis. None was entirely satisfactory, although there was a good clinical response in some patients. In 1917 he decided to induce tertian malaria as a controllable source of fever; patients were allowed to have up to 10 febrile episodes before the malaria was terminated with quinine. He reported improvement in half of those treated[34]. This result was so much better than had been obtained with any other type of treatment that malaria therapy was generally adopted, and became a special discipline available in major centres. Wagner von

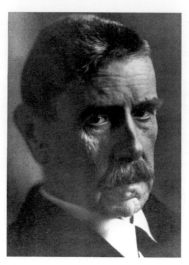

Figure 7.8. Wagner von Jauregg (1857–1940).

Jauregg received a Nobel prize in 1927 for his work on general paresis. In the 1930s various mechanical devices for the induction of fever such as hot baths, diathermy and heated cabinets were used, particularly in the USA (Figure 7.9). The British venereologist Ambrose King has described the procedure which he saw in use at the Kettering Institute, Dayton, Ohio during a visit in 1937:

> "The patient undergoing treatment was enclosed in an insulated cabinet with only his head protruding. Hot moist air was circulated over him at a temperature which was not sufficient to harm him but, by virtue of the moisture content which inhibited evaporation of sweat, his temperature

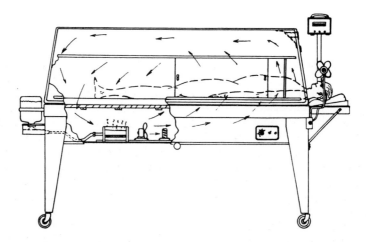

Figure 7.9. The Kettering Hypertherm. From Moore JE (1941) Modern treatment of syphilis. *(By courtesy of Baillière, Tindall.)*

had to rise. The object was to raise the rectal temperature to a level of 106 °F and to keep it constant at this level for eight to ten hours. At times the patient became very uncomfortable and some relief was given by opiates but care had to be taken not to overdo this. Fluid and salt loss in the sweat were replaced by infusions of saline into the veins. Sometimes the patient became light-headed and even delirious and much depended on the personality of the nurse in persuading him to continue[35]."

However, many physicians continued to rely on malaria therapy, which was still being used, in combination with antimicrobials, in the 1950s.

Intensive Arsenotherapy

The side effects of treatment with arsenicals could be formidable. Some of these, such as exfoliative dermatitis, haemorrhagic nephritis, polyneuritis and encephalitis, required the immediate withdrawal of arsenic, and even then could prove fatal. If reactions were less severe, treatment could cautiously continue. Because many patients did not complete courses of treatment lasting for a year or more, the possibility of short intensive arsenotherapy was reconsidered in the late 1930s, although earlier attempts – so-called "abortive treatment" – had been unsuccessful. Intensive therapy with neoarsphenamine was abandoned because of severe toxic reactions and mapharsen, a derivative of arsphenamine originally described by Ehrlich, was substituted. Large doses were given by slow continuous intravenous infusion over a five-day period. Although some patients developed major complications such as haemorrhagic encephalitis and peripheral neuritis, the incidence of infectious relapses was around 12 per cent, which was considered acceptable at a time when the exigency of the Second World War made it essential to conserve manpower[36]. Whatever one may think of this argument it was overtaken by events, because in 1943 the first report of the use of penicillin in early syphilis appeared.

Penicillin

The first clinical observation of the antibacterial action of *Penicillium* was made by the surgeon Joseph Lister in the 1870s. He used fungal culture extracts to treat some localised infections, but encountered the same problem which defeated Fleming 60 years later: the instability of penicillin in these extracts and the technical difficulty of concentrating the active substance[37]. Alexander Fleming (1881–1955) was a Scottish bacteriologist who worked at St Mary's Hospital, London. As a young man he had been involved in the early use of arsphenamine, which had been supplied to his chief, Almroth Wright, by Ehrlich. Subsequently, he became interested in natural defences against infection, and in 1922 discovered lysozyme, an enzyme with antibacterial properties which is present in many body fluids. His identification of penicillin came by chance six years later when he observed that a mould, later identified as *Penicillium notatum*, which had contaminated a culture plate appeared to have destroyed adjacent colonies of staphylococci. After some further work he published his findings, but they attracted little attention until 1938, when a team of scientists at Oxford headed by the pathologist Howard Florey and the biochemist Ernst Chain, began a study of antimicrobial substances. Eventually a method for producing and purifying penicillin was developed, and its antibacterial effectiveness was confirmed by early clinical trials. By this time the Second World War had begun, and the technology for the large-scale production of penicillin was not available in Britain. The work was undertaken in the United States, and a series of developments in manufacturing procedures led to accelerating production of the new antibiotic. In 1945 Fleming, Florey and Chain shared a Nobel prize for their work.

In early 1943 John Mahoney, of the US Public Health Service, was provided with some penicillin by the Oxford investigators. Having demonstrated a rapid cure of syphilitic rabbits, Mahoney and his colleagues treated four patients with primary syphilis; treponemes disappeared from the chancres within a few hours, and serological tests rapidly became negative[38]. Their paper was one of the most important in the history of syphilology (Figure 7.10). The engagement of the USA in a major war had led to many cases of early syphilis in the armed services, so it was essential to find the best way of using the new drug as soon as possible. It was decided to mount a co-ordinated study, and selected units of the US army and navy and the Public Health Service together with some university clinics explored

American Journal of Public Health
and THE NATION'S HEALTH

| Volume 33 | December, 1943 | Number 12 |

Penicillin Treatment of Early Syphilis[*]

A Preliminary Report

JOHN F. MAHONEY, M.D., R. C. ARNOLD, M.D., AND
AD HARRIS

U. S. Marine Hospital, Staten Island, N. Y.

THE number of diseases and infections which are favorably influenced by penicillin therapy continues to increase as experience in the use of the drug is gained. It is the purpose of the present report to record. in a preliminary way, certain observations which have been made in four patients with early syphilis (primary) who were treated with penicillin only.

A study of the usefulness of the drug in the management of syphilis was undertaken after limited animal experimentation indicated that penicillin

possessed some spirocheticidal activity. The plan of study embraced the concurrent carrying out of a complete delineation of the effectiveness of the drug in experimental syphilis in rabbits and the conduct of a small pilot study of the effects produced in patients with early disease. The prompt resort to the human being was sponsored by the general non-toxic character of the drug and by the knowledge that observations as to early effectiveness could be carried out without placing in jeopardy the patient's chance for ultimate recovery in event it became expedient to resort to conventional arsenic therapy.

The early results in the animal phase of the general study indicate that the time-dose relationship will prove to be as important in this therapy as in the use of other chemotherapeutic agents. Failures to sterilize experimentally infected animals with treatment schedules which utilize minimal amounts of the drug over a brief treatment period are predictable. The results from treat-

From U. S. Marine Hospital, Staten Island, N. Y. Medical Director William Y. Hollingsworth in Charge.

This study was undertaken at the request of the Committee on Chemotherapeutic and other Agents. Division of Medical Sciences. National Research Council, acting for the Committee on Medical Research of the Office of Scientific Research and Development. The penicillin was furnished through a contract between the Office of Scientific Research and Development and the Massachusetts Memorial Hospitals.

Presented before the Epidemiology Section of the American Public Health Association at the Seventy-second Annual Meeting in New York, N. Y., October 14, 1943.

[1387]

Figure 7.10. Title page of Mahoney et al.'s report in the American Journal of Public Health *(1943) of the first use of penicillin for the treatment of syphilis.*

a total of 26 regimens for the treatment of early, latent and neurosyphilis. The results of this massive exercise were analysed by the Office of Scientific Research and Development. This was a good arrangement; it was soon possible to lay down guidelines for therapy, and the shambles which followed the introduction of arsphenamine in 1910 was avoided. In 1947 detailed results of the treatment of a large series of cases of infectious syphilis were published[39]. It was clear that the new drug was highly effective: a course of intramuscular injections of soluble pencillin given three-hourly for 7–8 days achieved clinical and serological cure in over 90 per cent of patients. Furthermore, only 1–2 per cent of those treated had abnormal spinal fluids after therapy, a great improvement on the results previously achieved with metals, and side effects to penicillin were mild. In Britain the supply of penicillin was, in comparison with the USA, exiguous. Nevertheless, from 1943 onwards reports from venereal disease clinics and the armed forces confirmed the results of the transatlantic groups[40].

At first, soluble preparations, amorphous penicillin, then crystalline penicillin G, were the only ones available. The need for frequent injections meant that patients had to be kept in hospital throughout treatment. The development of "depot" preparations, which made once daily injections possible, was thus a major advance. Penicillin mixed with peanut oil and beeswax was followed in 1948 by procaine penicillin G and "PAM" (a formulation of procaine penicillin and aluminium monostearate). Various schedules of daily or twice weekly injections were followed, and the results were excellent. In early syphilis the clinical failure rate was reduced to 5 per cent (and most patients with treatment failure were cured by a second course of penicillin). In late benign syphilis the results were as good as any previously obtained with heavy metal therapy. Penicillin simplified and improved the treatment and outcome of many cases of neurosyphilis, and it was the best drug ever used for the prevention and treatment of congenital infections[41]. A still less soluble and therefore longer acting compound, benzathine penicillin, was introduced in 1952. In single dosage this cured early syphilis, and thus approached Ehrlich's *therapia sterilans magna*.

For several years after the introduction of penicillin some practitioners supplemented a course with a series of injections of arsenicals or bismuth, perhaps because they did not entirely trust the new remedy. Others, it is said, believed that prolonging the treatment would impress the patient with the gravity of the disease and the importance of returning for follow-up examinations. Eventually it was decided that penicillin had completely replaced arsenic, bismuth and mercury in all stages of syphilis, and adjuvant therapy was abandoned.

The Jarisch–Herxheimer Reaction

The overwhelming advantages of penicillin therapy were not only its effectiveness but the speed with which patients were rendered non-infectious, the simplicity of treatment and the relative freedom from side effects. Apart from occasional cases of allergy, these were minimal in comparison with previous forms of treatment. An exception was the Jarisch–Herxheimer reaction, which had been first described at the end of the nineteenth century and had been observed to occur with all forms of treatment for syphilis. In 1895 Adolph Jarisch (1850–1902), an Austrian dermatologist, described a phenomenon occurring in patients with secondary syphilis who were receiving mercurial inunctions: during the first few days of treatment the skin eruptions became worse rather than better[42]. A few years later the same reaction was recorded in more detail in a classical paper from Frankfurt by Karl Herxheimer (1861–1944) and his colleague Dr Krause[43]. They had seen 60 cases, all occurring after the first dose of mercury. They pointed out that the reaction was not only local; many patients felt unwell and developed fever and enlargement of lymph glands, but all these effects soon disappeared. Herxheimer (Figure 7.11) had been assistant to Neisser at Breslau, and later became director of the University Skin Clinic at Frankfurt. He was a handsome, gifted and energetic man who wrote well on many aspects of dermatology; it is sad to record that he died in a Nazi concentration camp at the age of 83.

The Course of Untreated Syphilis

Throughout the syphilis epidemic it had been observed that while some victims developed late complications others were unscathed. Curiously enough, a proper assessment of the fate of untreated patients was not made until the twentieth century, although such an assessment was important not only in its own right but to provide a yardstick with which the effect of treatment could be measured. A Norwegian syphilologist Caesar Boeck (1845–1913) was the first to attempt a prospective study. He was in charge of the Dermatological Clinic at Oslo between 1891 and 1910 and he had come to believe, like many of his predecessors, that the existing treatment of syphilis, predominantly with mercury, was toxic and ineffective and that patients might progress just as well if they were left untreated. Accordingly he initiated a long-term study of a group of subjects with early syphilis; they were kept in hospital until they were considered to be non-infectious, usually a period of about three months, and given general nursing care but no specific treatment. In 1929 Boeck's successor Bruusgaard published his reassessment of these patients, based on clinical examination and the study of

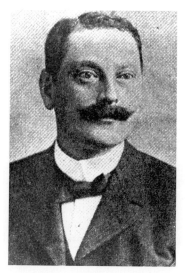

Figure 7.11. Karl Herxheimer (1861–1944).

100

clinical and autopsy reports, and in 1955 Gjestland performed a detailed study of all the available data[44]. About a quarter of the untreated patients had at least one infectious relapse. Gummatous disease affected 15 per cent of patients, usually within the first 15 years; cardiovascular disease developed in 14 per cent of the men and 8 per cent of the women, while neurosyphilis developed in 9 per cent of the men and 5 per cent of the women. In all, 30 per cent of the patients developed late complications of one sort or another.

A more recent study of the course of untreated syphilis was arranged by the US Public Health Service at Tuskagee, Alabama in 1932 and continued for 30 years. All the participants were black. Patients with early syphilis were treated with arsenicals but the remainder, who had a history suggestive of syphilis and positive serological tests, were left untreated. The results of follow-up examinations were similar to those reported from Norway; gummatous disease, cardiovascular and neurosyphilis were relatively common in the untreated group[45]. The Tuskagee study has been criticised as being unethical – written informed consent was not obtained from any of the participants – and possibly racist. Like many human experiments which have been performed during the long history of syphilis it was doubtless well intentioned, but the modern reader may think that it was unwise.

By the early 1950s the long search for an effective treatment for syphilis was over. No long-term study of the results of treatment was undertaken, perhaps because the spectacular success obtained with penicillin led to a consensus that the treatment of early and latent syphilis invariably prevented late complications. The possibility that this may not be true has caused some uneasiness in recent years.

Chapter 8
Chancroid and Donovanosis

Ruin on ruin, rout on rout,
Confusion worse confounded.

John Milton, *Paradise Lost*

Chancroid

Contagious ulcers of the genitals were well known in ancient and medieval times. Writing in 1306, the Italian physician Lanfranc described "ulcers arising from the rupture of hot pustules of young men ... from connection with an unclean woman", and went on to say: "If you wish to preserve the member from complete corruption, after connection with a woman whom you suspect of uncleanliness, wash it with water mixed with vinegar"[1]. A rapidly spreading necrosis of the external genitalia, called phagedenic ulceration or phagedenea, was often described in the early literature. In its destructive potential it resembled the synergistic bacterial gangrene which sometimes affects the genital area today. Phagedenea commonly followed genital ulceration, probably through superinfection by Vincent's or other organisms. The following report describing a case of the disease was written in 1810 by William Fergusson (1772–1846), inspector general of hospitals to the Portuguese army:

"It is certain that all changes of climate from a cold to a warmer temperature predispose the human frame to febrile affections or other forms of acute disease; and that the English, from their mode of life, always incautious and frequently intemperate, are exposed in a particular manner to suffer from this predisposition. And if, previous to this attack, they should have the misfortune to be affected with venereal ulceration, the elements of the disease which had previously been prepared within their bodies ... are diverted by this casualty into new channels, and make their exit as a local form of fever in the shape of *phagedaenic ulceration.*

To make this understood I shall endeavour to illustrate it by a short case. Shortly after the battle of Vimiera I was called by an officer, a friend of mine, who earnestly implored my assistance. I found him, four days after a connection in Lisbon, with the whole penis enormously swelled, of a deep red colour; malignant and ugly chancres on different parts of the prepuce, and two on the glans penis, the appearance of which I can compare to nothing but the holes made by a rusty nail in a piece of mahogany or logwood. The catastrophe, if left to nature, would inevitably have sealed his fate; but I caused him to be copiously blooded, applied the coldest acetous lotion to the part, purged him most freely with neutral salts, and enjoined every part of the anti-phlogistic regimen.

The success was perfect, the tumification speedily subsided; in a few days all the sores were in a state of the healthiest suppuration ... The woman who communicated the infection was an opera dancer in Lisbon, apparently in perfect health, who continued on the stage for many months afterwards, occasionally infecting others, without anything extraordinary, as far as I could learn, in the nature of symptoms[2]."

The earlier clinicians, for example John de Vigo, had differentiated syphilitic from non-syphilitic ulcers, but by the sixteenth century the distinction had been lost and both were attributed to the same "venereal poison". At the end of the eighteenth century it is clear from their writings that Hunter, Bell and their contemporaries were seeing cases of chancroid, but without recognising this as an independent venereal disease. Hunter thought that there were non-specific ulcers which could be mistaken for syphilis, but he did not characterise these any further, simply remarking that they could be distinguished by the response of a syphilitic chancre to mercury. He gave the incubation period of chancres as between 24 hours and several weeks, which suggests that some or many cases of chancroid, which has an incubation period of only a few days, were being included[3]. Bell stated that there was no fixed incubation period for chancres and that most appeared within three or four days of sexual contact. He recognised a "phagedenic chancre" which, through "neglect, peculiarity of the constitution or a virulent matter of infection", could rapidly progress and deepen so that much of the penis was destroyed within a few days; he had seen several such cases follow contact with the same woman, which certainly suggests the possibility of chancroid[4].

The nosography of these lesions was partly clarified by the Irish surgeon Richard Carmichael (1779–1849). He received his medical education in Dublin, where he later became surgeon to St George's Hospital and the Lock Hospital. He was interested in medical education and founded a medical school, and he also wrote several works about venereal diseases. Some of his opinions were distinctly controversial: Lancereaux described him as a "bold syphilographer". He was evidently a handsome man with a "stern cast of countenance"; he met his death by drowning while crossing an arm of the sea on horseback. Carmichael strongly supported Bell in separating gonorrhoea from syphilis. He did not agree with those who believed that all genital ulcers were syphilitic and that their variable clinical appearance was due simply to host factors: "It would be absurd to assert, as a general proposition, that the poison is always the same, and that the varieties of form which it assumes always depends on the constitution of the individual." He went on to argue the case for a "plurality of poisons", and proposed that only indurated chancres should be called syphilitic and treated with mercury; other genital ulcers which developed after an "impure connection" should simply be called "venereal"[5].

Ricord failed to recognise chancroid as a specific cause of genital ulceration; we have seen in Chapter 3 that his autoinoculation technique, by which he set great store, grievously misled him on this matter. In his younger days he was emphatic:

"There is only one syphilitic virus . . . The lesion produced is a pustule if the matter lodges beneath the epidermis, and ulcer if placed on an excoriated surface and an abscess if introduced into subcutaneous tissue – the virus being always one and the same[6]."

Despite his erroneous idea of aetiology, he made a clinical distinction between hard chancres, which were associated with non-suppurative adenitis and often preceded constitutional syphilis, and soft chancres, which were associated with suppurative adenitis and were rarely followed by generalised disease. The two kinds of lesion were so sharply characterised that it is surprising that Ricord failed to deduce that they were different diseases; his pupil Bassereau, however, saw that they were.

Léon Bassereau (1810–1887), a member of the noble family of Anjou, was born at Anduze, near Nimes. At first he read law but after a year abandoned this for medicine, which he studied in Paris. He received his MD in 1840, and having worked with Ricord he had already decided to concentrate on venereology, although he practised general medicine as well. He remained in Paris for the rest of his life. In his spare time he studied literature and the arts. Mme Récamier, the Parisian society beauty and wit, was his cousin and he was a frequent guest at her salon. Bassereau was too modest to seek titles and honours, although he was appointed Chevalier of the Légion d'Honneur in 1861. He married in 1841 and had five children. He was desolated by the death of his eldest son, also a doctor, in 1874 and effectively retired, passing his days quietly with his books and paintings and seeing only his family and a few old friends. He died in Paris in 1887, at the age of 77[7].

Bassereau's most important contributions to venereology were his identification of chancroid as an independent disease and the method of "confrontation" which he developed to study it. In a work published in 1852 he recorded a careful study of the history, symptoms and signs of a group of patients with genital ulceration and distinguished two types of chancre: *indurated chancres* were usually followed by constitutional symptoms and signs, while *non-indurated chancres* were a purely local disease, which could recur many times in some individuals. So far he was echoing Ricord, but he went on to say that by means of "confrontations" – contact tracing, as it would be called today – he had shown that each kind of chancre was associated with a similar lesion in the sex partners, both those who appeared to have transmitted the disease to the patient and those to whom the patient in turn had passed it on:

"If one confronts all the subjects who have had chancre followed by constitutional syphilis with the subjects who communicated the contagion to them or with those to whom they have transmitted it, one finds that all these subjects, without exception, have had chancres followed by constitutional 'accidents'. Never among them has the chancre limited itself to a purely local action . . . If, on the contrary, one confronts the subjects who have chancres which have not led to any symptoms of general syphilis with the people who have infected them, or whom they have infected, one finds that these, without exception, have chancres which have limited their action to the point of first contamination[8]."

Bassereau contrasted "Chancre précurseur de la vérole" with "Chancre a bubon suppuré", and proposed the concept of the "duality of the chancre", the fruit of what must have been an enormous amount of difficult clinical work; it ended the confusion which had surrounded the subject since the sixteenth century. His ideas were endorsed by another of Ricord's pupils, François Clerc, who pointed out that if people known to be syphilitic were inoculated with material from a syphilitic chancre no lesions would result, whereas inoculation of material from a soft sore was nearly always followed by the appearance of a similar lesion. Clerc introduced the word "chancroid". Nothing is straightforward in the history of this disease; he used the word to mean "related to chancre", because he believed that soft sores were caused by a modified syphilis virus[9].

Joseph Rollet (1824–1894; Figure 8.1) was another great French syphilologist who studied chancroid. He was born at Legnieu, not far from Lyon where, after a period of study of the classics, he entered the School of Medicine. He completed his studies in Paris, where he was awarded an MD in 1848. He returned to Lyon and in 1855 was appointed Surgeon-Major of l'Hospice de l'Antiguaille, which Paul Diday had made a major centre for patients with venereal diseases 20 years before. Rollet was tall, with a thin face, a long nose and thick eyebrows. He looked like the layman's idea of a philosopher: stooped, walking slowly with his hands behind his back, deep in thought. He has been contrasted with Ricord, charismatic, heaped with honours and decorations, a brilliant propagandist but with ideas which were often ill-conceived and sometimes wrong. Rollet was a careful observer who – perhaps because of his classical education – subjected his conclusions to a rigorous analysis. In debate he was calm, courteous and logical. His intellectual activity extended to the study of the history of medicine, particularly venereal diseases[10].

Rollet's contract at l'Antiquaille was for only nine years; in 1887 he was appointed professor of hygiene, a position which he occupied for the rest of his professional life, but his achievements in venereology during this time

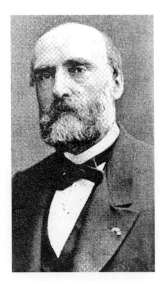

Figure 8.1. Joseph Rollet (1824–1894).

were remarkable. He established the incubation period of syphilis, showed that the secondary stage was contagious, and was among the first to observe that it could be transmitted by vaccination. He confirmed Bassereau's opinion that chancroid was a different disease. Chancroidal ulceration, he wrote, is repeatedly reinoculable in the same individual, but a syphilitic chancre is not; it is transmissible only to a recipient who is free from syphilis. Rollet found some cases which were hard to classify: the chancre was autoinoculable, yet signs of secondary syphilis developed later. He showed that these could be explained by the existence of a *mixed chancre* due, he said, to a simultaneous infection by the "viruses" of the two diseases[11]. Rollet's work finally convinced Ricord that Bassereau had been right, and he accepted the existence of chancroid and mixed chancres in a book which he published with Fournier in 1858.

By the time Lancereaux wrote his *Treatise on Syphilis* in 1866 he was able to give some data on the relative frequency of indurated and non-indurated chancres, and he reported that the latter appeared to be between two and four times commoner. He emphasised the progressive destructive qualities of chancroid and the severity of the phagedena which could complicate it, and he contrasted the suppurative adenitis which occurs in chancroid with the indolent indurated "true syphilitic bubo"[12]. Unlike Bassereau, many authors commented that although chancroid was known to affect women it was much less common than in men, and that many female partners of men with undoubted chancroid, including those who appeared to have transmitted the disease to them, showed no clinical abnormality. This is still a feature of chancroid, and is illustrated in the following case report, concerning patients of Ricord, needless to say:

> "A married pair invited a friend, an officer, to dinner. Everything went on in an unexceptional manner until near the close of the repast, when it was discovered that there was no cheese in the house, and the husband went out to buy some. The officer took advantage of his absence and abused the rights of hospitality. A few days after, the husband broke out with a chancroid, and applied to Ricord for advice. Ricord examined his wife and found her free from disease, but obtained a confession of her exposure with the officer, who happened at the same time to be under Ricord's treatment for chancroid[13]."

Bassereau's and Rollet's views on the "duality of the chancre" were widely accepted in France, particularly after they had been endorsed by Ricord, but those who may have thought that this ended the controversies about chancroid would have been wrong, as an unrewarding dispute over the identity and nature of the disease dragged on for another 20 years. Everybody joined in: Vidal de Cassis in Paris, von Baerensprung in Berlin, Hebra in Vienna, Koebner in Breslau, Hutchinson in England and Bumstead in the USA. The disputes surrounded the problem of whether, and in what circumstances, inoculated material from genital ulcers would induce similar lesions in the donor or in another person. Numerous experiments were performed, and eventually the inoculations included even pus from non-genital abscesses and the lesions of acne. As might be expected, these studies provided a mass of data which were, to say the least, difficult to interpret. But the results of one group of experiments, performed at about the same time by Bidenkap in Christiania and Koebner in Breslau, were disturbing. They reported that autoinoculation of material from an indurated chancre seldom "took", but if the chancre was mechanically or chemically irritated so as to suppurate more profusely autoinoculation yielded a pustule which could be transmitted in series. Although the modern reader might think that these experiments show that secondary pyogenic infection is indeed transmissible in series, at the time they were interpreted as indicating that "the soft chancre is an acute inflammatory manifestation of syphilitic contagion". As Zinsser aptly put it, Bidenkap's and Koebner's experiments "fell like a bombshell among the dualists, causing a great number of desertions from their ranks"[14]. Some of the doubters did not recant dualism completely; as was said of a recent Archbishop of Canterbury, they nailed their colours to the fence. For example, the American physicians Bumstead and Taylor wrote in 1883:

"Chancroid does not depend upon a specific virus of its own, incapable of being generated de novo. In most cases met with in practice chancroid is derived from a chancroid but it may arise, especially in persons debilitated by any cause, from inoculation of the products of inflammation, either simple or syphilitic, and subsequently perpetuate itself from one individual to another as a chancroid[15]."

The idea that genital disease could be due to non-specific irritation had already been used to explain gonorrhoea and condylomata acuminata. Indeed, Bumstead and Taylor went on to suggest an "interesting analogy" – false, as it turned out:

"We now know that [gonorrhoea] may be caused by any simple irritant, but more especially by the pus from the urethral and other inflamed mucous membranes . . . Such as the history of gonorrhoea has been, so, we predict, the history of chancroid will be."

The problems which genital ulceration gave to venereologists in the nineteenth century are not difficult to understand. Some of the lesions which they studied were due to syphilis, some to chancroid and some to neither of these. Even today, the cause of many genital ulcers is unknown, and the clinical features of those due to specific infections are very variable. The achievements of Bassereau and Rollet, working without laboratory aid, were considerable, but unfortunately the inoculation techniques which were so widely used were fundamentally flawed through an imperfect understanding of immunology. Further progress had to come through bacteriology, and in 1889 the cause of chancroid was discovered.

Augusto Ducrey (1860–1940; Figure 8.2) was born in Naples to a Swiss father and a Neapolitan mother. He studied medicine at Naples and made his discovery while working there as a young postgraduate. He later became professor of dermatology at Pisa, then Genoa and finally at Rome. His technique was ingenious. He had noticed that microscopy of pus from chancroidal lesions showed a multitude of different micro-organisms. He purified this material by inoculating it into each patient's own forearm. The resulting ulcer was reinoculated, and in this way he was able to passage the bacteria many times. The contaminants died out, and he was able to describe a short rod with rounded ends, later called *Haemophilus ducreyi*, which he concluded was responsible for the disease[16]. His claim was strengthened three years later when Unna (see pp. 151–152) described small clusters of similar Gram-negative rods, the characteristic "shoals of fish", in

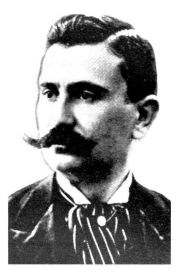

Figure 8.2. Augusto Ducrey (1860–1940).

chancroidal ulcers[17]. After this, for many years the organism was called the bacillus of Unna – Ducrey. Ducrey himself did not succeed in culturing the organism on artificial media, but by 1900 this had been achieved, and in the following year its pathogenicity was confirmed by animal inoculations[18]. Nevertheless, there were many problems in the laboratory diagnosis of chancroid. Gram-stained smears were widely used but subject to error, and culture was complicated and at best confirmed only two-thirds of clinical diagnoses. Some clinicians, remembering that chancroid was the only type of venereal ulceration which was autoinoculable, used this technique. Another diagnostic method was the delayed hypersensitivity test. This was introduced in 1913 by Ito, working with Bruck in Neisser's laboratory[19], and refined by Reenstierna in the Pasteur Institute in 1923. It involved the intradermal inoculation of a killed preparation of either chancroidal pus or a culture of *H. ducreyi*, the appearance of a raised papule signifying a positive result[20]. A commercial antigen was marketed for intradermal testing, and was still being used in the early 1950s. However, the Ito – Reenstierna test was of limited value; although it became positive in more than two-thirds of patients with chancroid this did not occur until late in the attack, and the test then remained positive for many years. This made the accurate diagnosis of subsequent attacks of genital ulceration very difficult.

The difficulties of laboratory diagnosis – which have still not been completely overcome – meant that long after the discovery of *H. ducreyi* chancroid was still being diagnosed on clinical grounds, as it had been in the nineteenth century. It is not surprising that the role of *H. ducreyi* was sometimes questioned. For example, a British Medical Research Committee reported in 1918 that it could find "no sufficient evidence that what is clinically known as soft sore is a special disease induced by a single species of micro-organism", and in 1935 a bulletin from the US Public Health Service came to much the same conclusion. In the 1940s and 1950s further efforts were made to define the growth requirements of *H. ducreyi* and to improve the bacteriological diagnosis of chancroid; this was particularly important because of continuing uncertainty about its epidemiology. Its predominance in men had been known for a long time, and it had been concluded that because of its constant association with intercourse symptomless infection of women must occur. Reliable culture for *H. ducreyi* would help to establish this, and if it was successful it could facilitate control, as had culture for *N. gonorrhoeae* in the case of gonorrhoea. Unfortunately, progress in this area was very slow, and to this day even the primary isolation of the microbes from genital lesions can be difficult. The epidemiology of chancroid remains obscure in many respects, but it is now believed that individuals who are capable of transmitting the infection to others have ulcers, although these may be symptomless; the existence of a carrier state without lesions is still hotly debated[21]. In the past few years chancroid has again become of major importance because of the association of genital ulceration with the transmission of the human immunodeficiency virus.

Before the advent of antimicrobials the treatment of chancroid was problematic. Exposure of the ulcers, by circumcision if necessary, was regarded as an essential first step, followed by regular bathing with antiseptics; buboes were aspirated. The course of the illness was often protracted, and recurrences after apparent cure common. Sulphonamides were first used in 1938. They greatly shortened the time needed for cure; they were used throughout the Second World War and for many years afterwards[22]. Although it remained common in tropical and subtropical countries, the incidence of chancroid in Europe and North America declined throughout the twentieth century; today, most cases in these localities are imported, although small localised outbreaks still occur. The reasons for the decline of what was once one of the commonest venereal diseases are obscure. It may be related to improved living conditions and better sexual hygiene; chancroid has always been more prevalent in lower socioeconomic groups, and in people who visit prostitutes. Perhaps for this reason it seems to have been regarded with some distaste by fastidious physicians, one of whom wrote in 1943:

> "It is a disease of the unenlightened and the common poor, of the dregs of society and of only the most indiscriminate and promiscuous men and women . . . It follows in the path of travelling circuses, marathon dance teams and carnival shows, vagabonds of the road and their ilk. With the advent of the 'trailer girl', the bawdy house on wheels, the itinerant whore and the camp followers it has become a disease of the byways as well . . . It is a disease of the unclean, of people who do not use soap and water with any degree of frequency, particularly when coitus is performed on the run[23]."

Donovanosis

This was the last major type of anogenital ulceration to be identified. It has received many names, including granuloma contagiosum, granuloma pudendi and sclerosing granuloma. In Europe it was formerly called granuloma venereum, but this was replaced by granuloma inguinale to avoid confusion with lymphogranuloma venereum. The word *Donovanosis* has been adopted during the last two decades. The disease has always been most prevalent in tropical and sub-tropical areas, and was first described in India. In the days of British sovereignty doctors working in the Indian Medical Service made many valuable observations. Kenneth MacLeod (1844–1922) was one of them. Born in the Outer Hebrides he studied medicine at Edinburgh University. He joined the Indian Medical Service in 1865, and in due course became professor of surgery at Calcutta Medical College. After his retirement from the service in 1888 he held various administrative posts in the British army, and in 1906 was appointed honorary surgeon to the King. He undertook a large amount of public work, and wrote extensively on public health and tropical medicine. MacLeod was a man "of fine stature", but inclined to be brusque and intolerant[24]. His description of donovanosis appeared in a summary of the operations performed in his department in Calcutta during 1881:

"The last series of two cases supply an illustration of a disease which is occasionally met with in India, namely serpiginous or lupoid ulceration of the genitals. The process commences with a venereal sore; from this as a centre or starting point, or from a bubo resulting from it, ulceration gradually and very slowly extends. The skin becomes tuberculated, the neoplasm breaks down and a circle of ulcer results, which is succeeded by an imperfect cicatrix. The scrotal and penile skin is destroyed, these organs get involved in a mass of cicatricial material, and the ulcer spreads by circles and bays into the groins, thighs and buttocks[25]."

This description makes very clear the combination of ulceration and fibrosis which characterises the disease. The same point was made by a British dermatologist, James Galloway, at a meeting of the Dermatological Society of London in 1896. He drew attention to a paper recently published in British Guiana entitled "The lupoid form of the so-called 'groin ulceration' of this colony" in which a disease similar to the one described by MacLeod had been discussed. Galloway remembered that a patient with this disorder had been seen in London in 1888 and had been examined by two of the best known dermatologists of the day, James Pringle at the Middlesex Hospital and Radcliffe Crocker at University College Hospital[26].

The early observers commented that donovanosis affected both men and women and that it was "locally contagious"; although it occurred in the region of the genitals, nobody suggested that it was a venereal disease. Its cause was discovered by another member of the Indian Medical Service, Charles Donovan (1863–1951). He was a student at Trinity College, Dublin, and joined the service shortly after he qualified. Most of his career was spent in Madras, where he eventually became professor of physiology and physician to Madras General Hospital. He was a skilled microscopist and draughtsman. In Madras he collaborated with William Boog Leishman (1865–1926), another Irishman in the Indian Medical Service, in the identification of intracellular protozoa (later called Leishman – Donovan bodies) as the cause of kala-azar; Leishman went on to become director general of the service, but Donovan remained at Madras until his retirement. He was evidently very popular, amusing yet sympathetic, and an outstanding teacher[27]. In 1905 he identified intracellular bodies, later called "Donovan bodies" (Figure 8.3), in stained tissue smears from patients with donovanosis, which he described under the heading "Ulcerating granuloma of the pudenda":

"In scrapings from the deeper parts of these growths small forms, oval in shape, about 1 to 2 μm in length, are found in the epithelial cells of the stratum malpighii or in macrophages, usually in large numbers, either scattered or in small round compact groups. They stain badly with methylene blue, haematoxylin and the different modifications of Romanowsky. By the last mode of staining, the cells possess a well-defined contour with a dark pink protoplasm therein, in the centre of which there exists a long flatly oval very dark pink chromatin mass. The epithelial cells containing the bodies bear a strong resemblance to mast cells, the presence of which has been brought to notice by Galloway in his lucid description of the histology of this particular granuloma[28]."

From the beginning there were arguments about the nature of these bodies. Donovan himself, and many others, thought that they were protozoa, but eventually they were shown to be capsulated Gram-negative bacteria. It was impossible to culture them on artificial media, but in 1945 members of Goodpasture's team at Vanderbilt University, Tennessee succeeded in propagating them in the yolk sac of fertilised hens' eggs[29]. The organism was named *Donovania granulomatis*, and later *Calymmatobacterium granulomatis*, but its bacterial affiliation remains uncertain.

As had happened with chancroid, it was difficult to study the epidemiology of donovanosis because of the lack of a good culture technique, and a further problem was that the areas of the world where the disease was most common had poor facilities for laboratory research. The mode of transmission was

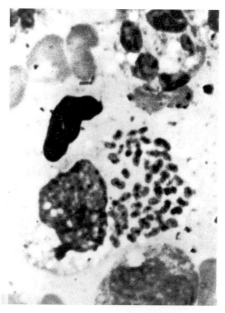

Figure 8.3. Donovan bodies. (From Anderson, de Monbreun and Goodpasture's paper in the Journal of Experimental Medicine *(1945) describing the propagation of* Donovania granulomatis *in the yolk sac of hens' eggs.)*

disputed. Because the majority of lesions affected the anogenital area most clinicians thought that donovanosis was a sexually transmitted disease, but it was pointed out that genital lesions in the partners of affected individuals were not often seen, and that the disease was uncommon in prostitutes[30]. Nothing could be discovered about the possibility of latent infections. Alternatively, since anal lesions were very common, it was suggested that the natural habitat of *C. granulomatis* was the bowel, and that transmission was predominantly through anal coitus[31]. A century after the first description of donovanosis these matters are still undecided.

In the nineteenth century it was found that the application of antiseptics was ineffective and that even cautery, scraping of the lesions with a sharp spoon or the application of caustics were often followed by recurrences. Many workers recommended complete excision of the whole affected area. Preparations containing antimony had been used in dermatology for centuries, and in the 1920s the systemic administration of antimony salts had been found quite effective for the treatment of some tropical protozoal diseases such as schistosomiasis, leishmaniasis and trypanosomiasis. This was the rationale for the use of antimony compounds for the treatment of donovanosis, which was still thought at that time to be due to a protozoal infection. It had some effect, particularly against early lesions. The sulphonamides and penicillin showed no specific activity against donovanosis, although they reduced secondary infection, but when streptomycin was introduced in 1946 it was found to be far superior to antimony, and became the drug of choice for many years. Although in the modern era treatment has greatly improved, in respect of its epidemiology and microbiology donovanosis has remained the least well understood of the venereal diseases.

Chapter 9

Gonorrhoea Virulenta

When I got home, though, there came sorrow.
Too, too plain was Signor Gonorrhoea.

James Boswell, *London Journal*

The violence of the original outbreak of syphilis moderated during the sixteenth century and gonorrhoea (which had no doubt been present all along, but over-shadowed by the more serious disease) re-emerged as a separate clinical entity. The symptoms of gonorrhoea were often clamant, "furious in their essence and rebellious in their course". Complications were common; many men developed epididymitis and became sterile and some, including Rousseau and Boswell, died of uraemia following urethral strictures. Treatment was needed not only to abate the severity of the disease but, since it was believed that syphilis and gonorrhoea were both due to the same venereal poison, to prevent the development of a full-blown pox.

There was no agreement on exactly how the "venereal poison" caused the symptoms and signs of gonorrhoea. To some, still clinging to Hippocratic and Galenic doctrines of humours, the discharge of gonorrhoea consisted of semen corrupted through humoral imbalance and focused in the prostates (as the seminal vesicles were then called). But an alternative idea was gaining ground, that the symptoms and signs of gonorrhoea were due to urethral ulceration. Meatal chancres were familiar to everyone, and it needed only a small step to believe that such sores could be small, multiple and endourethral. Writing in 1689 the French physician Louis le Monnier explained this idea:

"Virulent gonorrhoea or chaude-pisse ... is an involuntary flow of purulent and corrupted matter, accompanied by burning and painful ardour of urination ... This purulent matter, to my way of thinking, is neither the efflux of corrupted semen, nor of the glairy fluid contained in the prostates as has always been believed, but is rather the lymph which flows from its proper canals when they have been eaten away in several spots and torn by the power and activity of the venereal virus[1]."

The ulcer theory of secretion lasted for many years. It was accepted, for example, by Daniel Turner (1667–1740; Figure 9.1), one of the colourful figures with which the history of venereology abounds. A Londoner, he began his career as a member of the Barber Surgeon Company, but he was irritated by his low professional status and in 1711 resigned from the company and applied to the Royal College of Physicians for a licence. Although this was granted it was irregular, because he had no medical degree from any university; personal and pointed comments were made by his colleagues. Eventually he did obtain an MD. He applied to the president of the Academy of Yale, enclosing his portrait and a gift of books, and he was duly awarded an honorary doctorate. He had hoped that he would now be admitted to the Royal College of Physicians as a Fellow, but this was not to be[2]. Turner was a gifted clinician, and wrote well in a racy and readable style. His publications included *A Treatise on Diseases Incident to the Skin* (1714) and *A Practical Dissertation on the Venereal Disease* (1717), both of which were extremely successful and went through many editions. He accepted without question that the gonorrhoeal urethra was ulcerated, but carried the idea a stage further by applying it to women: "This thing resteth in their secret places, forming therein pretty little sores full of venomous poison, being very dangerous for those who unknowingly meddle with them"[3].

By the middle of the eighteenth century the ulcer theory had foundered. Morgagni had directed attention away from archaic ideas about body fluids towards pathological changes in individual organs. He showed that gonorrhoea in men was associated with neither a primary focus in the seminal vesicles nor with urethral ulceration, and in turn the English surgeon William Cockburn (1660–1736) pointed out that in men with gonorrhoea the urethra was inflamed rather than ulcerated. Finally, in 1753 John Hunter dissected the urethras of eight men hanged at Tyburn; two had had gonorrhoea when they died, but they showed only erythematous changes, without ulceration. He subsequently examined the urethras of many men who had had gonorrhoea at the time of their death, finding no ulceration, only congestion and occasional abscesses in the paraurethral glands. He believed that this erythema was a direct effect of the "venereal poison" on the urethral mucosa, "creeping along" from the meatus.

Hunter's *Treatise on the Venereal Disease*, was published in 1786[4]. Like others, he made a distinction between simple and virulent gonorrhoea. Simple gonorrhoea, he said, may begin after intercourse, but may also occur in

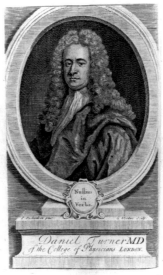

Figure 9.1. Daniel Turner (1667–1740).

association with rheumatism, gout, or even banal events such as cutting a tooth. In many cases there was no apparent cause. Although remarking that simple gonorrhoea was particularly common in men with a past history of urethritis, Hunter did not regard it as a venereal disease. It is difficult to know what to make of this; the term must have covered several different conditions, including today's non-gonococcal urethritis. In contrast, Hunter regarded virulent gonorrhoea as "due to venereal infection". He estimated the usual incubation period as between 6 and 12 days, although it could be less than this. Among the symptoms he included balanitis, mucoid or purulent urethral discharge, dysuria and, in severe cases, urethral bleeding. Chordee (a painful downward bowing of the penis due to periurethral inflammation) was listed as a sign of gonorrhoea by Hunter, as by all eighteenth century writers. He described inflammation of the paraurethral glands, sometimes leading to abscesses. Virulent gonorrhoea became more serious, and more difficult to cure, when the patient complained of pain in the perineum, frequency and urgency of micturition, and strangury. These symptoms indicated infection of Cowper's glands (which might suppurate), the bladder neck, prostate and seminal vesicles, and a correspondingly severe and prolonged illness.

Bell's *Treatise on Gonorrhoea Virulanta and Lues Venerea*[5] appeared seven years after Hunter's work. He devoted a whole volume to gonorrhoea. Again, he separated simple from virulent gonorrhoea. His description of the latter was more comprehensive than Hunter's, every symptom, sign and complication being discussed in detail. His vivid account of the involvement of the posterior urethra and adjacent structures reminds the modern reader how serious gonorrhoea could be in the pre-antibiotic era. The management of these complications clearly needed the greatest skill and judgment if permanent sequelae such as strictures and fistulas were to be avoided. Bell's summary showed his usual mastery of style and content: "Gonorrhoea is a local disease, proceeding from a specific contagion not necessarily connected with any other . . . The discharge of matter which takes place is not the effect of ulceration, but proceeds from an inflamed state of the urethra and contiguous parts . . . The disease is formidable in proportion to the depth of parts that are affected . . . In the cure of gonorrhoea no advantage is derived from mercury or any remedy acting solely on the constitution".

There was some disagreement about the relationship between gonorrhoea and swelling of the testicles. Hunter wrote that the swelling could follow any form of urethral inflammation – it was "only sympathetic", and should not be regarded as "venereal". He had observed that as the "irritation" was translated from the urethra to the testicle the urethral symptoms improved. Bell, on the other hand, thought that gonorrhoea was much the commonest cause of swelling of the testicle; it began in the epididymis, and later the scrotum might become red and inflamed.

Early Treatment Practices

The treatment of gonorrhoea in the eighteenth century was a mish-mash of established modalities such as bleeding and purging, the administration of herbal remedies, urethral lavage, the passage of medicated urethral sounds and, of course, prescription of mercury, the allegedly specific cure for "the venereal". Protagonists of a particular treatment were loud in their condemnation of those who suggested otherwise. All agreed on the importance of rest, the avoidance of alcohol and sexual continence. Le Monnier advised those treating patients with gonorrhoea to "commence by regulating their licentious and libertine life by having them shun those objects which set up and foment amorous feelings". This advice has been echoed by venereologists ever since but, needless to say, it was often ignored. The American diarist William Byrd (1674–1744) related that the day after he had consulted a surgeon about his "running" he and a friend "went to Spring Gardens where we picked up two women . . . about 10 o'clock we carried them to the bagnio, where we lay with them all night and I rogered mine twice and slept pretty well, but neglected to say my prayers"[6].

Then as now, the public had a touching faith in pharmacology – stronger than in religion, it was said – and many herbal remedies were prescribed for gonorrhoea. The function of these agents was conceived in humoral terms: to cool and sweeten the blood, hinder the flux by suspending its movement, and so on. Le Monnier suggested that the patient should take "at all hours of the day and night" a concoction of waterlilies, strawberries, lettuce and purslave leaves, maidenhair, pippins and flax". At night, "to procure for him a few hours of the sweetness of sleep" he recommended "an emulsion of melon and white poppy seeds, the roots of strawberries and marshmallow, leaves of dandelion, liverwort, maidenhair and lettuce, with the addition of syrup of violets, waterlilies and jujube". If these potions failed to improve matters, the patient should be advised to urinate with his penis in warm cow's milk, or soak the external genitalia in a bath of warm water for several days. A major problem which underlay treatment was the use of mercury. When there was genital ulceration as well as urethritis there was no doubt about it. Turner described how he handled such a case. The patient presented with a severe paraphimosis which he freed by a "fourfold incision." He continues:

> "It had been this fellow's misfortune, being drunk, to engage with a foul slut who had not only clapt him, but he unmindful to return the prepuce, in vain attempted it; and thereupon meeting with this pretender's bills [a quack's advertisements], or seeing them upon some pissing post, applies for relief; when after a fortnight's pain, well drain'd of his ready money, with his dripping rotten penis came to me; on whom, when I had thus taken off the symptoms, and not able by the common mercurials both inwardly and outwardly to obtain my ends, I hastened a salivation and thereby healed his sores; the glans incarn'd, and looks tolerably handsome; the extremity of the prepuce makes a sort of quadrangle, each corner, by reason of the cicatrix having a small knob which prevents it from playing freely over the glans; but from which he may at any time, if so minded, be freed by circumcision. As a martyr in the cause of Venus and unbridled lust, he thinks he has shed blood enough already; and if it now suffice to carry off his water, he talks (at least at present) that he has no other occasion[7]."

Towards the end of the eighteenth century it was acknowledged that systemic mercury was useless for the treatment of gonorrhoea, but unicist doctrine dictated that syphilis could follow gonorrhoea unless it was completely cured. What should be done? Some practitioners gave "a few light mercury inunctions" as soon as the acute symptoms of gonorrhoea had abated and Hunter, as might be expected, took the same view: "Whatever methods are used for the cure [of gonorrhoea] it is always necessary to have in view the possibility that some of the matter may be absorbed, afterwards appearing in the form of a lues venerea. To prevent this I would be inclined to prescribe small doses of mercury internally". Hunter's opinion prevailed, and well into the nineteenth century many surgeons prescribed a course of mercury either during or after the treatment of gonorrhoea. As we have seen, its side effects could be devastating and eventually, in 1824, the illustrious surgeon Astley Cooper was driven to declare that "a man who gives mercury for gonorrhoea deserves to be flogged out of the profession".

The doctrine of humorism had been that nothing should be done to check the flow of a urethral discharge, which was believed to chase the bad humours from the body, and in the eighteenth century many practitioners thought that uncomplicated gonorrhoea was a self-limiting condition – Hunter wrote of "time effecting a cure". Nevertheless, such masterly inactivity did not appeal to patients with acute urethritis, and urethral lavage was often employed. If complications such as epididymitis or prostatitis appeared, lavage was suspended and attempts made to reduce the inflammation by bleeding, vesication or the application of leeches. The timing of bleeding and the amount of blood to be withdrawn were regarded as matters requiring skilful judgment, and were the subject of many learned articles.

Bell gave a good account of the best contemporary practice. Accepting the dualist hypothesis, he was obviously writing from a wide practical experience. His approach was conservative. He condemned the emetics, purges and starvation diets currently in favour, which he regarded as debilitating and likely to prolong the disease. The mainstay of his treatment of uncomplicated infections was urethral lavage with a small elastic bag or syringe, self-administered by the patient 7–10 times a day. In an emergency Bell used as an irrigating fluid "port wine and claret, duly diluted ... a teaspoonful of brandy added to half an ounce of rosewater ... nay, rosewater itself, or even cold water directly from the spring", but for routine use he favoured a solution of white vitriol (zinc sulphate). Irrigation was not to be performed if the patient had developed epididymitis or there were signs of vesiculitis or prostatitis. If any of these were present he was advised to rest, given opium to relieve pain and treated with fomentations, bleeding, vesication or leeches. If there were signs of urethral obstruction, a sound was passed. Abscesses, for example of Cowper's glands, were opened early to avoid the formation of fistulas. Mercury was not to be used at all at any stage. It is quite clear from Bell's description that complicated gonorrhoea posed many difficult problems in treatment, but his optimistic conclusion was that in most cases "cure may be obtained at last".

Gleet

Although there were later modifications to the technique and apparatus, urethral irrigation remained the mainstay of the treatment of gonorrhoea in men until the advent of antibiotics. In Bell's hands many patients recovered from uncomplicated gonorrhoea after a course of treatment of three or four weeks; perhaps we should say "apparently recovered", because bacteriological confirmation of cure was, of course, not possible at this time. Gleet was a well-recognised sequel of gonorrhoea: a persistent, colourless, clear or cloudy urethral discharge without any symptoms such as pain or dysuria suggesting inflammation. It was axiomatic that it was, as Hunter put it, "perfectly innocent with respect to infection". However, there were some problems in the interpretation of post-gonorrhoeal urethral discharges. An imperfectly treated gonorrhoea might be infective even if the discharge was mucoid; alternatively, a persistent clear discharge might become intermittently yellow although remaining non-infectious. The whole matter required the nicest clinical judgment because, as Bell pointed out, "no precise marks have been discovered by which we can judge of this circumstance [i.e. infectivity] with certainty". We can sympathise with these dilemmas, because without laboratory tests it was impossible to decide whether a man was suffering from true chronic gonorrhoea or one of the varieties of post-gonococcal urethritis. Why gleet affected some patients but not others was obscure; there was talk of "relaxation and debility of the exhalants of the urethra", and "general weakness of the constitution", which disguised the fact that nobody really knew.

Gleet was treated both systemically and locally. Of course, the unicists insisted on a course of mercury if this had not already been given, while the dualists said that this was unnecessary. This apart, many practitioners prescribed balsams, turpentines and cantharides, although there seems to have been little confidence in their efficacy. Local treatment was by astringent or stimulant irrigations. The astringents commonly used were solutions of alum, white vitriol (zinc sulphate) and lead salts, to be "thrown up" frequently, not less than six or eight times a day according to Bell; predictably, treatment was often prolonged. If astringents failed to cure a gleet there might be recourse to intraurethral irritants with the object of inducing a brisk urethritis, as it had been observed that when this subsided the gleet often disappeared as well. One wonders how many patients persisted with this therapy for a complaint which was, after all, not particularly troublesome. Bell himself clearly had some doubts about it, and thought that "astringent injections, demulcents, cooling purgatives and in some cases the lapse of time alone" may be enough to bring about a cure.

In some cases, however, chronic gleet was due to urethral stricture or chronic prostatitis. Bell wrote that "it is our first duty to ascertain the real state of the urethra"; if a stricture was present "all other remedies are to be laid aside, and cure entrusted entirely to bougies". For chronic prostatitis neither injections nor-bougies were of any value, and dependence had to be placed on opiates. "Although they act chiefly as palliatives, the prevention of pain is of no small importance in a disease which otherwise is apt to make the patient miserable". Bell concluded his discussion of gleet by warning practitioners against "persevering with useless remedies . . . a practice which those not accustomed to this branch of business are very apt to fall into", words which should be engraved in letters of stone in every department of vencreology.

Urethral Stricture

Urethral obstruction following gonorrhoea was common in the eighteenth century, and there was much discussion about its cause and management. Its pathogenesis was obscure. Reviewing the matter in 1757 the German surgeon Lorenz Heister said that difficulty in voiding after an attack of gonorrhoea had been attributed to fleshy excrescences (caruncles or carnosities) in the urethra, tumours in the corpora cavernosa or enlargement of the prostate; he himself favoured the opinion that in some cases "a cicatrix ... remains after the cure of an ulcer in this part which had been caused by a Gonorrhoea"[8]. This opinion was in accordance with the "urethral ulceration" concept of gonorrhoea. Surprisingly, Hunter thought that strictures were "not commonly the result of venereal infection", he grouped them with strictures of doubtful origin such as those affecting the oesophagus or lacrimal ducts. Bell, however, having said that "urinary obstruction commonly follows clap", dismissed carnosities as a cause; he equated these with the "warty excrescences" (now called condylomata acuminata) seen on the glans and prepuce, which seldom extended more than half an inch into the urethra and caused minimal obstruction. Urethral strictures were another matter. They mostly affected the membranous urethra and could lead to difficult urination or even acute retention. Most surgeons now accepted that they were due to post-inflammatory fibrous tissue, but whether this was due to gonorrhoea itself or to its treatment was debatable. Strictures needed regular dilatation. Bougies were made of wax, lead, silver and other materials. In the eighteenth century the instrument, once passed, was left in place for several days, being removed only for urination. If this was not successful, attempts might be made to free the stricture by passing an "armed" bougie with a crystal of a corrosive at its tip. An English visitor to La Charité hospital in Paris described how silver catheters were often forced into the bladder "in spite of all opposition"; this was often followed by extravasation of urine, and there were fatalities[9]. Internal or external surgical division of strictures were usually unsuccessful, and in the last resort a trocar and cannula might have to be inserted into the bladder. As time went by the design of bougies improved; Clutton, Lister, Benique and other surgeons devised instruments with a single or double curve which were easier to pass into the bladder (Figure 9.2). Mechanical dilators, which were used for the treatment of both urethral strictures and "chronic gonorrhoea" were a later development which will be described in the next chapter. The successful management of these strictures required judgment and dexerity, and many surgeons became rich and famous for their ability to keep their patients' strictured urethras open.

Opinions on the Cause of Gonorrhoea

As it was gradually accepted that syphilis and gonorrhoea were different diseases there began a prolonged debate on the nature of gonorrhoea itself. Was it caused by a particular "virus", as Bell had suggested, or was it just a non-specific inflammation of genital mucosae? One of the first workers to address this problem was Swediaur in his *Traité Complet* (see Chapter 3). He was responsible for the introduction of the dire word *blennorrhagia*. His original definition was "a

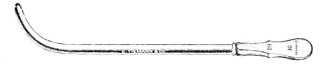

Figure 9.2. Urethral bougie. From Bumstead FJ, Taylor RW (1883) The pathology and treatment of venereal diseases: "An exceedingly graceful and useful sound which can be used with much delicacy of touch".

discharge of purulent matter through the orifice of the urethra in men and through that of the vagina in women accompanied by symptoms of local inflammation such as heat or smarting, particularly during the passage of urine". Blennorrhagia, he wrote, was produced by the action of either the syphilitic virus, in which case it was called syphilitic blennorrhagia, or of some other irritant matter applied to these parts. In expressing himself in this way Swediaur indicated that gonorrhoea could have causes other than the "venereal virus". To prove this he conducted a remarkable experiment. He injected an aqueous solution of ammonia, sufficiently strong to give it a "very piquant and burning taste" into his urethra twice, the second injection causing "the most severe pain I have ever experienced". The following morning he found "a considerable evacuation of purulent matter of the same yellow-green colour as that of a virulent chaude-piss". This convinced him that gonorrhoea could be caused by simple irritation of the mucous membranes[10]. Although he referred to his own "scepticism, supported by a healthy philosophy", Swediaur's final classification of "gonorrhoeas" became so complex that it is difficult for the modern reader to understand, but his idea that acute urethritis in men could be induced by non-specific irritation was taken up by others, and by Ricord in particular[11].

Ricord taught that gonorrhoea – "virulent urethral blennorrhagia" – was not a specific disease. In men, its *immediate* cause was the action of a variety of irritants (phlogogens) on the urethral mucosa; these included the vaginal fluid of women with leucorrhoea or who were menstruating, foreign bodies and gonorrhoeal pus itself. Among *predisposing* causes he mentioned temperament, climate, diet, alcohol, "an unnatural size of the male organ" and too frequent or prolonged intercourse. His conception of the interaction of immediate and predisposing causes resulting in gonorrhoea is epitomised in the following well-known passage, in typically Ricordian style:

> "Select a woman of pale lymphatic temperament – preferably a blonde – and the more whites [leucorrhoea] she has the better. Take her out to dine: oysters first, and don't forget to include asparagus. Drink a lot: white wines, champagne, coffee, liqueurs – they're all good. After dinner, dance with your friend. Get well heated during the evening, and quench your thirst with plenty of beer. At night, play your part valiantly – two or three times at least, but more would be better. The next morning, have a prolonged hot bath . . . if you don't get clap after all that, it will be a miracle[12]."

Ricord admitted that it was "extremely difficult to give a good definition of blennorrhagia", and eventually he used it to cover any inflammation of genital mucosae which followed intercourse. He thus referred to blennorrhagia of the glans, prepuce, anus and so on, with the result that the word became almost meaningless; the linguistic confusion helped to preclude any sensible discussion of the subject. However, Ricord was an experienced clinician and he could recognise gonorrhoea when he saw it. His treatment was straightforward. Mercury was, of course, forbidden, and astringent irrigations with silver nitrate or zinc sulphate were favoured. Ricord used a glass syringe and injected the fluid "suddenly, to take the mucous membrane by surprise, as it were" – the surprise being experienced not only by the mucous membrane, one might imagine. Cubebs, extracted from a Javanese pepper, and copaiba, a resin from leguminous trees in

Central America, were popular remedies for urinary tract disorders at the time, and were recommended by Ricord for the systemic treatment of gonorrhoea.

While Ricord's non-specific phlogogenic theory of the origin of gonorrhoea was widely accepted by his contemporaries, there were other voices. Rollet of Lyons for one said that the disease was caused by a specific virus; every individual with gonorrhoea had received this virus from another. This idea was supported by a series of the experimental inoculations of human subjects which were so common at this time. Sounds smeared with pus from non-genital abscesses and introduced into healthy urethras produced no disease, but if pus from cases of acute urethritis or ophthalmia was used, gonorrhoea invariably followed. The amount of pus used in the inoculations made no difference to the severity of the urethritis[13]. It was also observed that gonorrhoea acquired sexually had a definite incubation period, but urethritis due to physical or chemical irritants appeared almost immediately. These results certainly supported the ideas of the "virulists", but many eminent venereologists, including Fournier in France, Acton in England and Bumstead in the USA, continued to advocate the "non-specific phlogogen" theory. The controversy dragged on for 40 years until the development of bacteriology, and the discovery of the gonococcus, settled the matter.

Gonorrhoea in Women

The early writers had little to say about gonorrhoea in women, beyond expressing surprise that its manifestations were so much milder than in men. It was generally accepted that the disease principally affected the vagina. Any resulting discharge would be difficult to distinguish from *fluor albus* (leucorrhoea). In women, therefore, the diagnosis of gonorrhoea might be suspected mostly from the contact history – or, as Hunter put it, "the testimony of those whom we look upon as men of veracity". Bell thought that the urethra was often affected, as in men, in which case dysuria and urethral discharge would be helpful diagnostic signs. Several writers included inflammation of the labia and clitoris among the signs of gonorrhoea, and labial swellings and abscesses (presumably of Bartholin's glands) were well known. Pelvic infection in gonorrhoea seems to have gone largely unrecognised. Hunter said that "it has been asserted that the ovaria are sometimes affected in a similar manner to the testicles in men. I have never seen a case of this kind, and I should very much doubt the possibility of its existence". Bell disagreed: "In some cases the inflammation spreads to the bladder and even to the uterus and ovaria, or at least those parts become so much affected with pain as to give cause to suspect that they are in a state of inflammation. The parts become swelled and excessively painful, so that the slightest touch will create a great feeling of uneasiness". In this passage Bell was probably describing gonococcal salpingitis, but no more was heard of it for over half a century.

It is not surprising that throughout the first half of the nineteenth century ideas about gonorrhoea in women were confused. Since the disease in men followed sexual intercourse its causal agent, whether a specific virus or a non-specific phlogogen, must be situated in the female genital tract, but where? Most venereologists still favoured the vaginal cavity. Bell had written that gonorrhoea could affect the female urethra, but Swediaur strongly disagreed: "The least anatomical acquaintance with the parts which come into contact during coitus, or even common sense alone, will easily convince anyone of the falseness of this assertion"[10].

Many observers, including Ricord, remarked how often the lower genital tract of women whose partners had gonorrhoea appeared normal, using this as further evidence to support the "non-specific phlogogen" theory. Conversely, blennorrhagic vaginal discharges do not seem to have been regarded as very important, as the following quotation from Ricord shows:

> "In Paris, women may be said to have habitually a discharge, call it what you will, leucorrhoea, gonorrhoea, fleurs blanches etc; it affects all ages and stations. M. Lisfranc ... being called one day into the country to perform an operation on a washerwoman, amused himself out of scientific curiosity, while his associates were preparing the necessary apparatus, by examining the linen of Parisian ladies, a load having just arrived. He found evident signs of blennorrhagic discharges on nearly all. This shows how common this disease must be in the French capital[14]."

In these discussions the cervix, today recognised as the principle site to be infected in gonorrhoea, was hardly mentioned. It is not difficult to see the reason for this. Women were usually examined by inspecting the vulva and palpating the vagina, and sometimes even these simple procedures were omitted. In the nineteenth century a vaginal examination was evidently regarded as a very serious and solemn act (Figure 9.3). Writing in 1807, the Scottish obstetrician John Burns said "it is usual for the room to be darkened and the bed curtains drawn during an examination ... it should never, if possible, be proposed or made whilst an unmarried lady is in the room"[15]. According to Ricord, in France it was formerly necessary to have a consultation with three medical men before a vaginal speculum was passed, and although it came into common use (at least at the Midi) good clinical data were slow to accumulate. Ricord and Acton both describe the blennorrhagic vagina as showing erythema, erosions and granulations, which might also be present on the cervix. Ricord said that *Trichomonas vaginalis*, described in 1836, might be present, but he did not believe that this organism was the cause of vaginal blennorhagia, because it was not present in men with urethritis. He thought that blennorrhagia could reach the uterus and "run along

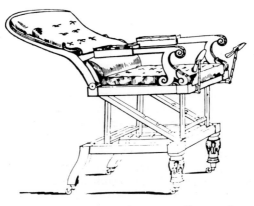

Figure 9.3. William Acton's "speculum chair", as illustrated in Ricord P (1849) A practical treatise of venereal diseases.

124

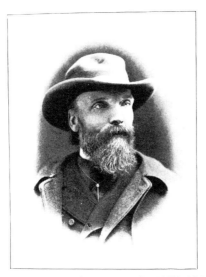

Figure 9.4. Emil Noeggerath (1827–1894).

the fallopian tubes"; affections of the ovary might result, although these were "very rare"[16]. The concept of infective cervicitis simply did not exist in Ricord's day. It was not until 1883 that the German gynaecologist von Bumm showed that "the most frequent site of gonorrhoea is the mucosa of the cervix uteri"[17].

In 1876, three years before Neisser discovered the gonococcus, Emil Noeggerath (Figure 9.4) made two of the most important discoveries in the whole history of gonorrhoea: its major role in the pathogenesis of pelvic inflammatory disease, and the existence of latent infections. Noeggerath was born in 1827 in Bonn, in the Rhineland. He received his basic medical education there, then proceeded to postgraduate study in Berlin, Vienna, Prague and Paris. By the time he returned to Bonn he had decided on a career in obstetrics and gynaecology, and was appointed assistant at the Obstetric Hospital. In 1857 he accepted the offer of a chair in obstetrics at St Louis University in the USA, only to find on his arrival that the appointment had been abandoned because of shortage of funds. He made his way to New York, and eventually obtained appointments at several hospitals and a chair in obstetrics and gynaecology at New York Medical College.

Besides being an accomplished clinician Noeggerath was interested in gynaecological pathology, and in the developing science of bacteriology. He published papers in the USA and Germany, and often returned to Europe. In a way he was a link between American and German medicine, although American doctors did not always welcome his Teutonic thoroughness while his German colleagues were sometimes suspicious of new ideas from across the Atlantic. He was a compulsive worker, apparently keeping himself awake at night not only by copious draughts of coffee but by immersing his feet in a bowl of cold water which he kept under his desk. Noeggerath was particularly interested in pelvic inflammatory disease. During the first half of the nineteenth century an inflamed pelvis meant an inflamed uterus: adnexal sepsis was regarded as secondary to this. To be sure, Ricord had thought that blennorrhagia could ascend and involve the fallopian tubes, and in 1857 the French gynaecologists Bernutz and Goupil had studied

125

at autopsy 99 cases which they thought showed that pelvic inflammation began with salpingitis, and that both conditions were related to gonorrhoea[18], but these opinions were largely ignored. The official view was that pelvic inflammation was due to obstruction of the lochia, uterine malposition, trauma and excessive intercourse: it was unrelated to gonorrhoea, which was centred in the vagina.

This was the situation when Noeggerath rose to address the inaugural meeting of the American Gynecologic Society in 1876. He has been portrayed as an "inordinately lean, tall man of saturnine mien, long-fingered and grim-thinking", surely one of the most unflattering descriptions of a gynaecologist ever written. His subject was "Latent gonorrhoea, especially with regard to its influence on fertility in women"[19]; it was an analysis of clinical data obtained from a large group of women with pelvic infection and their husbands. He began by saying that in men the "gonorrhoeic poison" typically causes acute urethritis, with obvious symptoms and signs, which was often followed by gleet. But there were other possibilities. The "gleety state" might be the *only* sign of gonorrhoea. Unaffected by treatment, it could persist as a "latent" condition, almost imperceptible, but infectious for a prolonged period. There might be exacerbations from time to time, or a complication such as epididymitis might develop, and some men with chronic gonorrhoea became infertile because of azoospermia.

Noeggerath went on to say that the wives of men in this condition were, with very few exceptions, also affected by latent gonorrhoea. They might not develop acute symptoms at first, but sooner or later would present with clinical evidence of either infection of the lower genital tract, such as a vaginal discharge, or pelvic inflammation. The latter was provoked by factors such as prolonged intercourse, parturition and pelvic examination or instrumentation, and then be wrongly attributed to these rather than to the underlying condition. An acute pelvic infection might settle down, but even so the gonorrhoea simply became latent again, and recurrences were possible at any time. Women with chronic gonorrhoeal pelvic inflammation were not only chronically unwell, but they were usually sterile. Examination "in the majority of cases will show a secretion which we may call mucopurulent, adherent to the mouth of the womb; this is surrounded by a circular highly coloured erosion". Here, he appears to be describing a condition which was to be defined as "mucopurulent cervicitis" a century later.

In essence, Noeggerath was presenting two complementary ideas: the existence of latent gonorrhoea in both sexes and a close connection between gonorrhoea, pelvic inflammation and infertility. Neither was well received by the members of the American gynaecological establishment who were present at the meeting. Unfortunately, Noeggerath had remarked that 60% of men marrying in large cities in the USA had had gonorrhoea at some time, and that 60% of the wives of such men would in turn become infected. The president of the society said that he regarded these estimates as not only offensive but an unwarranted attack on the moral standards of the American male. The reception of his presentation must have been humiliating for Noeggerath; all he could say was that he hoped that his colleagues might change their minds when they studied the matter further. This did not happen, and he was denounced by physicians and gynaecologists in many countries.

His views on latent infections had profound implications for clinical management. The convention at the time was that while intercourse was prohibited as long as a purulent discharge was present, it could be resumed when it had become

126

clear and mucoid. However, if gleet could be infectious – and Noeggerath showed that it could – the decision on when intercourse could be resumed after an attack of gonorrhoea became much more difficult. Following the discovery of the gonococcus in 1879 this decision could be based on laboratory rather than clinical findings, as Neisser himself strongly recommended. Neisser's discovery[20] came seven years after Noeggerath first presented his radical ideas, and within a few more years reliable culture methods became available. Noeggerath had thought that gonorrhoea probably had a microbial cause and had conducted some experiments himself in 1872, but without Koch's staining methods these had come to nothing. Happily, he lived long enough to see most of his ideas vindicated by the new technology, and accepted even by those who had so violently opposed them. In 1885 ill health forced him to return to Germany, and he lived in semi-retirement in Wiesbaden until his death in 1894 at the age of 67. He was now a forgotten figure, and his passing was largely ignored by the medical and scientific community.

Ophthalmia Neonatorum

The recognition of a connection between vaginal discharge in a mother and ophthalmia neonatorum in her baby was first suggested by the Leipzig surgeon Samuel Theodore Quelmatz (1696–1758) in 1740[21]; in accordance with current ideas, he thought the effect was mediated by the blood stream. Although some authors continued to attribute ophthalmia to exposure to bright light or cold air, a scrofulous constitution or a disordered state of the bowels, the association with maternal leucorrhoea was becoming accepted. Thus Benjamin Gibson (1774–1812), surgeon to the Manchester Infirmary, writing in 1806, described a child who had lost the sight of both eyes from ophthalmia. The mother said she had had *fluor albus* during her pregnancy. "It occurred to me that the eyes of a child, during their passage through a vagina where such a discharge was secreting, might receive the disease in question by contact between the fluid and the eyelids." Gibson made further enquiries "as far as the delicate nature of the case will allow", and found that in the course of a year 35 babies born in the Manchester Infirmary had developed ophthalmia; all of their mothers had had leucorrhoea[22].

In the early nineteenth century most doctors did not distinguish between syphilis and gonorrhoea, and the nature of leucorrhoea itself was uncertain; "mild" and "syphilitic" leucorrhoea were described, the latter being particularly associated with neonatal ophthalmia. But ideas about gonorrhoea were becoming clearer, and a series of the unprincipled inoculation experiments which were so common in the nineteenth century helped to clarify matters[23]. In 1820 the English surgeon John Vetch had inoculated a male urethra with ophthalmic pus, inducing gonorrhoea within 36 hours. In 1854 another surgeon, Pauli of Landau, placed the discharge from a baby with ophthalmia into the urethra of a young man, thereby giving him gonorrhoea in three days' time; unfortunately "despite warnings" the man subsequently transmitted the disease to his wife. In another experiment Pauli inoculated a prostitute's vagina with ophthalmic pus and she too developed gonorrhoea[24]. An association between gonorrhoea and at least some cases of ophthalmia neonatorum became widely accepted, although objections were raised that some babies born to women with leucorrhoea remained quite normal, and conversely that the mothers of some babies with ophthalmia did not have leucorrhoea. Noeggerath's work on latent gonorrhoea in men and women, published in 1872, answered the latter objection, and indeed illuminated the whole epidemiology of ophthalmia neonatorum.

By the second half of the nineteenth century ophthalmia neonatorum had become a serious problem. In European maternity hospitals it was occurring in up to 12 per cent of neonates; 20 per cent of affected babies developed corneal ulceration, and 30 per cent of these became blind[25]. This was the situation when Credé began his studies on the prevention of the disease, which were to revolutionise obstetric practice.

Carl Siegmund Franz Credé (Figure 9.5) was born in 1819 in Berlin, where his father, who was a French immigrant, worked in the Ministry of Health and Education. After attending the Friedrich-Wilhelm Gymnasium, Credé studied medicine at the University of Berlin. A period of postgraduate work in Belgium, Austria and Italy followed, then he returned to Berlin, where he was appointed assistant in obstetrics to Professor Johann von Busch. He became Privat dozent in 1850, and two years later was appointed physician in chief to the lying-in division of the Charité Hospital, where he established one of the first gynaecology departments in Europe. In 1856 he was appointed professor of obstetrics in Leipzig and remained there for the rest of his working life. His abilities as a surgeon, teacher and administrator enabled him to create a renowned department. His own clinical work was in obstetrics rather than gynaecology, and he wrote several textbooks and monographs on the subject. He was one of the ablest academic and practical teachers in Germany, and many of his students went on to distinguished careers. He himself had no desire to leave Leipzig, and he is known to have refused chairs in other universities, including Berlin. Personally he was modest, approachable and good-humoured[26].

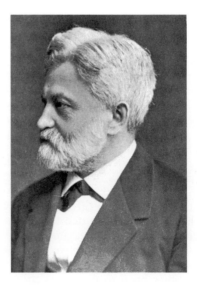

Figure 9.5. Carl Siegmund Franz Credé (1819–1892).

Credé began his studies on ophthalmia neonatorum in the early 1870s. The idea of prophylaxis was not new. As long ago as 1807 Gibson had made the following suggestions:

"First, to remove if possible the disease in the mother during pregnancy; second, if that cannot be accomplished, to remove artificially as much discharge as possible from the vagina at the time of delivery; and third, to pay particular attention to the eyes of the child by washing them immediately after delivery with a liquid calculated to remove the offending matter or to prevent its noxious action[22]."

These measures had been tried, but unenthusiastically and with little success, and it fell to Credé to devise a new regimen, and to demonstrate its efficacy in a large series of cases. He published only three papers on the subject. In the first, he described how thorough cleaning of the vagina of women in labour gave poor results. With vaginal douching and the application of borax solution to the baby's eyes after birth ophthalmia became less frequent, but did not cease. Finally, all eyes were wiped clean with cotton wool and plain water, then were treated with a single drop of 2 per cent silver nitrate solution applied with a glass rod; the vaginal douches were abandoned. He reported that in the three years since he introduced the silver nitrate technique in 1880 there had been only two cases of ophthalmia in 1160 live births[27].

The success of Credé's procedure was soon confirmed by others, and in the hospitals where it was used ophthalmia neonatorum virtually disappeared. Silver nitrate prophylaxis was a triumph of preventive medicine. Credé used to say that he was "only an obstetrician", but his eminence in this field meant that his work received proper attention from his colleagues. In this respect he was luckier that Semmelweis, whose ideas on the prophylaxis of puerperal fever, although right, were received with scepticism and hostility by the medical establishment of the day, and whose career suffered as a result. Like other pioneers, Credé made important discoveries about gonorrhoea without knowing its cause; he recognised that there must be an infective principle, but Neisser's discovery of the gonococcus came too late for him to apply to his own studies. Ill health forced him to retire in 1887. He developed carcinoma of the prostate, and ironically towards the end of his life became blind because of uraemia. He died in 1892 at the age of 73 years.

It has been shown in Chapters 3–5 that most of the features of syphilis had been discovered before its cause was known. This cannot be said of gonorrhoea. Some authorities denied a single specific causal agent, the concept of "blennorrhoea" was fundamentally flawed, the existence of subclinical infections was not generally acknowledged and it was often impossible to decide whether or not a patient had been cured by treatment. Neisser's discovery of the gonococcus in 1879 was therefore a most important event; it will be described in the next chapter.

Chapter 10
Gonorrhoea after Neisser

Every physician almost hath his favourite disease.

Henry Fielding, *Tom Jones*

Louis Pasteur and Robert Koch were the founders of bacteriology. Pasteur (1822–1895) was a chemist, and a brilliant innovative thinker. He ended the dispute about spontaneous generation, established that some microbes caused human disease and pioneered preventive inoculation. Koch (1843–1010) began his career as a general practitioner in East Prussia, and his interest in anthrax, a common disease in the locality, led him into bacteriology. Between 1881 and 1887 he developed many basic techniques, particularly the use of solid media for culture, and aniline dyes for staining bacteria; he also made full use of the major improvements being made in the design of microscopes. Koch's work made it possible to identify, culture and study many pathogenic bacteria, and he laid down a series of principles now known as "Koch's postulates". To prove that a specific bacterium causes a specific disease: (1) The bacterium should be present in every case of the disease; (2) it should be possible to grow it artificially in pure culture; and (3) the culture should then reproduce the disease when inoculated into a susceptible animal or human. These conceptual and technical advances led to a rapid accumulation of knowledge.

It was thought likely that gonorrhoea had a bacterial cause, but several attempts to discover this foundered through a lack of good staining and microscope techniques. Once these had been developed it was only a matter of time before the cause of the disease was discovered. The prize went to a young graduate student of dermatology working in Breslau. Albert Ludwig Sigesmund Neisser[1] (Figure 10.1) was born in 1855 at Schweidnitz, a small town near Breslau, which was then in Prussia but is now in Poland. His father was a prominent local Jewish doctor. Neisser received his medical education at the University of Breslau, obtaining an MD in 1877. He had wanted to be a general physician, but as there were no vacancies in the department of medicine he accepted a training post in the University Skin Clinic under Oscar Simon. Neisser had been interested in bacteriology as a student and was familiar with the new technology, including the use of aniline dyes. Using a Zeiss microscope with an oil immersion system and one of the new Abbe condensers (Figure 10.2) he embarked on his study of gonorrhoea. In 1879, at the age of 24, he published his best-known paper[2]. He had examined smears, stained with methyl violet by Koch's technique, from 35 men and 9 women with purulent urethritis and two patients with acute ophthalmia. He described how he had identified micrococci, mostly intracellular, in the smears:

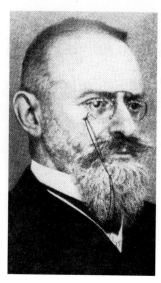

Figure 10.1. Albert Neisser (1855–1916). (By courtesy of the Wellcome Institute Library, London.)

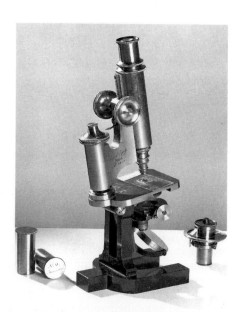

Figure 10.2. Zeiss microscope with Abbe-type illumination, 1878. This instrument is identical to the one used by Neisser in his discovery of the gonococcus. (Courtesy of the Optischen Museum der Zeiss-Werke, Oberkochen.)

"They are seldom seen as solitary individuals; almost always they appear as two micrococci packed close together so as to give the observer the impression of a single organism shaped like a figure of eight."

The organisms were not seen in specimens from patients with syphilis, chancroid or balanitis. Neisser concluded his short paper by reserving judgment about the significance of the organisms until culture and inoculation experiments had been performed.

This report was electrifying, and within a few years a flood of papers on the subject appeared. The majority of investigators reported similar results, finding the micrococci constantly present in gonorrhoeal pus and in severe ophthalmia neonatorum. Neisser himself returned to the subject in a paper published in 1882[3]. He now felt able to assert the specificity of the organism, which his friend Ehrlich had called the gonococcus:

"Gonococci are absolutely constant in every case of gonorrhoea . . . and they are not found in any other disease . . . furthermore, gonococci are the only organisms found in gonorrhoeal pus."

He went on to claim that he had successfully cultivated the microbe on a meat extract – gelatin medium, and produced some eminent witnesses, Cohnheim, Koch and Ehrlich, to agree that his cultures were pure growths of gonococci. However, human and animal inoculations failed, and there is some doubt about whether his claim was justified. Successful culture of "Neisser's gonococcus" proved to be elusive. The problem seems to have been not only to persuade the organism to replicate in vitro, but to avoid confusion with other non-pathogenic diplococci which were more easily cultivable. Leistikow, an assistant in the clinic for syphilis in the Berlin Charité Hospital, where there was abundant clinical material, was probably the first to culture the gonococcus[4]. In 1880 he reported that he and Löffler had successfully grown it on a blood serum – gelatin medium. Multiple animal inoculation experiments had been unsuccessful.

Many workers did not accept that the gonococcus was the cause of gonorrhoea. A few still clung to Ricord's "non-specific phlogogen" hypothesis, and remembered that there had been previous claims that this or that microbe was the cause of gonorrhoea which had come to nothing. It was pointed out that micrococci morphologically similar to gonococci could be found in the genital tract in some patients who showed no clinical evidence of gonorrhoea. There had been difficulty in cultivating the organisms, and their pathogenicity had not been established by inoculation experiments. In other words, Koch's postulates had not been satisfied. It is easy to understand these problems. There are non-pathogenic species of *Neisseria* and *Branhamella* in the human genital tract which are microscopically indistinguishable from the gonococcus, no animal model exactly reproduces human gonorrhoea and latent symptomless infections by *N. gonorrhoeae* are not uncommon. None of these facts was known in the 1880s.

Lingering doubts about the role of the organisms in gonorrhoea were eventually dispelled not by animal but by human experiments. These, which seem indefensible today, had been performed by doctors for many years without qualms, and in this case they certainly served their purpose. In Würzburg in 1883 Max Bockhart inoculated the urethra of a man with terminal general paresis with a pure culture of gonococci; he developed classical gonorrhoea after three days, and died from his paresis a week later. Post-mortem examination showed the presence of gonococci in the urethra[5]. Ernst von Bumm, who was later to become an eminent obstetrician and gynaecologist, was also working in Würzburg at the time. Having successfully cultured the gonococcus, he inoculated the urethra of a healthy woman with the culture, giving her gonococcal urethritis[6]. In 1891 Ernst Wertheim, another famous figure in the history of gynaecology, who was then working in Prague, inoculated pure cultures of *Neisseria gonorrhoeae* into the urethras of five men with general paresis and in every case induced typical gonorrhoea and recovered gonococci from the urethra[7]. Experiments of this kind gradually silenced the doubters, and *N. gonorrhoeae* was accepted as the cause of gonorrhoea.

Neisser's Later Career

Neisser used to say "What would I have been without the gonococcus?", but he was not a man to rest on his laurels, and at the end of 1879 he published the results of his studies on leprosy. The Norwegian physician Hansen had seen some bacteria-like bodies in wet preparations of leprous tissue; he gave some of this material to Neisser, who with modern staining techniques identified a new species of bacilli as the cause of the disease. Unfortunately this led to a dispute with Hansen over priority which dragged on for some years. Neisser himself thought that his work with leprosy was more important than his discovery of the gonococcus, and always felt resentful that he had not received the credit which he thought was his due. In 1882 Oscar Simon unexpectedly died of carcinoma of the stomach, and at the early age of 27 years Neisser was appointed associate professor and director of the Skin Clinic in Breslau, where he remained for the rest of his life. Thanks to his energetic fund raising, a new and imposing University Skin Clinic was erected, and opened in 1892 (Figure 10.3).

Neisser combined clinical and scientific skill with administrative ability, and the clinic soon became a major centre for clinical work, research and training in dermatovenereology. Neisser himself studied many skin diseases, but he never lost his interest in gonorrhoea. Time and again he stressed its serious potential, particularly for women, and he insisted that "cure" should be defined in terms of negative microscopic findings rather than by simple clinical examination. Neisser was instrumental in founding the German Dermatological Society in 1899, and the German Society for Combating Venereal Disease in 1902. Inevitably he became involved with syphilis; his work on this disease has been described in Chapter 6.

Neisser did not become a full professor until 1907, 25 years after his appointment as associate professor. This long delay could have been due to prejudice, antisemitism or simply to a feeling by the university authorities that dermatovenereology was not very important. Be this as it may, Neisser had become one of Germany's best known physicians, with an outstanding clinical, teaching and research record. He was happily married, loved literature and art, and played the piano well enough to appear in public with a chamber orchestra. His friends included such outstanding people as Gerhard Hoffmann, Gustav Mahler and Richard Strauss. His earlier abrasiveness mellowed as he grew older, and his many students regarded him with affection and respect.

Nevertheless, Neisser's professional life was not free from troubles. The worst of these came from his human experiments with syphilis in 1892. With the object of inducing passive immunity, he gave intravenous injections of sera from patients with early syphilis to a series of recipients aged 10–24 years, some of whom developed syphilis within a few weeks of the inoculations. When news of these experiments became known there was a public outcry. Neisser was accused of "maliciously infecting innocent children with syphilis poison", and the affair reached the Prussian Parliament. Neisser escaped with an official reprimand and a fine but he was deeply wounded, and felt that his honour as a scientist had been impugned. Today, these experiments (for which the subjects' permission had not been obtained) would be regarded as completely unethical, but this was not how Neisser or his colleagues saw it, and human experiments with dangerous pathogens continued for many years.

In later life Neisser became increasingly concerned with the public health aspects of sexually transmitted diseases, advocating free public clinics, voluntary examination of prostitutes and health education. He used to say that life without work would be unbearably dull, but by his mid-fifties he was tiring. In 1911 he fell down the stairs to the cellar of his house and fractured his femur. Recovery was slow, and he was found to have diabetes mellitus and renal calculi. When the First World War began in 1914 he shouldered a new burden, advising the German army on venereal disease control programmes. In the summer of 1916, although he had renal colic and a urinary infection, he insisted on attending an exhibition in Brussels. He had another attack of colic, and struggled as far as Berlin, where a calculus was removed from his bladder. Two days later, with a draining wound, he returned to Breslau; infection followed, and "the father of the gonococcus" died of septicaemia at the age of 61.

Non-gonococcal Urethritis

The discovery of the gonococcus was an important event in the history of venereology. Within a few years of Neisser's original paper the Danish microbiologist Gram had introduced the staining method which bears his name (although Neisser

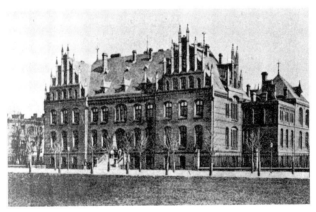

Figure 10.3. University Skin Clinic, Breslau, 1894. From Herzberg and Korting (1987) Zur Geschlichte der deutschen Dermatologie *(Courtesy of Grosse Verlag, Berlin.)*

himself preferred methylene blue), and reliable culture systems had been devised; in 1909 fermentation tests were reported which made it possible to distinguish *N. gonorrhoeae* from other neisseria[8]. With these improvements in the accurate laboratory diagnosis of gonococcal infections the stage was set for further clinical studies. The first of these was the identification of non-gonococcal urethritis.

For the first few years after Neisser's discovery it was assumed that all cases of sexually acquired urethritis were gonococcal, but once the initial excitement had died down and patients were examined more critically it became clear that this was not so. Several workers remarked that some men with urethritis showed no laboratory evidence of infection by *N. gonorrhoeae*; they were said to have "urethritis non-gonorrhoica"[9]. This was a revival of an old idea. The earlier writers had described "gonorrhoea simplex", evidently a milder disease than gonorrhoea virulenta, and in the first half of the nineteenth century many clinicians thought that gonorrhoea was not the only cause of a urethral discharge. However, although cases of non-gonococcal urethritis were repeatedly demonstrated by bacteriology there were diehards who continued to deny that the disease existed. As late as the 1940s some venereologists were still stating that virtually all cases of urethritis were gonococcal: those which appeared to be non-gonococcal had been either misdiagnosed or secretly treated with sulphonamides by the patient. For many years non-gonococcal urethritis was dismissed as a trivial disorder not deserving serious consideration, but from the 1970s on it became the object of intensive research (see Chapter 12).

Rectal Gonorrhoea in Men

In the mid nineteenth century there had been a suspicion that gonorrhoea might infect the rectum. Doyon, working with Diday in Lyon, had investigated the possibility in a rather unusual way:

> "Wishing to assure myself of the existence of these affections I have often conveyed on the end of my finger the urethral discharge of patients to their noses, lips and the folds within the anus, and rubbed it in! They, not suspecting what I had done, took no precautions to avert the consequences, and yet I have not seen any effect produced[10]."

Most venereologists did not believe that gonorrhoea could affect the male rectum, but after the discovery of the gonococcus scientific investigation of the problem became possible, and some cases were recorded; it was realised that the apparent rarity of rectal infections was because they were mostly symptomless. In 1883 the American physicians Bumstead and Taylor reported: "The existence of this affection appears now to be well authenticated, but its occurrence is extremely rare even in those countries, such as South America, where unnatural modes of coitus abound"[11].

During the first half of the twentieth century rectal gonorrhoea in men was regarded as rare; many standard textbooks on venereology did not mention it at all. It seems unlikely that it was not occurring, for primary syphilis of the anus was well known. It is more likely that some doctors were squeamish about taking specimens from the rectum, that the interpretation of Gram-stained smears from that area is notoriously difficult, and good culture techniques were not available then. Describing an outbreak of gonorrhoea in a residential boys' school in 1929, the author wrote that gonococcal urethritis was confirmed by microscopy of stained smears, but the rectal cases were diagnosed by the presence of "numerous papillomatous growths of a gonococcal origin". Nobody referred to homosexual infections in those days without expressing disapproval; in this case the doctor was surprised that "the boys who had fallen to these depths of degradation were not those in whom the stigma of physical and mental degeneration were apparent"; they included several athletes, and the head prefect[12].

Gonorrhoea in Women

By the end of the nineteenth century the location of gonococcal infection in the female genital tract had been decided. Von Bumm[6] had found that the cervix was the commonest site, followed by the urethra; he did not believe that gonococci infected the vagina. The last point was confirmed in the same year by Welander, who inoculated vaginal speciments from three women with urethral gonorrhoea into three men, none of whom became infected; subsequent inoculation of urethral specimens from the same women induced gonorrhoea in every man[13]. Although the importance of the cervix as the prime site for gonococcal infections in women was soon accepted, it took a long time to establish its clinical correlates, and confusion between endocervicitis and other cervical abnormalities such as ectopy ("cervical erosion") lasted well into the twentieth century.

In 1883 Arning, working in Neisser's clinic, discovered gonococci in eight women with infected Bartholin glands[14]. It is clear from the literature that many women with gonorrhoea had acute vaginitis; this was attributed to the irritating effect of gonorrhoeal pus descending from the cervix. A concurrent infection with *T. vaginalis* is now known to be common in women with gonorrhoea, and a potent cause of vaginitis, but at this time the organism was not thought to be a pathogen and its presence was not recorded. Gonococcal proctitis in a woman was first described by the American gynaecologist Orton in 1896[15]. The patient also had urethritis, cervicitis, endometritis and a husband with gonorrhoea. Later, it was pointed out that rectal infections were not uncommon in women. They could arise by contamination by material from the genital tract, but according to Norris: "In this country [the USA] the disease is most often met with among low class foreigners and is often due to the practice of sodomy"[16]. By the turn of the century, collated data indicated that in women with gonococcal infection the organisms were present in the cervix in 90–95 per cent, the urethra in 90 per cent and in the rectum in 30 per cent. These figures are not very different from those reported today. In these early studies the lack of a reliable laboratory test which would differentiate *Neisseria* species led to some faulty attributions. Thus Von Bumm[17] reported "gonococci" in the cervix of women where "the possibility of gonorrhoea was absolutely excluded"; however, culture from these patients yielded "milk-white plaques", and human inoculations were negative. These cases, and reports of "gonococci" in patients with ulcerative stomatitis suggest that non-pathogenic neisseria were being detected. The occasional cases of pharyngeal gonorrhoea following oral sex ("coitus illegitimus") which were reported may or may not have fallen into the same category.

Towards the end of the 1870s operative treatment of pelvic inflammatory disease – by the drainage of abscesses or the removal of diseased adnexa – provided material for laboratory examination. Gonococci were first found in tubal pus in 1880, and many workers were able to demonstrate the organisms in the tubes themselves. The pathogenesis of the accompanying peritonitis was disputed. Von Bumm claimed that the gonococcus could multiply in a columnar, but not a simple squamous epithelium; this meant that the organisms could not produce a true peritonitis. Wertheim conducted a series of experiments to settle the matter[18]. He obtained N. gonorrhoeae in pure culture from salpingitis tissue, confirmed it by human inoculation and then inoculated the material into mice, inducing a histologically and culturally confirmed gonococcal peritonitis. He concluded that the gonococcus can ascend from the lower genital tract and cause salpingitis and peritonitis, as Noeggerath had suggested. He did not find any experimental support for the idea, widely believed at the time, that secondary infection by other pyogenic cocci affected the outcome one way or the other; ascending gonorrhoea, with all its sequelae, was a disease of single aetiology. In the early years of the twentieth century N. gonorrhoeae was the commonest recognised cause of pelvic inflammatory disease.

Gonorrhoea in Children

Bacteriological tests helped to elucidate paediatric gonococcal infections. Gonococci were first identified in ophthalmia neonatorum in 1881, and within a few years it was shown that N. gonorrhoeae was present in about one-third of cases of ophthalmia neonatorum brought to hospital[19]. The aetiology of non-gonococcal ophthalmia was unknown at the time, but it was recognised as a milder disease, without the blinding potential of the gonococcal form. Its elucidation came after the discovery of Chlamydia trachomatis in 1907, which will be discussed in Chapter 11. Another problem concerned the aetiology of vulvovaginitis in young children. This had been recognised in the eighteenth century, but was not thought to be important. As time went by it received more attention, and there were occasional reports of the apparent communication of fluor albus from a mother to her daughter and of outbreaks of vulvovaginitis in orphanages and similar institutions, but for the most part the disease was attributed to non-specific factors such as anaemia, marasmus and skin disorders. Later, the occurrence of outbreaks in institutions where children were in close proximity to each other, associations between vulvovaginitis and conjunctivitis in children and between vulvovaginitis and maternal leucorrhoea led Pott to suggest that it was a specific communicable disease[20]. In 1885 Fraenkel, working in Hamburg, identified the "gonococcus of Neisser" in vaginal discharges from little girls[21] and it was soon realised that in children, unlike adults, the vaginal epithelium was susceptible to gonococcal infection.

An argument now developed about the natural history of gonococcal vulvovaginitis which has persisted into modern times. Some held that it was due solely to sexual contact with an infected person, but others that indirect infection from fomites was possible. The firm belief that gonorrhoea was invariably transmitted sexually impeded elucidation of the subject. In the nineteenth century sexual abuse of children in workhouses and other institutions was common, and child prostitution flourished; there was a superstition that an adult could cure his infection by transmitting it to a virgin. In these circumstances the sexual transmission of gonorrhoea to young girls could easily occur. On the other hand, the epidemics of vulvovaginitis among children in large families, hospitals and so on were often assumed to be non-gonococcal.

Even Fraenkel was doubtful about the pathogenicity of the organisms he had found in such cases, because he had failed to induce ophthalmia by rubbing the vaginal pus into the eyes of three moribund children. These problems were clarified by bacteriological studies. It emerged that many cases of "institutional" vulvovaginitis were gonococcal. The American paediatrician Holt, working in New York in the early years of the twentieth century, reported that gonococci were present in 2–10 per cent of inmates of institutions such as nurseries, orphanages and paediatric wards[22].

Gonococcal vulvovaginitis was regarded as highly infectious, and many well-documented epidemics occurred in children's wards following the admission of one infected patient; boys were relatively immune. The measures recommended to control these epidemics included screening of children on admission, and sometimes regularly throughout their stay, rigorous hygiene, scrupulous nursing care and isolation of those infected. Despite this, outbreaks sometimes made it necessary to close wards, and the danger to nurses from accidental eye infections was evidently considerable. With improved standards of infection control and nursing care these institutional epidemics became less frequent as the century wore on. Nevertheless, gonococcal vulvovaginitis was not uncommon in the general population: at one venereal disease clinic in London, 118 new cases were seen between 1925 and 1929[23].

Disseminated Gonococcal Infection

Gonococcal septicaemia was a common complication of gonorrhoea in the pre-antibiotic era, the patients usually presenting with acute arthritis of one or more of the large joints. Separation of this entity from non-gonococcal reactive arthritis only became possible after the discovery of the gonococcus. Isolation of the organism from the synovial fluid was difficult. At first, Neisser himself was unsuccessful:

> "Even if the gonococcus bacteria are responsible for the joint inflammations, they are probably localised in the synovial tissues themselves where they exert a constant irritation which periodically leads to effusions[3]."

In 1883 Petrone[24] reported seeing organisms resembling gonococci in the joint exudate of two men with urethritis and arthritis, but the first isolation of *N. gonorrhoeae* from an acutely inflamed joint was by Höck in 1893[25], whose patient was a baby with ophthalmia neonatorum. In the same year Neisser obtained isolates from two joints in an adult, and other workers soon recovered the organisms not only from the joints but from the blood[26]. In 1893 the French dermatologist Émile Vidal described a keratotic skin eruption sometimes associated with "blennorrhoea"[27]. For a time it was suspected that *keratoderma blennorrhagica* might be an unusual complication of gonorrhoea, but it was later shown to be non-gonococcal and linked with Reiter's syndrome (see Chapter 12). Neisser's pupil Abraham Buschke reviewed the subject of skin eruptions in disseminated gonococcal infection in 1899[28].

In the 1870s there were anecdotal reports of patients in whom an attack of gonorrhoea was followed by not only arthritis but signs of endocarditis or pericarditis; Neisser himself mentioned this possibility. Subsequently, several cases of endocarditis were described in which gonococci had been seen in stained smears from the heart valves, but the final proof of the association came in 1896 from Thayer, working at the Johns Hopkins Hospital[29]. His patient had typical bacterial endocarditis and *N. gonorrhoeae* was isolated in life by blood culture and at autopsy from vegetations on the mitral valve. As clinical awareness and diagnostic facilities improved, further reports on the cardiac complications of gonorrhoea followed, and in 1922 Thayer reported that since 1889 11 per cent of cases of bacterial endocarditis at Johns Hopkins Hospital had been confirmed as gonococcal; the illness lasted 4–9 weeks and was almost always fatal[30].

Treatment of Male Infections

By the end of the nineteenth century dramatic advances in the diagnosis of gonorrhoea had been made, but treatment had changed very little since the time of Ricord. In men, this had been based on rest, abstention from alcohol and sexual activity, systemic treatment with one or other of the balsams, and urethral instillations or irrigations. Local astringents such as zinc sulphate were now passing out of favour; they were regarded as irritating, and Neisser in particular preferred to use silver nitrate or one of the new silver protein preparations. Potassium permanganate irrigations, introduced by Weiss in 1880, became very popular. It was now known that the old favourites, culebs and copaiba, had no activity against *N. gonorrhoeae* in the laboratory, but they were still used; they were thought to relieve pain, reduce discharge and have a useful anaphrodisiac effect.

There were regional differences in the use of these modalities. The German and American schools favoured the instillation of silver salts or acriflavine into the urethra with a syringe; medicated bougies were sometimes used as well. The French, on the other hand, preferred urethrovesical irrigation – grand lavage – which had been introduced by Jules Janet in 1880. The principle was to wash out the urethra with large amounts of fluid (usually dilute potassium permanganate solution), delivered from a raised reservoir through a close-fitting nozzle. A stopcock regulated the flow. The original apparatus was refined by the American urologist Ferdinand Valentine[31] and in this form, with minor modifications, it was used throughout the world for more than half a century (Figure 10.4). As time went by the procedure developed its own mystique. Treatment was given one or twice a day. To begin with only the anterior urethra was irrigated, but if there was evidence of posterior urethritis the whole urethra as far as the bladder neck was treated. The distinction between anterior and posterior urethritis was made by examining the urine in the "two glass test" devised by Ricord; never a man to resist a *bon mot* he once said that "the posterior urethra drains into the bladder, but the anterior urethra into the shirt". It was important that the pressure of the irrigating fluid should not be too high. Harrison recalled that when he joined the British Military Hospital at Rotten Row in 1907 he had to reduce the pressure to a head of no more than three feet. Evidently his predecessor had thought differently:

"Being a man who believed in doing things thoroughly, he raised the irrigator vessels to a height of ten feet, and practically every patient in the ward had been laid out with epididymitis. He attributed this to their having been allowed turkey, etc. at Christmas and was very angry with me for suggesting that the cause was the fire hose he had turned down their urethras[32]."

For a successful posterior irrigation relaxation of the compressor urethrae muscle was essential. There were different techniques for achieving this; Valentine's was to encourage the patient to breathe deeply and to "divert his attention from the matter in hand by some witticism – not, however, one of which the patient himself is the subject". A course of treatment usually lasted for a week or two but longer periods, or repeated courses, might be necessary. After the discovery of antimicrobials, grand lavage was abandoned for gonorrhoea, but it was still used for recalcitrant non-gonococcal urethritis until the 1960s. A Janet, Valentine or Pelouze irrigator can still be seen in the corner of some of the older sexually transmitted disease clinics, like a disused reed organ now sadly silent and unwanted.

In earlier times the decision that an attack of gonorrhoea had been cured depended on clinical judgment alone, and it was recognised that mistakes could easily be made. After 1879 bacteriological confirmation of cure became possible.

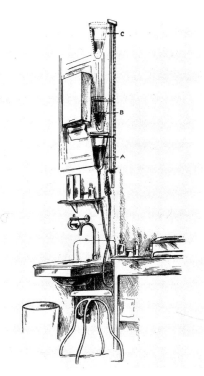

Figure 10.4. Apparatus for urethral irrigation. The patient stood in front of the basin. A, position of jar for anterior irrigation; B, position for posterior irrigation; C, dangerous pressure. From Pelouze (1931) Gonorrhoea in the male and female.

141

Neisser himself insisted that after treatment, microscopy for the gonococcus should be performed and repeated several times; only if all these tests were negative would the patient be told that the infection was cured and intercourse could be resumed.

The tests of cure recommended by Valentine[33] were typical of his time. Microscopy of urethral specimens for gonococci and examination of a centrifuged first-catch early morning urine specimen for leucocytes were performed. If these tests were negative, attempts were made to provoke a discharge by a large draught of beer or champagne (a procedure dating from the time of Ricord), passing a urethral bougie or irrigating the urethra with silver nitrate solution; any discharge produced was then examined for gonococci. Prostatic massage, with examination of the expressed fluid, was a further "test of cure". Urethritis often persisted after the treatment of gonorrhoea. Neisser found that 40 per cent of men with post-treatment urethritis still showed gonococci in the urethra. The remaining 60 per cent had "post-gonorrhoeal non-gonococcal urethritis", or post-gonococcal urethritis as it is called today; some of the patients might have conditions such as urethral strictures which required treatment, but the remainder could be left alone or given simple oral therapy. Persistent gonorrhoea was another matter altogether, because it posed a threat to the welfare of both the patient and his female partners.

There was never an agreed formal definition of chronic gonorrhoea, but an infection lasting for several weeks despite abstention from intercourse would generally fit into this category. Clinically, the patients had a slight mucopurulent urethral discharge, perhaps only in the morning (the "bonjour drop") and "threads" in the urine. Gonococci were not shed continuously, and it might take several attempts, perhaps with provocation by beer or irritating injections, to find them.

Chronic gonorrhoea was notoriously difficult to treat. Ricord said: "If I ever go to hell I know what I will be in for. I will find myself surrounded by patients with chronic gonorrhoea who endlessly implore me to cure them". It was generally ascribed either to inadequate treatment in the first place or to gonococcal infection persisting in follicles, ducts and crypts opening into the urethra or in patchy infiltrations of the submucous tissues. These lesions all formed what were sometimes called "feeding foci" for persistent infection. Treatment depended on either encouraging these foci to drain or destroying them. First, dilatation of the urethra by a series of straight or curved urethral sounds was undertaken, the procedure being followed by standard urethral lavage; treatment was continued regularly until tests of cure became negative. If this therapy was unsuccessful mechanical dilators were often used; the idea, according to Professor Oberlaender of Dresden, who devised many of these devices, was "to stretch or burst infiltrations, be they hard or soft, by means of superficial or subcutaneous injury". Mechanical dilators could also be used for treating strictures. Several different models were available; these dilators soon entered patients' folklore, and to this day some still ask whether "the umbrella" is going to be inserted (Figure 10.5).

The gonococcus is susceptible to changes in temperature, and some venereologists believed that heat applied to the urethra was often of considerable value, and devices such as hot water sounds, Kobelt's electrically heated bougie and Pollmann's electrode were used; others preferred ionisation or electrolysis of the mucous membrane through intraurethral electrodes. Merely to list these gruesome

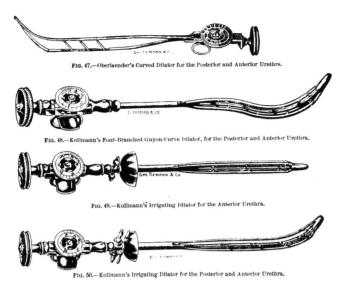

FIG. 47.—Oberlaender's Curved Dilator for the Posterior and Anterior Urethra.

FIG. 48.—Kollmann's Four-Branched Guyon-Curve Dilator, for the Posterior and Anterior Urethra.

FIG. 49.—Kollmann's Irrigating Dilator for the Anterior Urethra.

FIG. 50.—Kollmann's Irrigating Dilator for the Posterior and Anterior Urethra.

Figure 10.5. Urethral dilators, c. 1900. From Valentine (1900) The irrigation treatment of gonorrhoea. *"Kollmann's ingeniousnes seems to have no limit."*

instruments strikes a chill into the heart of the modern male reader. Although they were widely used it is difficult to know how much good they did.

Urethroscopy was an important part of management. The first practical instrument was made by Desormeux in 1853. Illumination of the urethra was a problem. In the early models sunlight was reflected into the tube by a mirror, but if this was not practicable an oil or petrol lamp, or even gaslight, were incorporated into the instrument (Figure 10.6 and 10.7). These were not satisfactory, and it was not until internal illumination with an electric light was introduced that the urethra could be clearly seen. Later, provision was made for inflating the urethra, and by 1913 Luys had devised an air urethroscope more or less in its modern form. Distended follicles, crypts and other areas of localised inflammation could be cauterised through the instrument, and it was also possible to diagnose incipient or incomplete strictures.

Chronic prostatitis was believed to be another important cause of chronic gonorrhoea. German and American writers were inclined to make a rather meaningless subdivision into catarrhal, follicular and parenchymatous forms, but the principle was the same: gonococci had infected the prostate and formed a "feeding focus" there. In practice, it proved very difficult to identify gonococci in the prostatic secretion, and it is possible that in many cases the prostatitis was non-gonococcal; present day investigators are having the same difficulty in deciding whether *Chlamydia trachomatis* causes chronic prostatitis. At all events, in the first four decades of the twentieth century it was thought that the treatment of chronic "gonorrhoeal" prostatitis was important, and this was undertaken by repeated prostatic massage, sometimes supplemented by diathermy.

Fever therapy, originally introduced by Wagner von Jauregg for the treatment of general paresis (see Chapter 7) was also used for the treatment of persistent or complicated gonorrhoea. In the 1930s the hyperthermia cabinet was employed

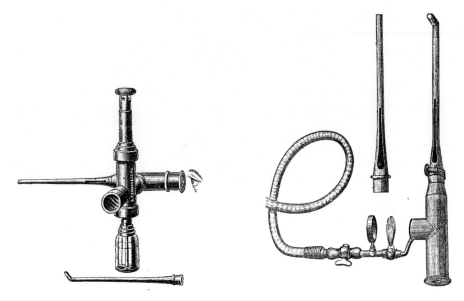

Figure 10.6. (left) Desormeaux's endoscope, 1853. Illumination was by sunlight, or by an oil-burning lamp.

Figure 10.7. (right) Endoscope illuminated by gaslight (1878). It is difficult to imagine this instrument in use.

for a time, a rectal temperature of 41 °C being maintained for several hours. Some patients, for example with gonococcal arthritis, responded dramatically[34], but fever therapy was demanding for both patients and medical staff and it was abandoned for gonorrhoea when the sulphonamides were found to be effective.

Treatment of Female Infections

Before the arrival of antimicrobial agents the treatment of women with gonococcal infections of the lower genital tract was laborious, and the results unsatisfactory. In earlier times frequent vaginal irrigation with lime water or mild astringents was thought to suffice but, after the discovery of the gonococcus, tests of cure showed that this treatment was virtually useless.

A regime gradually developed which involved treatment of all potentially infected areas. The vulva and vagina were thoroughly cleaned, and the ducts of the accessory glands treated with a silver salt, mercurochrome or acriflavine as these became available. Some venereologists irrigated the urethra with potassium permanganate, using a suitable nozzle attached to the male apparatus, while others preferred to instil an antiseptic. Finally, the cervix was cauterised with silver nitrate, or a medicated wick was inserted. Ideally, this treatment regimen was performed twice a day. If there was evidence of endometritis or pelvic inflammatory disease treatment became problematic. Complete rest was essential, although often not possible. Local treatment as outlined above was continued. Some venereologists irrigated the uterine cavity through a cervical catheter, and others used an apparatus which provided suction to the cervix, but these practices were generally frowned on.

For the most part the disease was left to run its course. In mild attacks complete resolution could occur – although reinfection was always possible – but more severe infections usually ran a prolonged course, with remissions and exacerbations. The formation of tubo-ovarian and other pelvic abscesses was common; these might drain into the vagina, bladder, rectum or even externally in the groin, or they might rupture into the peritoneal cavity with fatal results. Towards the end of the century operative intervention became safer and the drainage of abscesses, salpingo-oopherectomy, or even "pelvic clearance" were regularly performed. The plight of women with the pelvic complications of gonorrhoea in those days was never described better than by Neisser himself:

> "Should the infection reach the tubes, an acute febrile affection with severe attacks of pain, combined with tumour-like swelling of the tubes, occur which even in the most favourable cases keep the patient in bed for weeks and require the most careful treatment. Even after this, the condition usually is not entirely cured but leads to chronic persistent ill-health with frequent exacerbations. These recurrent attacks may become a danger to life, so that operative interference and removal of the collections of pus by laparotomy becomes inevitable. When both tubes are infected there is every prospect of lasting sterility[35]."

After treatment, stained smears of urethral and cervical specimens were repeatedly examined. At this time culture for N. gonorrhoeae was not much used for the initial diagnosis or follow-up tests because it was regarded as too difficult and unreliable for routine clinical practice. Tests of cure were very important. The difficulty of demonstrating gonococci in specimens from the female genital tract by microscopy, together with the acknowledged connection between latent gonorrhoea and pelvic inflammatory disease, led many venereologists to be very cautious about the resumption of intercourse. For example, Harrison[36] advised three full examinations at monthly intervals, and a final one six months later, before a woman could be pronounced cured. Then as now, it was difficult to persuade symptomless patients to reattend for examination and to secure compliance over abstention from intercourse.

Vaccine Therapy

Before the advent of antimicrobial drugs vaccines prepared from the causative organisms were often used to treat bacterial infections, with the idea of raising patients' resistance. Gonococcal vaccines were introduced at the time of the First World War. Most physicians who used them reserved them for the treatment of unduly prolonged, or complicated, gonorrhoea, but some used them for early infections as well, particularly in women. The vaccine could be "stock" or autogenous, and increasing doses were administered weekly for six weeks or so. Opinion on the success of gonococcal vaccines was divided, and many clinicians did not use them at all. "Protein shock therapy" by the injection of milk and other heterologous materials was even less successful.

The treatment of gonorrhoea in the pre-antibiotic period was obviously very difficult. Physicians using urethral lavage believed that it was an effective treatment for men provided it was started sufficiently early. The treatment of gonorrhoea in women, and of chronic infections in men, was much more difficult. Untreated, such infections, according to contemporary writers, could last for many years; with treatment the majority resolved eventually, although in some cases recovery may have been spontaneous rather than due to the doctor's efforts. Many men developed urethral strictures, and the regular dilatation of these was an important part of urological and venereological practice.

In both sexes gonorrhoea could cause infertility, and many women had to endure the misery of chronic pelvic inflammatory disease. "Single-child sterility" – the expression was Neisser's – was one of the features of Victorian gynaecology. Gonococcal infection of children – ophthalmia neonatorum or vulvovaginitis – was a constant possibility. Writing in 1900 Neisser rightly said that gonorrhoea was "a threat to society". In the years which followed his discoveries the disease itself became better understood and cure was more accurately defined. But although treatment improved it remained non-specific, and it was not until 20 years after Neisser's death that a specific treatment for gonorrhoea was developed.

The Sulphonamides

The use of synthetic compounds for treating infectious diseases began with the work of Ehrlich. His successors produced several drugs which were active against protozoa, but the common view was that bacteria were not susceptible to chemotherapy, the treponemata being a special case. The work of Gerhard Domagk (1895–1964) on sulphonamides changed these ideas. Domagk was a medical graduate of Kiel University, and later became professor of pathology at Münster. As a young man he became interested in chemotherapy, and like Ehrlich, but unlike Fleming, he had good chemical assistance, in his case from IG Farbenindustrie. In 1935 he reported that Prontosil, one of a series of azo dyes he had tested, was curative against haemolytic streptococcal infections in animals; he had also successfully treated a few human patients (including his own daughter). It was soon shown that the activity of Prontosil was due to the liberation of sulphanilamide, a relatively simple compound which could be easily manufactured. The drugs were then tried in other coccal infections and in 1937 the first studies of sulphonamides for the treatment of gonorrhoea appeared in Germany, Britain and the USA[37]. In this early work there were various treatment schedules involving Prontosil, sulphanilamide and standard irrigation therapy alone or in combination. The results were so successful that the sulphonamides were hailed as a breakthrough in the treatment of gonorrhoea, and many derivatives of the original compounds were marketed; venereologists observed with pleasure that the cure rate rose to 80–90 per cent as new sulphonamides were developed. Other forms of treatment, irrigations, vaccines etc., were abandoned. Although the sulphonamides were never one hundred per cent effective against gonorrhoea, they were a most important advance. Domagk was awarded a Nobel prize in medicine for his work, but he could not receive it because Hitler had prohibited any German from accepting this award. Domagk eventually received a Nobel prize medal, without the financial award, in 1947. In later life he studied the chemotherapy of other infections, particularly tuberculosis, and the chemical treatment of cancer.

Penicillin

Unfortunately, the clinical efficacy of the sulphonamides in the treatment of gonorrhoea steadily declined, owing to the appearance of resistant strains of *N. gonorrhoeae*. By 1944 this had become a serious problem: in some areas only 25% of men with gonorrhoea were being cured[38]. Adjuvant therapy with urethral irrigation had to be reintroduced, and some clinicians even advocated repeated courses of sulphonamides combined with fever therapy, a form of treatment which was also used for gonococcal arthritis. But relief for these problems was at hand. The first use of penicillin for the treatment of gonococcal infection had been in 1930. Cecil George Paine, a bacteriologist working in Sheffield, had read Fleming's early work and used a crude preparation of *Penicillium notatum* to treat two babies with gonococcal ophthalmia neonatorum; although the treatment was successful the study was not taken any further[39].

Penicillin was first used for the treatment of gonococcal urethritis in 1943 in the United States. To begin with, only sulphonamide resistant cases were treated, but penicillin soon became the standard treatment for all gonococcal infections. All reports concurred that this was the most effective drug for gonorrhoea ever tried[40]. Most of the early evaluation was performed in the Services, which had a prior claim on supplies of penicillin and plenty of cases of gonorrhoea, but as more supplies were made available civilians were treated as well. At first, multiple injections of an aqueous solution were required, but by 1945 repository preparations had been developed, and "one shot" treatment was possible; cure rates of more than 95 per cent were regularly achieved. Because the gonococcus was highly sensitive to penicillin, it was thought that resistance was unlikely. This was a case of being "fooled by hope"; the first evidence of resistance appeared in 1958, and during the following years penicillin-resistant gonorrhoea became a major problem. Streptomycin was introduced in 1944, and in single dosage was at first very effective. Besides being useful for the treatment of penicillin-resistant gonorrhoea it had the advantage of having little activity against *T. pallidum*, so that it was unlikely to mask incubating syphilis. Unfortunately, resistance of *N. gonorrhoeae* to streptomycin developed so rapidly that within a decade it could no longer be used. Since the 1950s clinicians and microbiologists, using a variety of antimicrobial drugs, have had a continuous struggle to maintain effective "one shot" therapy against developing resistance.

Chapter 11
Viruses and Chlamydiae

"Yes, I have a pair of eyes", replied Sam, "and that's just it. If they wos a pair o' patent double million magnifyin' microscopes of hextra power, p'raps I might be able to see through a flight o' stairs and a deal door".

Charles Dickens, *Pickwick Papers*

Genital Herpes

The word "herpes" has been in use for more than two millennia[1]. Derived from the Greek it means to creep, and was originally applied to any spreading ulcerative skin condition. The London surgeon Daniel Turner, writing in 1714, was among the first to use the word in its modern sense. He described the short and self-limiting course of facial herpes:

"The herpes is a choleric pustule breaking forth on the skin . . . On the face they arise with a sharp top and an inflamed base; having discharged the matter they contain the redness and pain go off and they dry away of themselves[2]."

Some of Turner's contemporaries mentioned "crystallines", small bullae on the prepuce and vulva which did not seem to be syphilitic. The English physician William Cockburn (1669–1739) described these lesions in his book *Gonorrhoea*, published in 1713. However, Jean Astruc is usually credited with the first full description of genital herpes, which appeared in his *De Morbis Veneris*, published in 1736: an English translation appeared in 1754[3].

"There frequently arise upon the surface of it [the glans] several hydatids, or watery and crystalline bladders which are filled with a lymph which is thin or thick, opaque or diaphenous . . . differing in number, size and degree of prominence, sometimes occupying the corona, sometimes the apex, sometimes the back, sometimes the sides of the glans . . . These disorders are not proper to men alone, but (mutatis mutandis) are common to women from the same cause. The labia pudendi, nymphae, clitoris and its prepuce, as also the caruculae myrtiformes at the orifice of the vagina being beset with malignant chancres, become swelled and inflated in the same manner as the prepuce or glans in men. Something of this kind is observed in catamites [boys kept for homosexual purposes] if they contract foul ulcers in the anus by the unnatural use of venery . . . the evacuation of faeces becomes difficult and painful, and . . . crystalline bladders frequently push forth at the margin of the anus."

After this, little more was heard about genital herpes for many years, until the founding fathers of dermatology included vesicular rashes in their laborious classification of skin diseases.

Thomas Bateman (1778–1821) was one of these pioneers. Born in Yorkshire, he studied medicine at Edinburgh; after qualifying, he moved to London, where he worked in the Carey Street Dispensary, a charitable group practice for the needy. Here he met the dermatologist Robert Willian, and as a result he developed a major interest in the subject. Bateman was a compulsive worker, his biographer says that "his pen was always in his hand when he came downstairs in the morning". His best known book was *A Practical Synopsis of Cutaneous Diseases*, published in 1813[4]. In it he discussed herpes zoster, herpes labialis and herpes preputialis – in those days herpetic infections were described according to their site. His account of the latter is excellent:

"The attention of the patient is attracted to the part by extreme itching and some sense of heat and on examining the prepuce he finds one, sometimes two, red patches . . . upon which are clustered five or six minute transparent vesicles . . . they commonly break about the fourth or fifth day and form a small ulceration on each patch."

Bateman went on to say that the ulcers took two weeks to heal completely, and that they were then liable to recur every six to eight weeks.

The history of dermatovenereology abounds with charismatic figures, and Jean Louis Alibert (1766–1837, Figure 11.1), who also advanced the study of genital herpes, was one of them. Born in Villefranche, he began his career as a teacher of classics and theology, but after the French Revolution he enrolled in the newly established École de Santé in Paris, and in due course was appointed attendant physician to l'Hôpital St Louis. At the time this was a run-down hospice for patients with chronic skin diseases, but it later became a "centre of excellence" under such luminaries as Bazin, Besnier, Sabouraud and Fournier. Here, Alibert embarked on a comprehensive study of dermatology. His extrovert personality was displayed in his famous teaching clinics held (like Ricord's) in the open air. He developed a classification of skin diseases, the *Monographie des Dermatoses*, which was published in 1832. In this he grouped herpetic diseases under the jaw-breaking generic term Olophlictide-olophlyticus, but unlike Bateman he mentioned lesions in women as well as men, saying that "it locates itself not only on the prepuce but also at the introitus vaginae; if we have fewer opportunities of observing it there, it is because of the natural modesty of the sex"[5].

So far there had been good clinical descriptions of genital herpes in men and women but nobody found much to say about its cause or natural history. A step forward was made by Francis Booth Greenough (1837–1904), who worked in Boston and was clinical instructor in syphilis at the Harvard Medical School. He was one of the first physicians in the USA to devote his career to venereology and genitourinary diseases, and his tall and commanding presence was well known to his contemporaries. At the annual meeting of the American Dermatologic

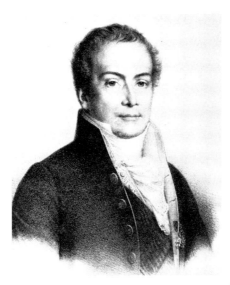

Figure 11.1. Jean Louis Alibert (1766–1837). (From Shelley and Crissey, Classics in clinical dermatology, 1953. Courtesy of Charles C. Thomas, Publisher, Springfield, Illinois.)

Association in 1880 he read a paper on herpes progenitalis[6]. His opening remarks could have been made in the 1960s. The disease was not serious, but "if we take into consideration the frequency of its occurrence, its tendency to relapse and the amount of mental anxiety it may give rise to . . . it assumes a much greater interest". The author then made several important points. Genital herpes was essentially a disease of young men and was very rare in women, there was often a past history of gonorrhoea, syphilis or chancroid, and it had a marked tendency to recur, some people having a fresh attack each time they had intercourse. An association with venereal diseases implied that genital herpes may itself be sexually transmitted. This had been suggested many years before by Boret[7], who described a male patient who developed his first attack 36 hours after intercourse and had many subsequent recurrences. Yet the idea of herpes as a sexually transmitted disease would be fatally weakened if, as Greenough stated, it seldom or never affected women. The matter of female infections was important, and was soon addressed by the redoubtable German dermatologist Paul Gerson Unna.

Unna (1850–1929, Figure 11.2) was born in Hamburg, the son of a general practitioner. His medical education began at Heidelberg, but was interrupted by the Franco-Prussian war, in which he was severely wounded. After the war he resumed his studies at Strasbourg. His thesis, on the development of the epidermis, was not well received and he had to re-write it. Disgusted with academe, he decided that after some further postgraduate work he would join his father's practice. While in Vienna he studied dermatology under Hebra and Kaposi, and undertook research on the histology of syphilitic chancres. In 1876 he returned to Hamburg and began general practice, but he was reluctant to abandon dermatology altogether and he opened a private clinic for skin diseases. This was so successful that he abandoned general practice and built a much larger skin clinic to which laboratories and accommodation for in-patients were added later, the whole forming an institute which he called "Dermatologicum." During the following 40 years Unna was active in clinical dermatology; he founded the science of dermatopathology and was tireless in writing, teaching and research. This was all without the power and prestige of a university department, so important in nineteenth century Germany; it was not until he was aged 68 years that he was appointed professor of dermatology in the new University of Hamburg. Unna was another workaholic. His only relaxation was to play the violoncello, and he would often invite professional musicians from Hamburg to join him in musical evenings at his house. He worked until a few days before his death at the age of 79.

Greenough's statement in 1880 about the rarity of genital herpes in women provoked a response from Unna which was published in an American journal two years later[8]. He was surprised at what Greenough had said, because personally he had seen at least 200 cases in the preceding four years. He suggested that the differences between Greenough's results and his own might be due to the composition of the groups they had studied. He himself had had four years service as the official examiner of prostitutes, in whom most of the cases had occurred. On the other hand, the disease might well be regarded as rare by dermatologists and gynaecologists in private practice. He went on to quote from the annual reports of the female syphilis clinic of the Hamburg General Hospital between 1878 and 1881, which showed that genital herpes was present in up to 8 per cent of the women admitted. He concluded that women are just as susceptible to herpes as men.

French venereologists were also interested in genital herpes in women. In 1869 Rollet had described a "blennorrhagic ulceration" of the cervix which was probably herpetic, and the association of herpetic vulvitis and cervicitis was discussed by Du Castel in 1901[9]. Recurrent attacks of herpes associated with menstruation

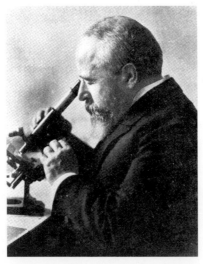

Figure 11.2. Paul Gerson Unna (1850–1927). (From Shelley and Crissey, Classics in clinical dermatology, *1953. Courtesy of Charles C. Thomas, Publisher, Springfield, Illinois.)*

– bouton de règle – were well known. Fournier distinguished "accidental" from "constitutional" herpes; the former followed events such as injury, attempted rape and blennorrhagia, while the latter were simply recurrences. In New York, Bumstead and Taylor were groping for an explanation of genital herpes (still described as a male complaint) when they wrote:

> "This affection must be regarded as neurotic in its nature, and its exciting cause a peripheral irritation of the nerves of the penis ... a long prepuce and the low grade of balanitis which quite often accompanies the condition, are quite common causes, while frequent sexual intercourse, excessive alcoholic indulgence and rich food are known to produce relapses. The vaginal secretion of some women has been known to cause outbreaks of this eruption[10]."

In France, Diday and Doyon published a book on genital herpes in 1886[11] in which they contrasted herpes associated with venery, as in prostitutes, with menstrual herpes, and suggested that they were two different diseases. The epidemiology of genital herpes remained obscure for half a century. Experienced clinicians in the nineteenth century had, like Greenough, obtained a history of venereal disease from many patients with genital herpes, but Fournier and others were reluctant to accept it as a venereal disease itself: first, because individual case histories to support this idea were lacking and second, because some attacks of herpes, for example during menstruation, were unrelated to intercourse. To escape from this dilemma some writers postulated a "herpetic genital fluxion", a predisposition to attacks which might then be precipitated not only by coitus and menstruation but by uncleanliness, hot weather, excessive venery, an attack of gonorrhoea and so on. Unna had concluded that the common factor was "excessive congestion of the genital organs ... universally found to be the true cause and basis of herpes progenitalis". There for the time being the matter had to rest.

Laboratory and experimental work resolved some of these difficulties. Unna[12] had been the first to describe the histopathology of herpes, and differentiate it from other vesicular eruptions. At the turn of the century filterable viruses causing disease in animals were discovered, and the possibility that herpes might be caused by a specific virus was soon considered. This was confirmed when a series of experiments showed that the inoculation of filtrates prepared from the lesions of facial herpes and herpetic keratitis could reproduce the disease in rabbits. In 1922 Levaditi showed that the viruses of herpes simplex and herpes zoster were different[13]. In 1921 Benjamin Lipschütz (1878–1931), working in Vienna, demonstrated intranuclear inclusion bodies in cells from the site of an eruption of herpes. He induced a vesicular eruption on the rabbit's cornea by inoculating material from herpes genitalis and herpes labialis; it was also possible, although more difficult, to produce lesions on human skin[14]. He thought that the viruses of "venereal herpes" and "herpes febrilis" were different, although most of his contemporaries thought that they were identical. During this time the natural history of herpes remained poorly understood. Many workers believed that recurrent attacks were due to fresh infections, but it was shown that in some patients these attacks could occur in the presence of circulating antibodies to the virus, with no rise in titre. Theory and practice did not match, and some virologists went so far as to suggest that the "virus" of herpes might not be a living infectious agent but a non-living toxic substance which could, in some circumstances, arise spontaneously.

Solution of the problem came from the work of the American virologist Ernest William Goodpasture (1886–1960). Goodpasture was born in Montgomery County, Tennessee. He received his medical education at Johns Hopkins Hospital, graduating in 1912. From the beginning he was interested in pathology and in 1924, after various appointments, he accepted a chair in the subject at Vanderbilt School of Medicine which he occupied until 1955. He has been described as quiet, serene and scholarly. Today, he is best remembered for the discovery that many viruses will grow well in fertilised hens' eggs, which led the way to the development of vaccines against several diseases. But he also made a major contribution to the study of herpes through his work on experimental herpes in rabbits, which led him to expound the important principle of latency:

"Following the primary infection, if invasion of nerves occurs in the human as in lower animals, it seems quite probable that the virus remains in a latent state within the ganglia after the local lesions have healed. A second cutaneous eruption then may result from autoinfection[15]."

Later it was shown that some patients with an acute attack of herpes developed rising titres of antibody, proving that at least some attacks were truly primary; it was becoming clear that the events which preceded a first and a recurrent attack of herpes were quite different.

The possibility of sexual transmission had been considered by some of the early workers, but in 1940 Sharlit published an unequivocal report of one adult infecting another[16]. It is hard to understand why such an event, which is commonplace today, had not been described before. Nevertheless, despite intervening discoveries, the authors of textbooks of venereology continued to attribute genital herpes to "neurasthenia", "irritation", or they ignored it altogether except as a differential diagnosis for primary syphilis. It was not until the 1950s that it was fully accepted as an independent viral sexually transmitted disease. Although it had been widely believed that the viruses of genital and non-genital herpes were identical, it was shown in the 1960s that there were two viral types. The use of typing methods, together with improved serological tests, were of crucial value in unravelling the complex epidemiology of these infections.

In 1853 Legendre gave the first description of genital herpes in a child, a seven-year-old girl who had been sexually assaulted[17]. The first report of neonatal herpes appeared in 1934, when an Italian ophthalmologist described an infant with conjunctivitis followed by a dendritic corneal ulcer, its aetiology being confirmed by animal inoculation[18]. In the following year there was a case report from the US of a premature infant who died of an acute illness characterised by hepatic and adrenal necrosis. Intranuclear inclusions were seen in parenchymatous cells from these organs, and it was suggested that these might be herpetic, although the route of infection was not determined[19]. Other reports of fatal disseminated disease in infants followed, and the whole subject became of great importance when the incidence of genital herpes in adults began to rise in the 1960s.

During the 200 years since genital herpes was first recognised treatment has been unsatisfactory. In the early days most physicians confined themselves to prescribing bland applications such as talc, starch poultices and zinc sulphate solution, but some resorted to bizarre and even desperate measures, particularly in attempts to prevent recurrences. The affected epithelium might be destroyed by escharotics or excised, and male patients were sometimes circumcised. Systemic treatment had a few advocates – Hutchinson claimed success with courses of Fowler's solution (potassium arsenite) – and during the 1940s and 1950s small-pox vaccination had a vogue, despite sometimes calamitous side effects. Other ineffective treatment modalities used at this time included inactivated herpes simplex virus vaccines, vaccination with BCG, "photodynamic inactivation" (the application of neutral red followed by fluorescent light to the affected area) and topical application of antiviral agents. Acyclovir, introduced in the early 1980s, was the first drug shown to influence the course of genital herpes.

Genital Papillomavirus Infection

Penile and anal warts were well known in the ancient world. The word condyloma (from the Greek *kondylos*, a knuckle) was used to describe warts and other lesions at the anus. The name *thymion* was applied by Celsus and others to warty lesions of the penis; the Byzantine physician Aetius (*fl.* AD 550) explained its origin:

> "The name thymus arises from the similarity of the lesions to the tips of the plant of the same name . . . this complaint occurs around the anus and pudenda and between the legs."

Another word *ficus*, a fig, was also widely used, but both these words have now vanished[20]. The term *Condyloma acuminatum* came into use towards the end of the nineteenth century.

Treatment in the early days consisted of simple destruction or excision of the lesions. Patients with anal warts did not receive much sympathy, because the condition was widely regarded as being due to sodomy. The satirists Martial and Juvenal made much fun of these unfortunates, and according to Dionysius (sixth century AD), at a clinic in Rome:

> "The surgeons spared neither iron nor fire and were not moved to pity by the cries of the patients, because they had brought the disease on themselves by their unnatural conduct[21]."

After the fall of the Roman Empire there were occasional descriptions of penile lesions which were probably warts. Writing at the beginning of the fifteenth century Lanfrance of Milan described *Ficus* as "an excrescence of a peculiar nature which grows in the prepuce and sometimes on the head of the penis"[22]. It seems likely that anogenital warts still existed in the medieval world, but their identification was submerged when the pandemic of syphilis began, and recognisable descriptions did not reappear until the eighteenth century. In his *Treatise on the Venereal Disease* (1786) Hunter wrote:

> "Another disposition which these parts acquire from the venereal poison is the disposition to form excrescences called warts . . . perhaps the parts acquire this disposition from the venereal matter having been long in

155

contact with their surface . . . These excrescences are considered by many
as not simply a consequence of the venereal poison but possessed of its
specific disposition, and therefore have recourse to mercury for the cure
of them[23]."

Hunter evidently believed that warts arose when the "venereal poison" lingered
in contact with the genital epithelium. Although he said that he had never known
mercury to cure them, it was widely prescribed. The sometimes tragic results of
this are described in a report published in 1776 by Dease[24]. Two young men
with urethral discharge and penile warts were assumed to be "poxed" and were
repeatedly "salivated"; they succumbed to chronic mercury poisoning, the warts
remaining unaffected until their death.

Benjamin Bell's opinions were different. The belief that warts were syphilitic
was, he said, "by no means well founded". In 99 of 100 cases they appear to be
entirely local; treatment by mercury was inappropriate and could cause "much
mischief". The aetiology of the disease was unknown, but:

"Whatever tends to excite the flow of an unusual amount of blood to
the penis seems to create a disposition in these parts to formations of this
kind. Hence they succeed to various forms of irritation[25]."

Among these irritants was gonorrhoea. He had often observed them appear "on
the termination of gonorrhoea when the patient, having considered the cure
complete, is surprised by the appearance of this new symptom". Bell was one
of the first surgeons to discuss the differentiation of extensive genital warts from
cancer. Warts, he said, could spread to cover the whole glans, and if they become
ulcerated:

"the whole mass assumes such a diseased appearance as, with those
not accustomed to this branch of business, gives suspicion of their
being cancerous. Of this I have met with different instances where the
penis, after being doomed to amputation, has been saved and the warty
excrescences removed."

Condylomas affecting the labia pudendi were mentioned by both Hunter and
Bell. The French surgeon Antoine-Jacques-Louis Jourdan (1788–1848) described
their appearance on the labia, clitoris, perineum and anus[26]. They could follow
gonorrhoea, or indeed any irritation "light but prolonged"; they could also
occur during pregnancy or after "l'abus du coit" (this intriguing expression
was unexplained). In the mid nineteenth century venereologists were familiar with
penile, vulval and anal condylomas which by this time, according to Lancereaux,
were also called "warts, vegetations, cauliflower excrescences, figs, cocks' comb
etc"[27]. Although vulval condylomas and their enlargement during pregnancy
were known, condylomas of the cervix were not described until the twentieth
century. This may have been partly due to infrequent speculum examination, yet
in 1921 it was stated that this was "one of the rarest of gynaecological disorders
. . . the cervical type is as rare as the vulval type is common"[28]. This observation
is difficult to understand, since today cervical condylomas are not uncommon.

By the early nineteenth century all but a few clinicians had abandoned the early
idea that genital warts were related to syphilis. The consensus was now that they

were caused by the action of irritants. They often followed gonorrhoea – for a time, they were called "gonorrhoeal warts" – but many patients showed no sign of this infection and it was then maintained that gonorrhoeal pus was simply one of many irritants which could provoke the formation of condylomas, the others being dirt, decomposed sebaceous matter and secretions "disordered by venery", hence the name "venereal warts" which is still sometimes used today. The idea of non-specific irritation had also been employed to explain the pathogenesis of male urethritis and genital herpes; in the case of anogenital condylomas the hypothesis was accepted by such eminent figures as Hebra, Kaposi, Von Bumm and Hutchinson, and lingered until well into the twentieth century. Anal condylomas in women were attributed to "the flow of discharges backwards from the vagina", and in men to "chronic irritation".

By 1905 the causes of gonorrhoea, chancroid and syphilis had been discovered, and there were now efforts to find a microbe which caused anogenital warts. Several workers reported spirochaetes in the lesions, and some claimed to have found protozoa and other organisms, but none of these suggestions was confirmed and they were soon forgotten. A more profitable idea was that the disease might be related to skin warts. A hint of this had come from an early case report by Astley Cooper (1768–1841, Figure 11.3). An ornament of Guy's Hospital, he was renowned for his skill in diagnosis and his brilliant operative technique. It was said at the time that George IV and Astley Cooper were the two best known men in London. In 1835 he wrote:

"Mr Chandler removed some warts from a patient in this hospital which were of a very large size and, as he was returning the knife, this gentleman [his dresser] put his hand forwards and it entered just under the thumb nail. He left Town for the south-west part of England; in a little time he had an irritation about the nail, and a wart grew out from the spot where the puncture had been made[29]."

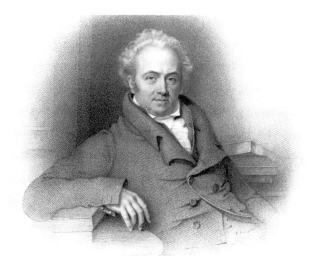

Figure 11.3. Sir Astley Paston Cooper (1768–1841). (Courtesy of the Royal Society of Medicine Library.)

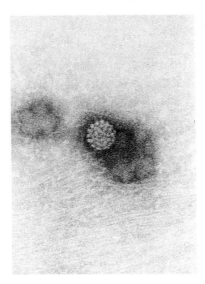

Figure 11.4. First (1970) electron micrograph of a virion from a vulval wart. (Negative staining, × 181 000.)

In 1893 the French dermatologist Gémy had been struck by the histological similarity between skin warts and genital condylomas[30], and during the next few years several authors pointed out that many patients with condylomas had common skin warts as well. Was it possible that both diseases were caused by the same parasite? The viral aetiology of skin warts had been proved early in the twentieth century, when it was shown that the disease could be transmitted by the inoculation of cell-free filtrates of excised warts; attempts were now made to extend these experiments by inoculating extracts of skin warts into the genital epithelium, and of genital warts into the non-genital skin. Not surprisingly, it proved difficult to obtain volunteers for these studies; some prostitutes were persuaded to participate, and in one disgraceful experiment a virgin was inoculated. In some cases the inoculation of extracts of penile warts into non-genital skin was followed by the development of common warts at the inoculated site. There were not many of these experiments, but enough to secure acceptance of the hypothesis that anogenital condylomas were caused by a virus identical to that which caused common skin warts. The evidence for this opinion was summarised by the Swiss dermatologist Frey in 1924[31], and was not seriously questioned.

There was no further progress in studying the viruses for many years. Virus particles were seen by electron microscopy in extracts of common skin warts in 1949, and virions of identical appearance were seen in low concentration in extracts of anogenital warts in 1968 (Figure 11.4). Papillomaviruses cannot be propagated in cell culture, so the methods of classical virology could not be used to study them. In the late 1970s it became possible to prepare cloned viral genomes and thereby to compare viruses extracted from different anatomical sites. It was found that papillomavirus types from genital condylomas were different from those from skin warts, and the "unitary" hypothesis which had been accepted for so many years was therefore incorrect.

158

The sexual transmission of genital warts was always contentious. In 1826 Jourdan had thought that although they could occur in both sex partners it was difficult to decide their contagiousness, adding (quite rightly) that "the declarations of the patient are not sufficient when a long interval has elapsed since the suspect coitus"[26]. Astley Cooper, however, had no doubt about the matter:

"Warts ... are a local disease, yet when I say local I must observe that they frequently secrete a matter which is able to produce a similar disease in others. A gentleman in Sussex was called to a lady in labour; he felt something in the vagina, and found it to be a crop of warts. In conversation with the husband, he told him that his lady had a number of warts. The gentleman stated that at the time he was married he had a wart on the penis, and that he had no doubt but that he had communicated them to his wife[29]."

The United States venereologist Freeman Bumstead disagreed. He thought that the supposed contagiousness of condylomas was apparent rather than real:

"Warts are most frequently observed in men and women who have had gonorrhoea, balanitis, chancroids or syphilis, but this is simply because the skin or mucous membrane has for a time been moistened by an acrid secretion which has favoured abnormal development of its papillae. It is often said that they are contagious, but such instances are readily explained on the ground that the acrid secretions from the vegetations ... when transplanted to another individual, act in the manner already explained and give rise to others[32]."

Three years after this was written an experiment performed by Kranz in Munich showed that, after all, genital warts might be contagious. Condylomata acuminata were transferred to the genital regions of normal individuals by the application, after scarification, of small fragments of tumour or fluid expressed from a genital lesion[33]. Nonetheless, by the end of the nineteenth century genital warts were not regarded as "of venereal origin", they were still held to be due to irritation. This view was modified after the discovery of the alleged viral identity of genital and skin warts. A history, or the current presence, of skin warts provided a simple explanation for the development of genital warts: the accidental transfer of the virus from these to the genitals. Sexual transmission of the virus was thought to be very unusual. Reviewing the literature in 1921, the German dermatologist Heller could find records of only 11 cases[34].

During the 1920s and 1930s some venereologists began to question these assumptions, as their clinical experience was that in many cases genital warts appeared to have been sexually transmitted. The disease, like the venereal diseases, became commoner during the Second World War than in peace time, and in 1950 the English venereologist Harkness wrote that despite their apparent causal identity with skin warts "in a large percentage of cases the genital variety is spread venereally", and that in his experience it was extremely rare to find them associated with warts in other parts of the body[35]. As had been found with genital herpes, it was difficult to establish infectivity by the examination of sex partners of people with the disease, particularly since warts had a long incubation period, but this was eventually achieved by Barrett and his colleagues in 1954[36]. They examined a large number of soldiers returning from the war in Korea who had developed genital warts, and they also examined their wives, many of whom had developed lesions after their husbands' return. They concluded that the condition was highly contagious, and should be classed as a venereal disease. The reaction of the dermatological establishment, particularly in the United States, to this suggestion was one of outrage. Indeed, one dermatologist went so far as to circularise colleagues in various countries to ask "Do you believe that it is correct to consider condylomata acuminata a venereal disease?", and 94 per cent of those who replied answered "No." For some years the idea of sexual transmission was quietly dropped and belief in the less disturbing "unitary" hypothesis maintained. But later studies were to show that Barrett and his colleagues were right; the prevalence of skin warts in patients with genital condylomas had been overestimated, and in the majority of patients the disease had been transmitted sexually.

Extragenital condylomas were described from time to time, the commonest site of these being the anus. In discussing such "venereal excrescences" Bell distinguished between those which appeared by spread from warts on the genitals, which he regarded as a local disease requiring local treatment, and those which developed in early syphilis and were often accompanied by a generalised rash. The latter were undoubtedly syphilitic, and needed treatment with mercury; they were later called *condylomata lata* by Ricord. By the end of the nineteenth century anal warts in both sexes were attributed to irritation from discharges, uncleanliness and other non-specific factors. There were occasional case reports of associations between anal warts and anal coitus, as had been discussed by the ancients, but male homosexuality was an emotive subject and the matter received little attention until 1929 when Parnell, who had had an extensive experience of venereal disease in the Royal Navy, made the following comment, whose obliquity is characteristic of references to male homosexuality at the time:

> "Altruistic persons have commonly attributed anal warts to excessive perspiration; for such a belief there are no grounds, nor are they seen in patients suffering from slight anal discharges such as are present with fissures. Their actual origin must remain obscure, but that they are associated with certain forms of sexual inversion is patent to anyone with a large clinical experience[37]."

Many venereologists believed that there was a strong association between anal warts and anal intercourse, but the truth of this idea had to await epidemiological studies, which became much easier to perform after the decriminalisation of most homosexual practices in industrialised countries in the 1960s. It soon emerged that 80 per cent of men with warts confined to the anus admitted anal coitus.

Anogenital warts in children were mentioned only occasionally in the early literature. A case of condyloma acuminatum in a neonate was described in 1903 in the USA[38], and a report of a three-year-old girl with genital and lip lesions, with associated gonorrhoea, appeared in 1940[39]. Between then and 1980 only 18 other cases were reported, but today the disease is not uncommon, and there has been much discussion about its epidemiology and association with sexual abuse.

The treatment of anogenital warts has always been problematical, and recurrences common. Bell said that they could be removed by a knife, scissors or

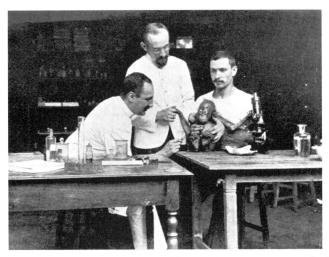

Figure 11.5. Java, 1906. Left to right: Halberstaedter, von Prowazek, Leschner (a technician). From Neisser, Beiträge zur Pathologie und Therapie der Syphilis, *1911.*

ligature, but "few patients will submit to the use of the scalpel for the extirpation of numerous warts." He believed that the tumours could be ablated by the application of irritants such as cantharides. Nevertheless, surgical destruction by knife, cautery or acids was used throughout the nineteenth century. Cocaine became available as a local anaesthetic in the mid-century, but was not always used; one clinician, having evidently lost patience with such niceties, thought it preferable "simply to cut them off without any anaesthetic whatever." In the early twentieth century some venereologists thought that they would often regress if they were simply kept clean and dry, although one disdainfully added "it is difficult to carry out this treatment in the class of patients among whom venereal warts are most prevalent". A new treatment by the application of podophyllin was introduced by Kaplan, a US army doctor, in 1942[40]. This drug had been used by American Indians for treating skin diseases and Kaplan, who was interested in ethnic medicine, decided to give it a trial. It proved to be effective, and has been widely (perhaps too widely) used by venereologists ever since, with surgical extirpation reserved for extensive or recalcitrant lesions. There have been no real advances in treatment in the 50 years since Kaplan's work, and permanent cure is as elusive as ever.

Chlamydia Trachomatis Infections

Oculogenital Infection

The discovery of *Chlamydia trachomatis* was an unexpected by-product of Neisser's expedition to Java in 1903 to study experimental syphilis in monkeys. The members of the team included Ludwig Halberstaedter (1876–1949) and Stanislaus von Prowazek (1875–1915; Figure 11.5). Halberstaedter had been assistant in Neisser's department of dermatology in Breslau, and von Prowazek was a microbiologist seconded from the Imperial Public Health Administration in Berlin. Once in Java, they became interested in trachoma and asked Neisser's permission to do some research on the disease. This was refused, but fortunately they went ahead with their studies and identified inclusion bodies in conjunctival scrapings from orangutans whom they had infected with scrapings from patients with trachoma (Figure 11.6). They published their results in 1907[41]. Within the next few years these were confirmed, and they and other workers reported similar inclusions in conjunctival cells from some infants with non-gonococcal ophthalmia and in cervical cells from their mothers[42]. In 1910 Lindner reported inclusions in urethral specimens from 3 of 10 men with non-gonococcal urethritis[43], and in the same year typical inclusion conjunctivitis was induced in monkeys' eyes by the inoculation of specimens from these ocular and genital sites[44]. These experiments suggested that the same inclusion-forming agent could cause non-gonococcal urethritis, cervical infection and non-gonococcal ophthalmia neonatorum. Halberstaedter and von Prowazek suggested a family name Chlamydozoa for the organisms, from the Greek *chlamys*, a cloak. At first they thought that they might be protozoa, but when it was discovered that they could pass through bacteria-proof filters they were (wrongly) regarded as viruses.

Halberstaedter did no further work on Chlamydozoa after 1910. His major interest was now radiotherapy, first of skin diseases but later of malignant tumours. After the First World War he became director of the radiotherapy department of the Berlin Cancer Institute. When the Nazis came to power in 1933 he left Germany and took charge of the radiotherapy department of the Hadassah Hospital in Jerusalem. Sadly, his department was destroyed in the fighting of 1948, and he died soon afterwards. He was described as a fine teacher, with a ready wit and a gift for repartee. Von Prowazek continued his career in microbiology, and was appointed to a chair at Hamburg University. He was active in research, with a particular interest in insect-born diseases. He identified the causal agent of epidemic typhus, later named *Rickettsia prowazekii*, in 1914. While investigating the louse vector von Prowazek, like Ricketts before him, contracted typhus himself, and he died at the early age of 39.

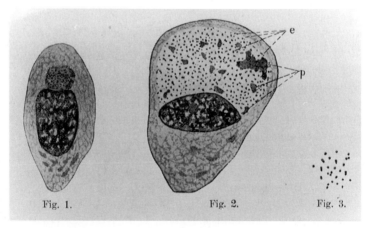

Figure 11.6. Chlamydial inclusions (Figs. 1 and 2) and elementary bodies (Fig. 3). From Halberstaedter and von Prowazek's first paper (1907).

The intensive studies triggered by the discoveries of Halberstaedter and von Prowazek lasted for only a few years, but during that time the clinical and epidemiological groundwork of oculogenital chlamydial infection had been laid. Attempts were made to define some of the clinical features of these infections. In 1904 Ludwig Waelsch, working in Prague, had described a "rare form" of non-gonococcal urethritis which had an incubation period of 10–14 days, ran a mild but protracted course and was very difficult to cure[45]. Ten years later several workers described the urethroscopic features of "Waelsch urethritis", a reddened mucous membrane with multiple soft infiltrates "like the nodules in trachoma". Inclusions were described in urethral scrapings from some men with the condition and Lindner, one of the pioneers who remained active in the field for many years, conjectured that there might be a "genital trachoma;" however, inclusions were also found in specimens from men with non-gonococcal urethritis without the Waelsch features[42]. There the matter rested until 1934, when an American ophthalmologist, Philip Thygeson, added adult inclusion conjunctivitis to the canon of oculogenital chlamydial infection[46]. He also described the life cycle of the organism, and made a substantial study of non-ocular infections. In a series of papers he expanded the observations of the early workers by examining larger numbers of patients; he confirmed the presence of the chlamydial agent in the cervix of mothers of babies with inclusion conjunctivitis and in the urethra of men with non-gonococcal urethritis. He concluded that mild urethritis in men and cervicitis in women were a "reservoir" of chlamydial infection[47].

In the early 1930s both psittacosis and lymphogranuloma venereum were found to be caused by inclusion-forming agents. The Frei reaction, produced in the skin of patients with lymphogranuloma venereum by injection of a killed preparation of the infecting agent, was described in 1925. In 1932 there was a flurry of excitement when it was found that urethral discharge from patients with "Waelsch urethritis" acted like the Frei antigen, and that the Frei antigen gave a positive reaction in patients with "Waelsch urethritis"; there was speculation about a possible connection between the urethritis and the causal agent of lymphogranuloma venereum[48]. The uncertainty of the relationship between the inclusion-forming agents of trachoma, inclusion conjunctivitis, genital tract infections, lymphogranuloma venereum and psittacosis led to a protracted argument about their taxonomy which was eventually resolved in the 1960s by Moulder. He showed that chlamydiae are intracellular bacteria and introduced the present classification of a family Chlamydiacae, genus *Chlamydia*, with two species *C. psittaci* and *C. trachomatis*, the latter comprising ocular, genital and lymphogranuloma venereum strains[49].

Venereologists had taken little part in these matters, but interest in non-gonococcal urethritis reawakened in the 1940s. It was common, its cause was unknown and while sulphonamides appeared to cure some cases, penicillin was completely ineffective. The disease needed a complete reappraisal, and this was initiated by an English venereologist, Arthur Herbert Harkness (1889–1970; Figure 11.7). Harkness was born in South Africa and received his medical education at Guy's Hospital, London[50]. When he returned to England after service overseas in the First World War he found himself responsible for some thousands of sailors suffering from various venereal diseases. This aroused his interest in venereology, and although he did not receive a formal training in the speciality – which was not available in England at that time – he gained experience through a series of junior hospital appointments and was eventually

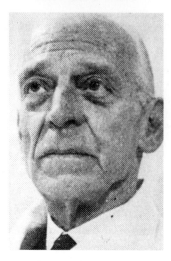

Figure 11.7. Arthur Herbert Harkness (1889–1970).

appointed director of the venereal disease clinic at St Peter's Hospital, a major London urological centre. He subsequently received honorary appointments at other hospitals, and developed a large private practice. He was a genial, popular and generous member of the developing speciality. Unusually for the time, he studied non-gonococcal urethritis and its complications for many years, his efforts culminating in a classical monograph on the subject, which was published in 1950[35] and won him an honorary Fellowship of the Royal College of Surgeons.

Harkness revived the concept of "Waelsch urethritis", and confirmed the urethroscopic findings reported 30 years before. He identified and illustrated undoubted chlamydial inclusions in urethral scrapings from men with non-gonococcal urethritis, particularly the Waelsch form. Like his predecessors he was severely handicapped by the lack of sensitive and specific diagnostic methods, and his view that scattered cytoplasmic "elementary bodies" also indicated infection by "Chlamydozoon" is not accepted today. Nevertheless, Harkness was influential in reviving interest in non-gonococcal urethritis and genital chlamydial infection at a time when they were often overlooked.

By 1950 non-gonococcal urethritis was generally recognised as an independent sexually transmitted disease. Its cause remained obscure; it was variously attributed to infection by a range of organisms which included *Trichomonas vaginalis*, "pleuropneumonia-like organisms" (now known as genital mycoplasmas), and an assortment of other bacteria. The role of *Chlamydozoon* remained controversial, and the only way it could be identified was by a laborious search for inclusions. But in 1957 T'ang and his colleagues[51] devised a technique for isolating chlamydial agents in the yolk sac of hens' eggs, and with this more sensitive method progress became possible.

The first reported isolation of *Chlamydia* from genital material was in 1959, when the agent was recovered from the eyes of a baby with inclusion conjunctivitis and from the mother's cervix[52]. The first isolations from the male urethra were in 1964, the subjects being the fathers of babies with inclusion conjunctivitis, men with adult inclusion conjunctivitis and the male sex partners of women with inclusion conjunctivitis[53]. Dunlop and his colleagues used the same technique to investigate men with non-gonococcal urethritis, and recovered the organisms from 4 of 10 cases[54]. The yolk sac method was cumbersome and unsuitable for screening large numbers of specimens, but in 1965 a more easily manageable cell culture system was introduced by Gordon and Quan[55]. Francis B. Gordon, a graduate of the University of Chicago, had a long and fruitful career in medical microbiology, particularly chlamydial infection; he died in 1973 from accidental drowning at sea. His cell culture procedure made it possible for many large surveys on chlamydial genital infection to be performed and, together with the immunotyping of *C. trachomatis* strains by microimmunofluorescence which followed in 1970, marked the beginning of the modern era of the study of chlamydial infection.

Since its cause was then unknown, the treatment of non-gonococcal urethritis was empirical, and it was not directed at *C. trachomatis* or any other specific micro-organism until the last decade. Sulphonamides were widely prescribed, but the cure rate barely exceeded 50 per cent; Penicillin was found to be ineffective. Many venereologists followed Harkness and continued to use urethral irrigation, and a combination of streptomycin and a sulphonamide was prescribed in some British clinics; it had been originally proposed as a catch-all treatment for infective urethritis, both gonococcal and non-gonococcal. In the early 1950s the tetracyclines were introduced and soon became the treatment of choice. Although other organisms, particularly the genital mycoplasmas, are now known to cause some cases of non-gonococcal urethritis, *C. trachomatis* is accepted as the commonest cause, and since it is responsible for all the complications in men, women and babies treatment is now directed primarily at its eradication. Working in the heat and discomfort of Java, Halberstaedter and von Prowazek might have been surprised to know that they were to have a lasting influence on venereology.

Lymphogranuloma Venereum

The recognition of lymphogranuloma venereum as an independent disease came through the convergence of several groups of clinical observations. In 1786 Hunter described a suppurative inguinal bubo which arose without apparent cause and was unaffected by mercury. He wrote that buboes of this kind:

> "are generally preceded and attended by a slight fever . . . they are generally indolent and slow in their progress. When they suppurate . . . the matter comes slowly to the skin, and the colour is different from that of the other [syphilitic] bubo, being more purple[56]."

Hunter was puzzled by these buboes. He did not think that they were syphilitic, and was inclined to think that they might be "scrofulous". In 1833 William Wallace of Dublin described an "indolent primary syphilitic bubo". It is, he says, painful and accompanied by fever and a "general feeling of indisposition". As the inguinal nodes enlarge, "the matter slowly approaches the skin . . . the vitality of a large portion of the integument is often destroyed, from whence there result . . . numerous fistulous openings"[57]. Although he called the disease syphilitic, Wallace admitted that there might be other causes – in fact, he had given an excellent description of early lymphogranuloma venereum.

Writing in 1867, Philippe Ricord described a "bubo d'emblée," which was not preceded by a primary chancre or followed by any signs of secondary syphilis[58]. This particular kind of "poradenitis" was subsequently described by many authors; intuitively, they thought the disease was venereal, but not syphilitic. In 1890 Hermann Klotz[59] said that he had personally seen more than 100 such cases in hospital and private practice, nearly all of them in men; he had noticed that a small genital lesion was usually present, and thought that the buboes were the result of the absorption of septic material, but he did not believe that this was syphilitic or tuberculous. He had a greater personal knowledge of the disease than most observers, having developed axillary adenitis himself after operating on a patient with suppurating buboes. The superficial penile lesion which Klotz described was mentioned by some other clinicians, but remained controversial for many years – some denied that such lesions existed, and others simply mentioned that the inguinal adenopathy was preceded by balanitis. Finally, in 1913 Joseph Durand, Joseph Nicolas and Maurice Favre, working in Lyon, gave a full clinical and pathological description of the disease as it was then understood[60]. They believed that the buboes were due to a specific but unknown sexually transmitted infection, the portal of entry being the inconspicuous genital lesion already described. The histology of the buboes showed resemblances to Hodgkin's lymphoma, which led them to call the disease "lymphogranulomatose inguinale." This unfortunate and confusing name was the first of many to be suggested. Eventually, the majority of venereologists came to favour "lymphogranuloma inguinale", but because this was easily confused with granuloma inguinale (donovanosis), this was changed to lymphogranuloma venereum in the late 1930s.

The next thread in the skein was the matter of "climatic bubo". Since the middle of the nineteenth century suppurative inguinal adenitis was familiar to clinicians working in warm climates, and it was also seen in sailors returning from the tropics. The disease seemed to affect only men, and a penile abrasion was often present; it was variously attributed to venereal disease, malaria and even plague. In 1896 a British naval surgeon, Charles Godding, called it "climatic bubo", and argued that since there was often a history of intercourse in a tropical country it was probably a venereal disease[61]. The descriptions of climatic bubo and lymphogranuloma inguinale so closely resembled one another that it is hard to understand that it was not until the late 1920s that it was realised that they were the same disease. In 1925 Wilhelm Siegmund Frei, a lecturer in the Department of Dermatology at Breslau (which had been directed by Neisser at one time), inoculated a preparation of pus which had been aspirated from a bubo of a patient with lymphogranuloma venereum intradermally into subjects with various forms of inguinal adenopathy. A delayed skin reaction developed in patients with lymphogranuloma but not in those with syphilis, tuberculosis or Hodgkin's lymphoma[62]. This was a valuable discovery. Not only was it now possible to confirm that lymphogranuloma venereum and climatic bubo were the same disease – although this idea was only slowly accepted – but to identify the late manifestations of lymphogranuloma.

Elephantiasis of the vulva, sometimes accompanied by inguinal adenopathy, had been recorded by Desruelles in 1844[63], and a few years later Pierre Charles Huguier (1804–1873) described a chronic vulval swelling with ulceration which he called "esthiomene," from the Greek "eating away"[64]. More case reports of this condition followed, and in 1873 Fournier firmly called it "vulval syphilides"[65]. During the next half-century clinicians struggled to understand the aetiology of esthiomene and vulval elephantiasis; they were attributed to syphilis, chancroid, lupus and even chronic irritation. It was noticed that some of the patients also developed inflammatory strictures of the rectum; these had been known since the middle of the nineteenth century and were regarded by many clinicians, including Fournier, as due to tertiary syphilis. But although some of the patients had undoubtedly had syphilis, antisyphilitic remedies were valueless.

In the early years of the twentieth century there were suggestions that since the "ano-rectal syphilome" and esthiomene often occurred in the same individual they might be related, and the term "genito-anal-rectal syndrome" came into use[66]. The syndrome was described as affecting mainly women, particularly prostitutes, and as comprising combinations of vulval elephantiasis, esthiomene, proctitis and rectal strictures. Its cause remained unknown, but light dawned in 1927 when Frei had the idea of using his skin test on patients with the "genito-anal-rectal syndrome". He obtained positive reactions, and although he was initially cautious in linking the syndrome to lymphogranuloma venereum his results were soon confirmed by others, and it seemed increasingly likely that the pathogenesis of this strange group of diseases, which had defeated clinicians for three-quarters of a century, had at last been decided. Direct proof that the lesions were all caused by the same agent came in the early 1930s when this was isolated from bubo pus and infected anorectal tissue by inoculation of mouse brain and the yolk sac of hens' eggs[67]. Its development cycle was found to be similar to that of the psittacosis agent, and its final identification as a member of the Chlamydiae was made in the 1940s.

Before the development of antimicrobial drugs the only possible treatment for lymphogranuloma venereum was to attack its various manifestations surgically. At one time surgical extirpation of the buboes was recommended, but many patients treated in this way developed postoperative elephantiasis. It was possible, with care, to dilate soft rectal strictures, but advanced strictures needed major surgery. Esthiomene and elephantiasis required plastic surgery; without antibiotic cover these operations were hazardous, and patients had long and miserable illnesses. The sulphonamides were first used for the treatment of lymphogranuloma venereum in 1945[68]. They were quite effective if the disease was confined to the lymph nodes, but neither the sulphonamides nor the tetracyclines, introduced later, could by themselves cure its late manifestations, and surgery was still often required. Throughout its long and complicated history lymphogranuloma venereum has been a most difficult disease to treat.

Reiter's Syndrome

The history of Reiter's syndrome and reactive arthritis is second only to syphilis in its complexity and capacity to generate controversy. The association of arthritis with genital infection was observed for many centuries. Discussing *Gonorrhoea simplex* Bell wrote in 1793 that he had no doubt that a urethral discharge and rheumatism could occur together:

> "Of this I have met with different well-marked instances where a flow of matter from the urethra has alternated with pains in the knees and other large joints[69]."

The condition was fully characterised by Brodie in 1818. Sir Benjamin Collins Brodie (1783–1862) was a surgeon at St George's Hospital, and the acknowledged head of the medical profession in London for 30 years. He had a particular interest in orthopaedic surgery, and wrote a classic work "Pathological and surgical observation on diseases of the joints," in which he described five patients with urethritis and polyarthritis[70]. In subsequent reports he mentioned that these features were sometimes accompanied by conjunctivitis or iritis.

Brodie and other commentators loosely referred to the urethritis which accompanied arthritis as "gonorrhoea" or "blennorrhagia," but it could not be characterised until after Neisser's discovery of the gonococcus in 1879. This made it possible to separate the septic arthritis of gonococcal septicaemia from the aseptic arthritis which accompanied *Gonorrhoea simplex*. Soon afterwards, the French physician Pierre-Émile Launois demonstrated an association between non-gonococcal urethritis, arthritis, iritis and keratoderma blennorrhagia, the skin eruption already described by Vidal[71]. In those days culture for *N. gonorrhoeae* was insensitive, and many physicians had a lingering suspicion that the laboratory diagnosis of their "non-gonococcal" cases might be erroneous.

In 1916 another case was described by Hans Reiter (1881–1969); he had studied medicine and hygiene at many of the leading European schools and was now professor of hygiene at the University of Berlin. His patient was a young Prussian soldier who developed non-gonococcal urethritis, polyarthritis and conjunctivitis after an attack of diarrhoea. Reiter mistakenly thought that it was a hitherto unknown spirochaetal infection, "spirochaetosis arthritica". On the strength of this report the syndrome has born Reiter's name ever since, although in the French literature it is called "Syndrome de Fiessinger – Leroy", after two workers who recorded an identical case, also in 1916; curiously enough, their patient and Reiter's fought on opposite sides in the Battle of the Somme. Subsequent studies indicated that the syndrome, whose nature was unknown, seemed to be initiated by an infection, enteric or venereal, the latter being non-gonococcal or (perhaps) gonococcal; the clinical features were the same whatever the nature of the preceding infection. Because of the two epidemiological forms of Reiter's syndrome, and the involvement of multiple organs and tissues, studies were inevitably piecemeal and distributed among many specialities; the result was a massive and rather unrewarding literature. It was unfortunate that from the beginning clear definitions were lacking, and the term Reiter's syndrome was sometimes applied to the complete triad and sometimes to cases of sterile reactive arthritis. The two syndromes are now generally considered together, although they may not have identical causes.

The first reports linking Reiter's syndrome with *C. trachomatis* appeared in the early 1960s; chlamydial inclusions were seen in urethral biopsies, the organisms were recovered by urethral culture, and there was serological evidence of recent infection[73]. It was later shown that more than one-third of patients with acute "venereal" Reiter's syndrome had a urethral chlamydial infection; there has been a continuing controversy about whether, or in what form, the organisms are present in affected joints. The role of *N. gonorrhoeae* continued to puzzle investigators. After the introduction of antibiotics it was observed that some patients with arthritis and gonococcal urethritis who were treated with penicillin had persistent urethritis and arthritis, although gonococci had been eliminated from the genital tract[74]; some, but not all of these men had a synchronous infection with *C. trachomatis*.

Studies performed during the last three decades have established that Reiter's syndrome/reactive arthritis can be initiated by *C. trachomatis*, and possibly *N. gonorrhoeae*; whether other sexually transmitted factors are involved remains unknown. The issue is complicated by the occurrence of the syndrome after enteric infections, inflammatory bowel disease and in some patients with no sign of any precipitating infection[75]. Twenty years ago it was shown that predisposition to the syndrome is strongly linked to the possession of the HLA B27 antigen. It has so far been impossible to make a coherent whole from these diverse factors.

Chapter 12
Venereologists and Others

All professions are conspiracies against the laity.
George Bernard Shaw, *The Doctor's Dilemma*

The first venereologists were probably surgeons. In the Middle Ages, barber surgeons provided much personal care: besides trimming hair and beards they extracted teeth, opened abscesses and set fractures. They were trained by apprenticeship, and organised into guilds. Physicians had a higher status. They had a long academic university training, and they saw themselves as observers and consultants rather than as practical medical workers. It was therefore natural that barber surgeons and surgeons should deal with genital ulcers and discharges, dilate urethral strictures and so on, while the physicians held themselves aloof from such mundane matters.

The situation changed when syphilis appeared in the late fifteenth century. Physicians asserted that since this was a systemic disease requiring internal medication with mercury, guaiacum and other drugs they, rather than surgeons, should have the responsibility[1]. This restrictive policy had no hope of success in the middle of a major epidemic when physicians were relatively few in number, and surgeons continued to prescribe internal medication for their syphilitic patients. As time went by surgeons objected to being associated with barbers. They developed a more elaborate system of training and eventually their own professional bodies, and barber surgeons disappeared. In many European countries venereology was linked with with dermatology; syphilis then became the concern of physicians, while surgeons continued to treat gonorrhoea and its complications. In Britain, the practice of venereology remained predominantly in the hands of surgeons until well into the nineteenth century, and they did not finally quit the speciality until modern times.

In the medieval world the Church bore the main responsibility for providing shelter and care for the sick in hospitals and almshouses; both St Thomas' and St Bartholomew's hospitals in London began as monastic institutions in the twelfth century. In the following centuries many large European cities, believing that medical care should also be a secular responsibility, built hospitals for their own citizens. The idea of a hospital as a place for curative treatment did not exist then. These institutions provided shelter and nursing care for people who were old, chronically sick or insane. Syphilis was then a florid disease, and its sufferers were often acutely ill and in great pain; many had widespread offensive skin ulcers. Hospitals were reluctant to admit these patients, and a system of "lock hospitals" was devised for them.

Lock Hospitals

In the early Middle Ages lazarettos had been built for the custodial care of lepers, and with the decline of leprosy these became available for the care of syphilitics. They became known as "lock hospitals" or "locks", a name which may have been derived from the French *loques*, rags used by lepers to wipe their sores before they entered. It was thought to be in the public interest that the "venereal" patients should be segregated from others, because they might be a source of infection or even moral corruption, and some new lock hospitals were built. One of the best known of these was the London Lock Hospital at Hyde Park Corner (Figure 12.1), which was opened in 1746[2]. This became a major centre for the treatment of venereal disease in the capital. A chapel was added to the main building in 1764. Many of the patients were prostitutes; their "reformation" was regarded as an important part of their management, and was encouraged by chapel services, sermons, tracts and so on. The area around the London Lock Hospital later became fashionable as Belgravia, and there were complaints about the presence of a hospital for venereal diseases. In 1841 the female beds were moved to Paddington and the male beds and out-patient department to Soho. The hospital survived until the advent of the National Health Service in 1948.

Lock hospitals run along similar lines were opened in many of the major cities of Britain and continental Europe. Their ambience was often punitive and coercive. For example, in 1864 the regulations for female patients in the "lock wards" of the Edinburgh Royal Infirmary laid down that those not confined to bed were expected to be in the work room by 10 a.m., with a cup of tea at 4 p.m. if they had been "diligent", letters not from relatives were opened by the matron and no visitors were allowed[3]. Nevertheless, although they were far from ideal

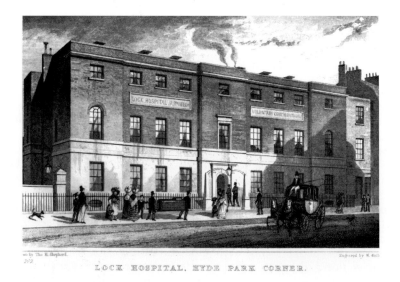

Figure 12.1. Lock Hospital, Hyde Park Corner, London. From a nineteenth century engraving. (By courtesy of the Wellcome Institute Library, London.)

the lock hospitals did provide care and treatment at a time when it was otherwise unavailable for many people.

Services for Venereal Diseases in General Hospitals

In the sixteenth century the facilities in most cities for the treatment of the large number of infected patients were sparse. In London, for example, St Thomas' Hospital had four "sweat wards"[4]. St Bartholomew's Hospital owned several locks, and in the main hospital William Clowes recorded that three-quarters of the beds were occupied by syphilitics. Many people were treated outside hospitals by individual doctors or by quacks, but some had no treatment at all. The situation dragged on in this way until the eighteenth century, when the modern hospital system began to develop. In Britain and the USA hospitals were built with private funds and managed by independent boards, but in continental Europe public funding and central government control were more usual. In London, several "voluntary" hospitals – whose consultants were unpaid – opened; these included Guy's, St George's, the Westminster and the Middlesex hospitals. Voluntary hospitals were pre-eminent in general medical and surgical care, but they were financed by private beneficiaries, and boards of management were uneasy about the disapproval which the provision of a venereal disease service might provoke. In London, some of the hospitals were prepared to treat small numbers of patients, but there was no consistent practice; the Middlesex Hospital opened and closed its "venereal" wards several times as opinions fluctuated[5]. Matters were even worse in provincial cities; for example, no beds were available in any of Liverpool's three hospitals. In Edinburgh, the first public hospital opened in 1729, and although the admission of infected patients was prohibited a "salivation room" for mercurial treatment was provided. A larger hospital, opened in 1750, had beds in a lock ward for female patients, although men were not admitted until 1884[3].

The Nineteenth Century

By the middle of the nineteenth century the incidence of infection was approaching its peak. There were not enough voluntary hospitals to care for the needs of patients with general medical and surgical conditions, let alone those with venereal diseases. The venereologist William Acton estimated that in 1856, when the population of London was 2.5 million, there were fewer than 300 hospital beds for these patients[6]. The lock hospitals were chronically underfunded and always running into financial difficulties; moreover, they were built only in some cities. Under the Poor Law Acts workhouses – public institutions in which the indigent received board and lodging in return for work done – were built. Some of these in larger towns had venereal wards; in others, infected patients were placed in the general sick wards. Many prostitutes who were destitute, infected or both had to be admitted – at one time it had been the custom to insist that they wore a distinctive yellow dress. Conditions in workhouses were dreadful, and medical care rudimentary[7].

Patients with venereal disease who could afford it had private medical treatment. Those who could not, or who felt too guilty and embarrassed to

173

see a doctor (or who wondered what reception they would get if they did), consulted quacks[8]. An advertisement for LEAKE's Patent Pills stated that the sole proprietor would give advice in his home to those taking the pills, observing in all cases "the most inviolable secrecy". It added reassuringly: "N.B. A back Door, and Lights in the Passage at Night". It is not difficult to see the attraction of quacks: they were discreet and uncensorious, and if their treatment was largely ineffective, at least their patients were not mercurialised; indeed a promise not to use mercury was often given in advertisements (Figure 12.2). Only a minority of practitioners treating patients with venereal diseases had any special knowledge or experience of the subject. For the most part they were surgeons whose major interests lay elsewhere, parish doctors and general practitioners. They have had a bad press, being presented as medical Sarah Gamps – ignorant, punitive and uncaring. Prostitutes in lock hospitals were certainly treated harshly, although doctors were sympathetic towards women who had been unwittingly infected by their husbands.

The ambivalence of the Victorians towards sex has been endlessly discussed in

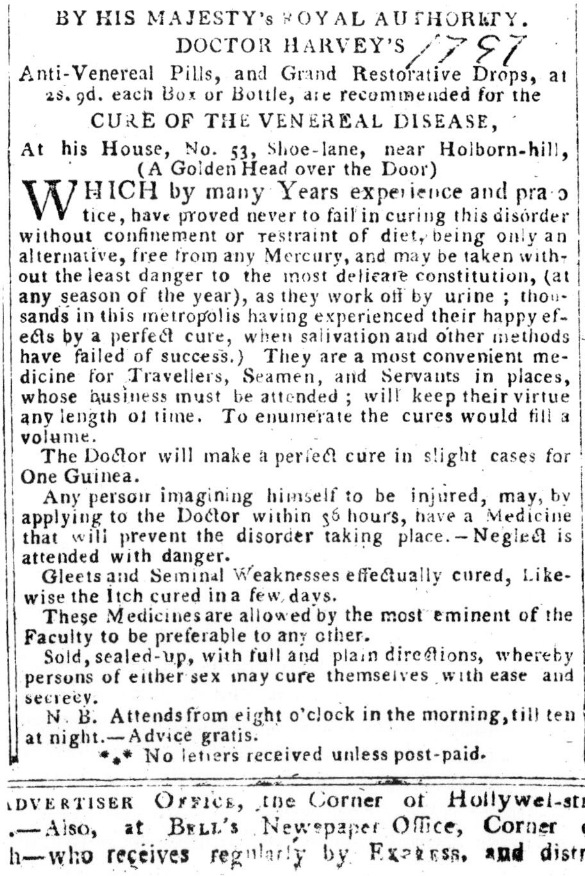

BY HIS MAJESTY's ROYAL AUTHORITY.
DOCTOR HARVEY'S *1797*
Anti-Venereal Pills, and Grand Restorative Drops, at
2s. 9d. each Box or Bottle, are recommended for the
CURE OF THE VENEREAL DISEASE,
At his House, No. 53, Shoe-lane, near Holborn-hill,
(A Golden Head over the Door)
WHICH by many Years experience and practice, have proved never to fail in curing this disorder without confinement or restraint of diet, being only an alternative, free from any Mercury, and may be taken without the least danger to the most delicate constitution, (at any season of the year), as they work off by urine; thousands in this metropolis having experienced their happy effects by a perfect cure, when salivation and other methods have failed of success.) They are a most convenient medicine for Travellers, Seamen, and Servants in places, whose business must be attended; will keep their virtue any length of time. To enumerate the cures would fill a volume.
The Doctor will make a perfect cure in slight cases for One Guinea.
Any person imagining himself to be injured, may, by applying to the Doctor within 56 hours, have a Medicine that will prevent the disorder taking place. – Neglect is attended with danger.
Gleets and Seminal Weaknesses effectually cured, Likewise the Itch cured in a few days.
These Medicines are allowed by the most eminent of the Faculty to be preferable to any other.
Sold, sealed-up, with full and plain directions, whereby persons of either sex may cure themselves with ease and secrecy.
N. B. Attends from eight o'clock in the morning, till ten at night. – Advice gratis.
. No letters received unless post-paid.

ADVERTISER OFFICE, the Corner of Hollywel-str
.—Also, at BELL's Newspaper Office, Corner o
h—who receives regularly by Express, and distri

Figure 12.2. Handbill advertising a proprietary medicine, 1797. (By courtesy of the Wellcome Institute Library, London.)

modern times. A part of this was to regard venereal disease as a moral rather than a medical problem, patients having brought their infection on themselves. This view was undoubtedly taken by many doctors, and reflected in their handling of patients who had infringed the current moral code. Nevertheless, a sweeping condemnation of the medical profession in this matter seems unfair. The doctors were struggling to cure their patients and contain an epidemic with no laboratory tests, little effective treatment and virtually no support from the authorities or indeed from their own colleagues. It is charitable to assume that, like other doctors, they did the best they could with the resources available. A Victorian surgeon called Samuel Solly (1805–1871), not a venereologist, made a notorious remark to a government committee investigating syphilis that it was "intended as a punishment for our sins and we should not interfere in the matter"[9]. This was typical of the puritanism of the time. We may reflect that in other eras both before and after the nineteenth century the general attitude towards sex and venereal disease was much more tolerant. In 1662 the vicar of Stratford-on-Avon treated some of his parishioners for gonorrhoea and apparently thought nothing of it[10].

British venereology never developed the close links with dermatology which occurred in other European countries, and attempts made in a few hospitals to combine the two were unsuccessful. Jonathan Hutchinson, one of the greatest nineteenth century syphilologists, mastered both disciplines. He was one of the "big five" of dermatology in London at the turn of the century, the others being Radcliffe Crocker at University College Hospital, Colcott Fox at Westminster Hospital, Malcolm Morris at St Mary's Hospital and John James Pringle at the Middlesex Hospital. These men had a large experience of syphilis in their hospital and private practices, but none of them was interested in gonorrhoea. Syphilis was a fascinating disease, presenting major clinical and intellectual challenges, but the great syphilologists found gonorrhoea, genital sores and discharges too "venereal"; they were happy to leave the management of these to surgeons and gynaecologists.

The inevitable result of the fragmentation of venereology and the lack of beds in teaching hospitals was that instruction of medical students in the subject was lamentable. Louis Wickham, a French dermatovenereologist, visited London in 1889. He remarked that students appeared indifferent to the subject; for prudish reasons patients were separated and put to one side, and were little used for teaching. He added that English specialists were unanimous in wanting to change this state of affairs[11]. Their concern at a time when so much venereal disease was being treated by practitioners who knew very little about the subject is understandable; it was obviously important that medical students should be well taught, but this did not happen for many years.

In England there were no consultants in venereology or syphilology, and no academic departments devoted, directly or indirectly, to these subjects. A writer in 1851 was "at a loss to point out what science has gained by the writings of the London surgeons on syphilis since the commencement of the present century"[12]. This remark was made in an unfavourable review of "A practical treatise of the urinary and generative organs of both sexes" by William Acton (1813–1875), a prolific and successful author of books on venereology and related subjects: sexual behaviour (in men), illegitimacy and prostitution. Acton had studied under Ricord and had an appointment at the Female Venereal Clinic in Paris. In London, he was at one time surgeon to the Islington Dispensary, and he had a large private practice. He was an experienced physician and a gifted social observer, but he did not engage in research or scientific enquiry; perhaps this is why his name is now forgotten. Indeed, in Britain there were no notable figures in the subject between Benjamin Bell, who died in 1806, and Jonathan Hutchinson, who published his first paper on syphilis in 1857. The management of patients was rooted in tradition and inhibited by moral stigmas, and no serious scientific research on the subject was done until the turn of the century.

The Twentieth Century

The sombre and depressing state of British venereology was much improved after the report of the Royal Commission on Venereal Diseases was published in 1917 (see Chapter 13). One of its major recommendations was that special clinics for the free and confidential treatment of venereal diseases should be established by local authorities in all large towns, and venereal disease officers appointed to run them. The administrative problems of creating and staffing these clinics and blending them with existing facilities were immense. Hospital management committees did not welcome the arrival of large numbers of "venereal" patients, and often provided accommodation of poor quality, located in out-of-the-way corners and dingy basements. The staffing of the clinics became easier after the war when doctors and technicians who had had experience of treating the diseases in servicemen became available. Physicians in charge of the larger clinics were assisted by doctors from other branches of medicine employed on a sessional basis, and by members of a new grade of technicians in venereology, derived from the special treatment assistants of the Royal Army Medical Corps, who undertook most of the routine microscopy and treatment. Some hospitals made no more than a gesture at providing a venereal disease service, a dermatologist treating syphilis, a surgeon gonorrhoea in men and a gynaecologist infections in women, often on different days and in different parts of the hospital; it is hard to imagine a more unsatisfactory arrangement.

The new service was greatly influenced by the appointment in 1919 of Colonel Harrison (Figure 12.3) as adviser on venereal diseases to the new Ministry of Health. Lawrence Whitaker Harrison (1876–1964)[13] was born in Lancashire and received his medical education in Glasgow. Two years after qualification he joined the Army Medical Serivces, where he was taught and perhaps influenced by Almroth Wright, who was professor of pathology in the Army Medical School at the time. He saw active service in South Africa and India, and on his return to England in 1909 was appointed bacteriologist to the military hospital at Rochester Row. This was an old military hospital now devoted entirely to the treatment of infected soldiers and the education of army medical officers in venereology[14]. Harrison soon developed a major interest in venereal diseases; he improved the sensitivity of the Wassermann reaction and studied the treatment of syphilis with mercurials and the new arsenicals. When the First World War began in 1914 he served at the front until in 1915 he was ordered to command a hospital in France assigned to the treatment of venereal diseases which was being badly run by officers with no knowledge or experience of the subject. In 1916 he returned to England to command Rochester Row Hospital and was appointed adviser on venereal diseases to the War Office. He continued in these duties until the end of the war, when he retired from the army.

Harrison's clinical, scientific and administrative experience made him ideal for

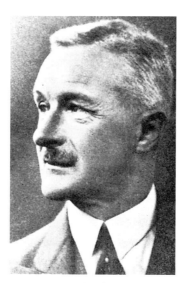

Figure 12.3. Lawrence Whitaker Harrison (1876–1964).

the Ministry of Health appointment, but before accepting it he insisted that he should also direct one of the new treatment centres, so that his advice would be based on first-hand experience. This was agreed, and a model centre to his design was built at St Thomas' Hospital[15]. There were separate male and female clinics, and at a later date in-patient facilities and a maternity ward were added. The centre was intended to ensure rapid diagnosis and treatment under conditions of privacy; it was open from 8 a.m. to 8 p.m. for six days a week and on Sunday mornings. Harrison was aware from personal experience of the importance of microbiology, and a laboratory was attached to the clinic in which two full-time pathologists worked until the outbreak of the Second World War. He retired from St Thomas' in 1936, but continued his work at the Ministry of Health until 1947; Like Ricord, he maintained his interest in venereology into old age. During his formative years Harrison had been a soldier. He was slow to adapt to the idea of peaceful persuasion, and although he was courteous and approachable his rigidity and single-mindedness did not always endear him to his colleagues. On the other hand, the young speciality needed leadership, and he provided it. He visited clinics throughout the country, suggesting improvements and giving advice and help. In his heyday he was a formidable figure – the first British physician to devote virtually his whole career to the speciality – and the influence of "Colonel Harrison" can be detected even today, 45 years after his death.

During the 1920s the quality of the new venereal disease service in Britain was gradually improved by better out-patient accommodation and some provision for in-patients. Laboratory services were expanded, and a central Venereal Disease Reference Laboratory established in 1924. This progress was marred by the conditions in some of the lock hospitals, which had been allowed to deteriorate by their boards of management. The surgeon in charge of the Edinburgh lock in 1918 described it as "an awful place"; as late as 1920 all treatment of men was done in one small theatre so overcrowded that privacy, asepsis and detailed examination were impossible[3]. Harrison, supported by many eminent

177

people, including the Archbishop of Canterbury and the chief medical officer to the Ministry of Health, made repeated complaints about conditions in the London Lock Hospital: poor facilities, indifferent medical management and a repressive moralistic regime. Eventually, after 10 years of pressure, some improvements were grudgingly introduced[16]. The venereal disease service was improved when the Poor Law was reformed in 1928. Many of the old Poor Law hospitals were upgraded to become municipal hospitals which provided medical care comparable with that of the large voluntary hospitals, and venereal disease clinics shared in this process.

The layout of the clinics changed very little between the wars. Their walls were tiled in white or painted in "hospital green". In the male clinics the apparatus for urethral irrigations were conspicuous (Figure 12.4), and in the female clinics the examination couches were fitted with various types of stirrup to facilitate pelvic examinations. Otherwise, the equipment was minimal[17]: "record" or glass syringes for taking blood or giving injections, hypodermic needles (periodically sharpened on a whetstone), a set of urethral sounds and perhaps a urethroscope, and vaginal speculae. All this equipment was sterilised on the premises. In addition, most clinics had apparatus for light-field and dark-field microscopy. Although some laboratories claimed good results with simple media, culture for *N. gonorrhoeae* was generally regarded as unreliable until selective media were introduced in the 1960s. Serological tests for syphilis were available everywhere. In those days treatment made heavy demands on the clinic staff. The intravenous injection of arsenicals needed time and skill (although one venereologist claimed that he could administer 25 doses of arsphenamine in an hour); toxic reactions were common, and could be serious. Urethral irrigations for urethritis needed care, and complications such as epididymitis and urethral stricture gave many problems. The treatment of women was delicate, difficult and time-consuming. As time went by venereology became the main interest of doctors working in clinics rather than a supplementary source of income for those with main commitments elsewhere. At the same time, more physicians were attracted into the speciality and the predominance of surgeons as venereologists, which had continued for

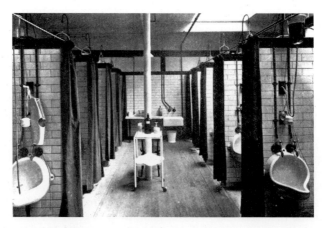

Figure 12.4. Seamen's Dispensary, Liverpool, opened in 1924. The curtained cubicles were for irrigation and other treatment. (By courtesy of Dr O.P. Arya and Dr J.B. Plumb.)

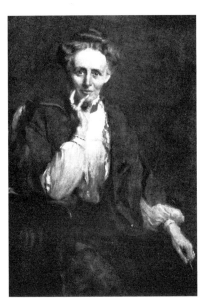

Figure 12.5. Mary Scharlieb (1845–1930). (By courtesy of the Wellcome institute Library, London.)

hundreds of years, began to decline. Despite this, in the 1930s the London Lock Hospital still maintained a strict rule that members of the consultant staff should be Fellows of the Royal College of Surgeons. In 1948 the National Health Service came into being, and the venereal disease service became a national rather than a local responsibility. Venereologists now received the appointments, pay and status of physicians and surgeons in other specialities, the culmination of the slow progress which had begun, centuries before, with the medieval barber surgeons.

Until the middle of the nineteenth century the medical profession was reserved for men. The first woman doctor of modern times was Elizabeth Blackwell, who obtained a degree in New York in 1849. In England, Elizabeth Garrett Anderson was licensed in 1865. The Women's Medical College in Pennsylvania opened in 1850, and medical courses for women began in London in 1866. Despite immense difficulties some women graduates began to practise obstetrics and gynaecology, and inevitably became involved to some extent in the problems of venereal disease. A distinguished example was provided by the career of Dame Mary Scharlieb (1845–1930; Figure 12.5). She worked first in India, then at the New Hospital for Women (now the Elizabeth Garrett Anderson Hospital) in London as a consultant gynaecologist[18]. Her concern for the effects of venereal diseases on the health and fertility of women was expressed not only in her clinical work but in her interest in the social aspects of the infections and in their prevention by health and sexual education. Although she did not operate until she was over 40 she became a skilful and resourceful surgeon. She was immensely popular, and the word was that a woman with a difficult gynaecological problem would always be wise to "see what Mrs Scharlieb thinks". Tactful and sympathetic, she would have been an excellent venereologist. Female doctors were slow to take up venereology; for a long time it was unthinkable that a woman should examine

179

a male "venereal" patient, although the reverse situation was quite acceptable. During the 1930s women began to practise in the speciality, often after beginning their careers in public health. Their number increased during the Second World War, when many servicewomen required specialist treatment, and from the 1950s onwards women doctors began to adopt venereology as their first career choice.

Continental Europe

In continental Europe venereology pursued a different course. Venereal diseases were seen as a public health responsibility earlier than in Britain. In Russia, Catherine the Great established the world's first hospital exclusively for the care of patients with these diseases at St Petersburg in 1770[19], and a few years later Denmark became the first country to provide free treatment from public health medical officers[20]. In many European towns there were lock houses and clinics for the examination of prostitutes. The relationship between dermatology and venereology in Europe is long and complex. In the eighteenth century skin and venereal diseases were, as in Britain, handled mostly by surgeons. In France after the Revolution, medical services were reorganised; dermatology then became a part of internal medicine, but venereology remained the concern of surgeons. Since dermatologists saw many patients with syphilis it was inevitable that the two specialities should coalesce, and departments of dermatovenereology were established in some of the reformed or newly built hospitals[21].

In Paris the ancient l'Hôpital St Louis became a hospital which specialised in skin diseases. Jean Louis Alibert (1766–1837) was appointed to the staff, and set out to study the "uncharted ocean of disease"; through him the hospital became a major centre for clinical services and study. The dermatology service expanded under a series of masters who included Bazin, Vidal, Besnier and Sabouraud. All of them, although primarily dermatologists, had experience of syphilis, but in due course a section for venereal diseases was added (Figure 12.6); its most illustrious director was to be Alfred Fournier (1842–1914), a pupil of Philippe Ricord. Ricord himself had been appointed in 1831 to l'Hôpital du Midi, a run-down institution for venereal diseases in rue St Jacques; he transformed the hospital, and with it the practice of venereology. It was financed by the civil authorities, not – as in Britain – by charitable donations. At its peak it had 400 beds, all for men[22]; treatment of in-patients was free, but out-patients were expected to pay for their medicines. Ricord's scientific work, his teaching skill and his personal charisma made venereology a valuable discipline in the eyes of his colleagues; as well as Fournier his pupils included Bassereau, Clerc, Diday and Rollet, who were active not only in Paris but in Lyon and other cities.

These events in France were paralleled in other countries. In eighteenth-century Vienna, syphilitics were treated at the Spital zu St Marx, evidently a dismal place where "in one part of the building the insane lie in chains, and in another there is a room with an inscription over the entrance 'For women rendered unfortunate by love'"[23]. Nevertheless, there was the beginning of a school of dermatovenereology under van Swieten, who occupied the chair of medicine and Josef von Plenck (1733–1807), a surgeon turned venereologist, whose treatise on the subject featured a new mercurial with the strange name *mercurius gummosus Plenckii*.

The next generation of Viennese masters in the field was headed by Ferdinand

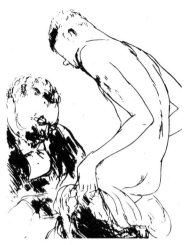

Figure 12.6. Medical examination at the Hôpital St Louis: André Dunoyer de Segonzac. From Vogt H (1960) Medizinische Karikature von 1800 bis zur Gegenwart. (By courtesy of Springer-Verlag, Heidelberg.)

Hebra (1816–1880). He began his career in dermatology in the "rash room", an annexe of the Allgemeine Krankenhaus where patients with intractable dermatoses were housed. Like Alibert, Hebra was fascinated by the diversity of skin diseases. He studied them systematically and in due course became renowned as a clinician and teacher, and was appointed to a chair in 1849. Although he was a strong advocate of mercury he was not much involved with syphilis, but in 1849 a syphilis clinic was formed under Carl Sigmund (1810–1883), an energetic, witty and charming physician. Unusually for the time, he was interested in gonorrhoea as well as syphilis; he was another strong advocate of mercurial treatment for syphilis, both by inunction and with Zittmann's decoction, a weird mixture of sarsaparilla, aniseed, senna and mercury sublimate. Hebra was succeeded by his son-in-law Moriz Kaposi (1837–1902), a clinician of immense skill who wrote a treatise on syphilis, and Sigmund by Isidor Neumann (1832–1906), another pupil of Hebra. It was said of Neumann that he knew more about syphilis than any of his contemporaries with the possible exception of Fournier, and he was a firm believer in the unity of the specialities, saying that it was impossible to be a good dermatologist without a knowledge of syphilis, or a good venereologist without a knowledge of dermatology[24]. He was not the first, and by no means the last, to hold this opinion. Ernest Finger (1856–1939; Figure 12.7) succeeded Neumann as director of the University Syphilis Clinic. Although he wrote extensively on other diseases, his *magnum opus* was his book on gonorrhoea (*Die Blennorrhoe der Sexualorgane und ihre Complicationen*), a classic which first appeared in 1888. Short and slender, he gave an impression of "delicacy and gentleness"[25]. Under this succession of eminent physicians, the Viennese centre was enormously influential and attracted visitors from all over the world – to the chagrin of the heads of departments and clinics in northern Europe, particularly France.

In Germany, the treatment of patients with venereal diseases was shared between private practitioners, municipal clinics and, in major cities such as Berlin, Bonn, Breslau, Munich and Wurzburg, at university centres of dermatovenereology. The Charité Hospital in Berlin was founded in 1727, and in 1844 Carl Simon (1810–1857) established a successful syphilis clinic there, which was followed by a department of dermatology. Simon died at the age of 46 years of general paresis, and was succeeded by Friedrich von Baerensprung (1822–1864)[26], who was a true dermatovenereologist, dermatology occupying the beginning and syphilology the end of his professional life. Like Neisser, he incurred public hostility for some experiments with syphilis inoculations, and he was unlike most of his contemporaries in completely forbidding the use of mercury in his clinic. He too died of general paresis. His successor was Edmund Lesser (1852–1918), who is best remembered as being director of the department when *T. pallidum* was discovered by Schaudinn and Hoffmann in 1905. Lesser was in charge of both the skin and venereal clinics at the Charité Hospital, and under him at the turn of the century Berlin reached its peak as a centre of teaching and research in both these subjects.

Vienna had been the centre most favoured for training doctors in dermatovenereology, but the skin clinic at Breslau, founded in 1877 by Heinrich Kobner, soon became no less influential under the direction of Oscar Simon and his successor Albert Neisser. Many of Neisser's pupils went on to become directors of skin clinics and university departments, among them Jadassohn (his successor), Buschke and Herxheimer. Neisser believed that every university should have a clinic for syphilis and skin diseases, so that undergraduates and postgraduates could be properly taught. The two disciplines should be closely united, and if the workload became too heavy for a single clinic he would sooner duplicate the clinic than divide the subjects[27]. This opinion was not uniformly held. Unna thought that the practice of combining dermatology with syphilology diminished the effectiveness of teaching programmes, because the size of the syphilis problem and the intense interest of government in its suppression might monopolise the professor's time. A similar problem has occurred in the late twentieth century when, particularly in large cities, the size of the AIDS problem threatens to

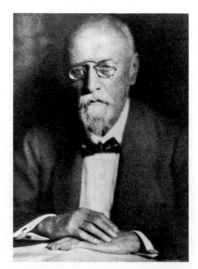

Figure 12.7. Ernest Finger (1856–1939).

182

diminish the care and resources required for the treatment of "traditional" infections. In Europe, therefore, clinical studies by the great French, German and Austrian physicians prepared the ground for the advances in bacteriology of the late nineteenth century. Although relations were sometimes strained, the linkage of dermatology and venereology in university departments provided not only a secure academic basis for the work (which was never achieved in England) but also many clinical departments of the highest quality, adequate teaching and a reasonable uniformity of clinical practice.

In the New World

In its early days American venereology was greatly influenced by European practice. Translations of the works of the British, French and German masters – Hunter, Bell, Ricord, Fournier, Neisser and Neumann – were available soon after their original publication, and American dermatologists often studied in European centres. In the expansion of medical services after the Civil War (1861–1865) many medical schools founded departments of dermatology, where syphilis occupied part of the teaching programme; in others skin diseases, syphilis and genito-urinary surgery were combined as a single speciality. Sometimes, clinical services and teaching for venereal diseases were scattered between departments of internal medicine, surgery and obstetrics and gynaecology, and suffered accordingly.

The first true venereologist in the United States was Freeman Josiah Bumstead (1826–1879)[28]. He studied medicine at Harvard Medical School and in Paris, then took a circuitous route to venereology via general practice, ophthalmology and otology. He was appointed visiting dermatologist to the New York City Hospital in 1866, and subsequently professor of venereal diseases at the College of Physicians and Surgeons. In 1861 he wrote a monumental textbook, *The Pathology and Treatment of Venereal Diseases*, which went through many editions and was much admired in Europe. At the age of 45 years, although he was by now an experienced and successful physician, he felt the need to improve his knowledge of dermatology and returned to Europe, where he was to be seen sitting with several of his former pupils on the front bench in Hebra's clinic in Vienna. Bumstead was a handsome man with a full dark beard; his appearance was dignified and scholarly, but he was relaxed and genial with his friends. He died at the early age of 53 years.

Bumstead's colleague and later successor Robert William Taylor (1842–1908) had an unusual career, even for a venereologist. He was born in Coventry, in England, and emigrated to the United States as a child. He first became a licensed pharmacist and ran a highly successful business before studying medicine in New York. In due course he became professor of dermatology at the New York Postgraduate Medical School, and in 1879 joined Bumstead as co-author of a revised edition of his textbook; in later revisions he became sole author. Taylor made his name in venereology as the first to describe neonatal syphilitic dactylitis, but he was an expert dermatologist – more so than Bumstead – and published a massive *Atlas of Venereal and Skin Diseases* in 1889. He wielded a sharp pen at times, and his former colleague G.H. Fox summed him up succinctly: "Bob Taylor – a man of strong antipathies and fond of scraps, but he had a warm heart"[29].

The third member of this trio of notable American venereologists, and in some ways the most influential, was Prince Albert Morrow (1846–1913)[30]. Morrow's first name, like that of a distinguished modern venereologist, did not mean that he was of royal blood. He was born in Kentucky and received his medical education in New York. He then spent two years studying dermatology in Europe before starting practice in New York, and soon became professor of dermatology and genito-urinary diseases at New York University. Morrow was a dermatovenereologist of the European kind, with a major interest in syphilis. Like Fournier, whose *Syphilis and Marriage* he translated into English, he became increasingly involved in the social aspects of venereal disease, and in 1905 he founded the American Society of Sanitary and Moral Prophylaxis. Morrow had a magisterial and dictatorial manner which some attributed to his early days as a school teacher.

These serious and dignified physicians were, on occasion, able to relax. Fox has left an irresistible account of meetings of the New York Dermatological Society in the 1870s, at a time when Bumstead, Taylor and Morrow were members:

"In the early days of our Society, the collation or supper which followed each meeting was a much more elaborate affair than the simple "spread" of the present day. Midnight invariably found us eating and drinking, while the discussion of various topics and the telling of stories by members and guests often lasted through the night. I remember Dr Allan McLane Hamilton in particular used to pop in after the adjournment of our regular meeting and entertain us by the hour with his brilliant stories and vaudeville impersonations, while Dr William T. Bull favoured us with a song on many occasions . . . Of one member who never showed any cases nor uttered a word in the discussions of those shown by others Dr Otis once made a remark which I can never forget. He said he had never known this quiet member to open his mouth except to put in an oyster[29]."

Between the end of the Civil War and the turn of the century immense progress in American dermatology and venereology was made: new specialised journals and textbooks were published, new academic departments established, and a group of enthusiastic and dedicated physicians, many with European training, prepared the ground for the later flowering of the specialities. The obverse of this rosy picture was the state of clinical services for patients with venereal diseases during this time. A basic hospital system had been established by the middle of the nineteenth century, largely financed by subscriptions and public donations. Unfortunately, there was the same partial or complete exclusion of "venereal" patients as occurred in England. In 1822, for example, the Massachusetts General Hospital prohibited their admission, and similar policies were in force in other cities[31].

There were some institutions which cared for patients with venereal diseases, alcoholics and others regarded as socially undesirable; in its early days the New York City Hospital was one of these, and at one time was considered as a possible venereal disease hospital[32], although facilities were poor. The advent of arsenicals for the treatment of syphilis forced a reconsideration of the situation, and from 1910 onwards increasing numbers of patients were admitted to the medical wards of hospitals for treatment. Many doctors, while accepting the need for in-patient beds, were bitterly opposed to the establishment of out-patient clinics by boards of health. Their motive may have been partly financial, as patients attending public clinics would be lost to private practice. In 1914 the New York Department of Health succeeded in opening a clinic, but this was for the diagnosis of venereal diseases only; treatment was expressly forbidden.

Between the end of the 1914–1918 war and the early 1930s public services for venereal diseases in the United States were in the doldrums. Clinics were scarce, of poor quality, crowded and unpleasant. Some "pay clinics" were established in which the cost of treatment was less than that charged by private practitioners, but patients still felt that they were being stigmatised and the clinics were not popular. Investigation and treatment of high quality was provided by university departments of dermatology and venereology, but these were few and far between. In effect, most venereal disease was treated by private practitioners, but many doctors were poorly trained in venereology because the university authorities did not think the subject was important; many clinicians, like their colleagues in Europe, regarded the subject as uninteresting and unlikely to improve their professional standing. The result was that even patients who could afford to pay might find themselves lobbed between dermatologists, urologists and gynaecologists, nobody having overall responsibility for their management. As in Europe, many turned to quacks or home remedies. Matters remained in this unsatisfactory state until the crusade of Thomas Parran and his associates in the mid 1930s forced a revision of national policy (see Chapter 13). Ironically this period, when clinical services for patients with venereal disease were often of poor quality, was distinguished by a series of outstanding syphilologists.

In 1915 Johns Hopkins Hospital established a clinic entirely devoted to the clinical and experimental study of syphilis; it was called "Department L" ("L" standing for lues), because at that time the word syphilis was taboo. The clinic grew rapidly, and in 1929 Joseph Earle Moore (Figure 12.8) became director. He was a general physician, but syphilis was his greatest interest and the subject of all his research. He established a system of treatment with alternating courses of arsenic and bismuth lasting for 70 weeks, elucidated the natural history of

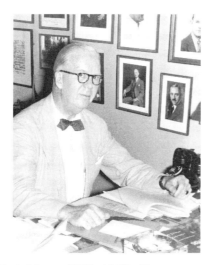

Figure 12.8. Joseph Earle Moore (1892–1958). (By courtesy of Mr Ambrose J. King.)

neurosyphilis and recognised the association of false-positive serological tests for syphilis with various acute and chronic diseases. Towards the end of his career he was involved in the development of penicillin therapy. He was equally well known on both sides of the Atlantic, particularly in Britain where he influenced a whole generation of venereologists. Although of a warm and generous nature he had a sharp wit, defining an expert as "a son of a bitch from some other city, usually Washington"[33].

Doctors and Patients

Doctors have been attending to patients with venereal diseases for a very long time. What did they think of each other? To answer this question we must turn not only to medical literature but to lay writers. Society's attitude to venereal diseases reflects its attitude to sex. In the sixteenth century the English surgeon William Clowes spoke of this "pestilent infection of filthy lust", and it is hard to imagine that he was very sympathetic to his patients. Yet by the time of the Restoration in the following century venereal disease was taken as a matter of course, and the dramatists of the day brought it into many of their comedies. In the eighteenth century venereal disease was seen by lay writers as a misfortune, but no disgrace; doctors tried to help their patients, but as so often in the history of medicine they were suspected of having one eye on the financial reward they could expect. James Boswell described a consultation with his surgeon friend Andrew Douglas:

> "After breakfast Mrs Douglas withdrew and I opened my sad case to Douglas, who upon examining the parts declared I had got an evident infection . . . I joked with my friend about the expense, asked him if he would take my note for what I was unable to pay, and bid him visit me seldom that I might have the less to pay. To these jokes he seemed to give little heed, but talked seriously in the way of his business[34]."

Needless to say, Boswell's jokes did not stop Douglas from submitting an account. Even university professors were not beyond reproach. In a letter written in 1763 the Scottish novelist Tobias Smollett (1721–1771) described "The celebrated Professor –, the Boerhaave of Montpellier", who had a large practice in venereology. "I have reason to think", he said, "that Professor – has cured many patients who were never infected"[35].

A rather different picture was painted by those who knew the great Scottish surgeon and venereologist Benjamin Bell (1749–1805). His contemporary James Wardrop wrote:

> "His manner was devoid of every kind of affection – simple and unostentatious. He was of a kindly disposition, and in stating his opinion made use of plain but very accurate language . . . giving great assurance and confidence to the sick[36]."

Bell certainly seems to have taken endless trouble with his patients, making no distinction between those with venereal diseases and those with other conditions. He related that on one occasion he rode 20 miles on horseback to see a worried newly wed man with a mild non-specific urethritis. He was entirely tolerant of his patients' sexual peccadillos and passed no judgments. Philippe Ricord (1800–1889), the greatest clinical venereologist of his time, was a man of the world: he understood and sympathised with his patients' problems. The American doctor and litterateur Oliver Wendell Holmes (1809–1894), who had met him in Paris, wrote:

> "When an inexperienced youth visits Paris for the first time, succumbs to temptation and awakes in trouble one fine morning, he can hardly do better than take a cabriolet and drive to the residence of M. Ricord. No man will handle his feelings or his person more tenderly . . . no man will send him away in a state of such philosophical acquiescence[37]."

No doubt Ricord's easygoing attitude to venereal diseases was one reason for his large hospital and private practice. He became well known not only to his colleagues but to the man in the street, as this story shows:

> "During the Commune in 1871, as Ricord was driving one day to Passy in his elaborate coach with a gold-liveried coachman he was stopped by a squad of Federals intent on maltreating a rich bourgeois. Asked his name, Ricord replied 'I am Ricord! Who did you think I was?' At this name, well known and popular with the masses, the affair took a comic turn. 'Well, well', said one of the comrades, 'is he really Ricord?' 'Do you believe him?' asked another. A third man, all excitement, cried out 'Yes, that's Ricord, I recognise him!' Then, while they all shouted 'Hurrah for Ricord,' one man wrote the words 'Property of the Nation' on the back of the coach, and Ricord drove off[38]."

To be sure, there were many well-known venereologists after Ricord, but they lacked his persona and charm. In any case, times were changing. By the end of the nineteenth and the first decade of the twentieth centuries the venereal diseases were the same, but the attitude of society – shared by many medical men – was completely different. The indulgence of Bell and Ricord had disappeared. The diseases were now seen, if not as a punishment, at least as a stigma of moral transgression. Hence Solly's notorious remark that syphilis was a self-inflicted punishment for sin and that "we should not interfere in the matter". It was inevitable that in this climate of opinion the relationship between doctor and patient should suffer. It is tiresome to read of people striking moral attitudes, and perhaps a visit to Ricord's clinic may provide an antidote. William Acton went to the Midi on Easter Monday, 1850, and described the master in action:

> "The brotherly feeling of Ricord towards his patients is seldom abused: he will laugh at, or with, one patient, and ridicule another's fears. Students will participate in his mirth, and the patient will smile . . . Let a patient, however, fail to follow the prescribed routine, the light raillery gives place to just indignation, and he receives such a public admonition as serves as a warning to the inmates of the whole ward, who equally respect the kindness and talent of the Professor[22]."

Undoubtedly some venereologists were inclined to pass judgments on their patients' behaviour, but most were content to do their best "to repair the misdeeds of Venus Vulgivata", as Vertue has charmingly put it, and to leave moral strictures to others. Of course they grumbled – all professional people do – but their complaints were not about moral issues. They complained of being overworked, of poor facilities and of the behaviour of their colleagues. There were other problems. Wansey Baily, a well-known specialist in his day and a consultant at St George's Hospital, wrote to *The Lancet* in 1932 about a financial problem:

> "Because treatment at clinics is free, the [private] practice of many specialists is reduced to vanishing point, so that the state loses their income tax as well as funding unnecessarily large and numerous clinics ... The venereal specialist sees ruin staring him in the face[39]."

In the days before the need for antisepsis was realised, doctors did not protect their hands in the post-mortem room or the operating theatre and some contracted syphilis, as their successors contract hepatitis B or HIV infection today. Among the unwitting victims were several well-known figures. Friedrich von Baerensprung died of general paresis, an unfortunate father and son, Herman and Maximilian von Zeissl, who practised venereology in Vienna, both died of neurosyphilis which followed infections contracted during minor surgery, and James Lane, a surgeon at St Mary's and the London Lock Hospitals, died of tabes dorsalis after many years' suffering.

Professional Colleagues

How did the venereologists' colleagues regard them and their speciality? Undoubtedly to many of them venereal diseases were distasteful, their treatment stereotyped and those who practised this branch of medicine inferior people. John Bloxam (1844–1926) was a surgeon at the London Lock Hospital who specialised in the repair of nasal deformities caused by tertiary syphilis; his obituarist observed that "it has been regretted that a man with such gifts for general surgery should have early specialised in venereal disease"[40]. Despite his distinction in the field, Harrison was never elected a member of the medical committee at St Thomas' Hospital. Writing in 1930 the distinguished American syphilogist John Stokes put the matter in this way:

> "Have you ever leaned over the rail of a liner at sea as the captain, resplendent in gold braid and flanked by his aides, comes down the deck? And, leaning out further, have you seen the grimy head of a stoker pop through a scuttle just above the water line? In the contrast you can see the status of venereology[41]."

Some venereologists accepted their lot and, as one put it, "went about their business in an aura of subdued anonymity". Others simply denied their calling. Sir Alfred Cooper (1839–1908) was a surgeon at St Bartholomew's and the London Lock Hospitals. He became "the best kind of society surgeon", and was well known for his skill and tact in treating venereal diseases, particularly among the aristocracy. He co-authored a book on syphilis which went into two editions, married well and left a fortune. Yet his obituarist in the *British Medical*

Journal could not bring himself to call Cooper a venereologist, almost as though this was something shameful:

> "For many years he was surgeon to the Lock Hospital, where he acquired great practical experience in the treatment of the important class of disorders for the relief of which that institution was designed[42]."

William Acton was well known in his day, but the British Medical Journal published only a report on the circumstances of his death (from coronary thrombosis), and nothing about his career. Continental venereologists also suffered from their colleagues' disapproval. Even in Paris, where the attitude to sex was quite tolerant, Ricord had to wait for 20 years before he was admitted through the portals of the Academy of Medicine, while Neisser did not become a full professor in Breslau for 25 years after being appointed assistant professor.

In an issue of *The Tatler* in 1710 the essayist Richard Steele (1672–1729) referred to Gaspare Tagliacozzi, a sixteenth-century pioneer in the surgical repair of nasal defects caused by syphilis, as "the earliest clap doctor in history"[35]. Steele was confusing gonorrhoea with syphilis, and "clap doctor" became "love doctor" in later editions. Its final version was "pox doctor", a term which has irritated many generations of venereologists. However, better times were coming for those ministering to patients with "the scars of Venus".

Chapter 13
Public Health Matters

Can love be controll'd by advice?
John Gay, *Acis and Galatea*

During the last century there has been a spectacular control of infectious diseases. Smallpox is now extinct, and in developed countries cholera, malaria, diphtheria, poliomyelitis and other diseases which formerly caused many deaths have been virtually eliminated. This has been achieved first, by improving the environment through sanitary action and second, by protecting the individual by immunisation or personal hygienic measures. Venereal diseases, however, are not adequately controlled. A comprehensive review of the history of this complex matter throughout the world cannot be attempted here; instead, we will consider some key points, successes and failures, in the long struggle.

Europe from the Twelfth to the Eighteenth Century

Efforts to control the spread of venereal diseases began in the Middle Ages. In Southwark, near the City of London, an ordinance of 1162 prohibited the owners of brothels from keeping any woman "who hath any sickness of *brenning* but that she be put out upon the peyne of makeit unto the Lord a fine of a hundred shillings"[1]. The "lord" in this case was the Bishop of Winchester, whose palace was then at Southwark and who owned the land on which there were no less than 18 brothels. How the bishop felt about his role in these matters is not recorded, but the expression "bitten by a Winchester goose" to describe someone who had contracted a venereal disease was still in use in Shakespeare's time. A comparable decree was issued by Joan I, Queen of Sicily, in 1343:

> "The Queen commands that the Superintendent and a surgeon appointed by the authorities examine, every Saturday, all the whores in the houses of prostitution. And if one is found who has contracted a disease from coitus, she shall be separated from the rest and live apart, in order that she be prevented from conveying the disease to the young men[2]."

During the epidemic of the fifteenth and sixteenth centuries the sequestration of syphilitics was enforced under the old quarantine laws. The rich had to stay in their houses and the poor were driven away, threatened with death and abandoned, even by their doctors. A law of James IV of Scotland in 1497 required patients affected with *Grandgore* (syphilis) to leave Edinburgh for the island of Inchkeith, on pain of being branded on the cheek[3]. In the sixteenth century some communal baths were closed by the authorities because they were thought to encourage promiscuity and the spread of infection (Figure 13.1). Prostitutes, believed to be the source of most infections, were an early and persistent target for sanitary regulation. Attempts to close brothels were usually unsuccessful – they simply reopened at new addresses. In many eighteenth-century European cities, Paris for example, the proprietors of "tolerated houses" were made responsible for the medical condition of their girls. There were frequent raids by the police, accompanied by surgeons who examined them; those judged to be infected were detained in special hospitals until they were better. Measures of this kind continued in a desultory way, but they had little impact on the levels of infection.

England: The Contagious Diseases Acts, 1864–1869

By the early nineteenth century towns had become larger and more prosperous, travel was easier and the incidence of infection had steadily increased, with particular concern about the number of people with syphilis. It was estimated that during the 1830s and 1840s half the surgical out-patient attendances at one London hospital were for venereal disease[4]. The high levels of infection in

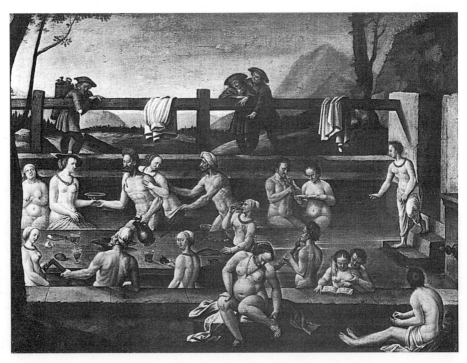

Figure 13.1. Communal bath at Louèche, from a painting by Hans Bock the Elder, late sixteenth century. (Öffentliche Kunstsammlung, Basel.)

European armies prejudiced their military efficiency, and further efforts were made to regulate prostitution. In Britain there were demands, supported by many doctors, for government intervention. It was argued that the state had the same duty to deal with women who had venereal disease as it had to deal with those with smallpox or typhus. William Acton (see Chapter 12) took this view. His experience in London and Paris had convinced him that although prostitution could not be extirpated it was nonetheless a social evil which could not be ignored. He thought that prostitutes should be subjected to regular medical inspection, as in France; there, those working in brothels who were registered and regularly examined (les filles a numéro) were much less likely to be a source of infection than street walkers (les filles en carte)[4].

The British government, responsible for a far-flung empire and seriously alarmed by the prevalence of venereal disease in the armed forces, gave way to pressure. There was no question of adopting the French system of licensed brothels, which was regarded as sponsoring immorality, but the government was willing to consider compulsory medical examinations. But when it introduced the Contagious Diseases Act in 1864, amended in 1866 and 1869, it ran headlong into trouble.

The object was to identify infected women and remove them from circulation until they were cured. The original Act applied only to a few major ports and garrison towns in England and Ireland, but the number of these was increased in later amendments. A woman named as a prostitute was obliged to undergo a medical examination, and if she was found to be infected could be detained for treatment in a lock hospital for up to three months. The police were to keep a list of prostitutes and decide who should be on it. There was little difficulty over women who were full-time professionals working in brothels, but those who resorted to prostitution only occasionally were much more difficult to identify; the evidence against them might be little more than hearsay or malicious rumour, and there were many false accusations.

The medical examination itself left much to be desired. In some places it was far from private or confidential and was witnessed by prurient bystanders peering through the window. In the original Act the use of a vaginal speculum was specified, but when it was found that many doctors did not know how to pass the instrument, and indeed were injuring some women in their attempts to do so, this requirement was withdrawn. The examination thus consisted of a naked-eye inspection of the pudenda for signs of ulceration, rashes or discharge. At this time the causes of venereal diseases were unknown and no laboratory tests were available, so there was no possibility of diagnosing infections in "carriers" with no signs of disease. The examination of servicemen for signs of infection was avoided. Witnesses to the Select Committee on Venereal Diseases [in the army and navy] in 1867 testified that periodic genital examination of servicemen would be "an extremely difficult thing to carry out on account of the prejudices of the men", and that in any case would "destroy the men's self-respect"[5].

The Contagious Diseases Acts provoked a public outcry, particularly from a group of highly placed women led by Josephine Butler (Figure 13.2) a clergyman's wife and evangelical Christian deeply committed to moral reform[6]; she was supported by prominent people such as the progressive writer Harriet Martineau and Florence Nightingale. They thought it outrageous that women who had been corrupted for the satisfaction of men should then be treated like criminals; compulsory vaginal examinations, they said, were an affront to

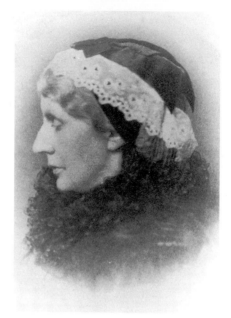

Figure 13.2. Josephine Butler (1828–1906).

personal liberty and human decency. Proposals that the legislation should be extended to industrial towns in the north of England provoked a struggle which has been hailed as a landmark in the nineteenth-century women's movement. The Acts were suspended in 1883 and repealed three years later despite vociferous protests from the medical establishment, many venereologists, *The Lancet* and the *British Medical Journal*. For the next 30 years there was no more legislation directed at prostitutes in Britain, although their licensing and medical examination continued in many European countries.

It may be asked whether the Contagious Diseases Acts succeeded in reducing the incidence of venereal disease. They had little effect, because they were not only impossible to enforce but wrongly conceived. The spread of these infections cannot be curtailed by action against prostitutes, or indeed any other single group; measures directed against all who are at risk are needed. This was not realised for many years, but in the mean time the repeal of the Acts, and the agitation which preceded it, had far-reaching consequences, some of them unforeseen. Concern about the fate of young prostitutes led to the Criminal Law Amendment Bill of 1886, which raised the age of consent to 16 years and introduced stringent penalties for keeping brothels. The effect of this legislation was simply to drive prostitution underground, so that it became clandestine and entirely uncontrolled. A further clause, inserted at the last moment, made any form of male homosexual activity illegal.

The Victorian age in England abounded in agonised debates about such sexual issues, and another soon arose over the Notification of Diseases Act of 1889, which allowed local authorities to impose restrictions on people suffering from certain infectious diseases. There was a move to include venereal diseases among these, which was strenuously opposed by many doctors who argued that compulsory notification would lead to the concealment of infections and thus defeat its own object. The notification of venereal diseases was not adopted, but the matter was raised and debated again at the time of the Royal Commission on Venereal Diseases in 1916 (see below). Another problem came from the desire of many doctors to spare the feelings of relatives by using evasive terms on the death certificates of patients who had died of a venereal disease. Osler pointed out that as a result syphilis was being seriously under-reported in the national statistics: "even in death, a stigma was associated with it"[7].

International Conferences, 1899–1902

The late nineteenth century saw the formation of various "purity" organisations which condemned not only prostitution but homosexuality, masturbation and other sexual activities regarded as offences against morality. There were public meetings, and tracts and pamphlets were published. These populist groups had links with the contemporary temperance and evangelical campaigns. A more direct attack on the problems of venereal disease came when the First International Conference for the Prophylaxis of Syphilis and of Venereal Diseases was held in Brussels in 1899 and a second three years later, attended by luminaries such as Fournier, Neisser, Morrow and Pringle.

Other meetings and conferences followed. The recommendations which emerged formed the basis of action by the authorities of many countries in providing clinics, teaching doctors, undertaking health education and so on. National organisations were formed, among them the German Society for Combating Venereal Disease, the French Society of Moral and Sanitary Prophylaxis and the American Society for Sanitary and Moral Prophylaxis. Their resounding titles at least indicated a desire to tackle some of the problems rather than ignore them.

The need for action was clear, because at the turn of the century the venereal disease problem was out of hand. In Berlin in 1900 16 000 people were treated for gonorrhoea or syphilis; it was claimed that more than one-third of men in Hamburg had had syphilis at some time and that on average *every* man had had gonorrhoea at least once. In New York Prince Morrow reported that 80 per cent of men had had gonorrhoea and nearly 20 per cent syphilis[8], and in England it was estimated that there were 40 000 cases of syphilis a year in London and 130 000 in the whole country[9]. There was also concern about the effect of gonorrhoea on the birth rate, which was falling; Noeggerath had described the connection between gonococcal infection and both male and female infertility as long ago as 1876.

How much public understanding there was of these problems is a moot point; discussion was blanketed, and the diseases referred to only obliquely. For example, in his "Round the red lamp", published in 1894, Conan Doyle wrote a short story about a man who consulted a doctor "whose patients did not consider his seclusion a disadvantage, in view of his speciality". The patient had abnormal teeth and eye disease, and he was told that he had a "strumous diathesis", inherited from his father; he had to cancel his wedding, and later killed himself. It is clear that the doctor was a venereologist and the patient had congenital syphilis, but syphilis was a forbidden word then; we may wonder how many of Doyle's readers knew what the story was about.

England: Royal Commission on Venereal Diseases, 1913–1916

Action by the British government was long overdue, and in 1913 Sir Malcolm Morris developed this point in a letter to *The Lancet* in which he proposed a Royal Commission to investigate the whole problem[10]. This call was echoed in a letter to the *Morning Post* in July 1913, signed by many well-known doctors. Morris (1849–1924, Figure 13.3) was an influential figure. He had studied dermatology in Berlin and Vienna before being appointed consultant physician to the new department at St Mary's Hospital. Like Hutchinson and Neisser he had a particular interest in the skin conditions due to leprosy, tuberculosis and syphilis, all diseases with important social aspects. He was impatient with the "conspiracy of silence" which surrounded syphilis. His efforts were successful, a Royal Commission on Venereal Diseases was appointed, and he was asked to be a member. A stern and self-disciplined man, Morris had been knighted by Edward VII in 1908; like many Englishmen of his generation he was interested in church architecture and devoted to cricket[11].

The Royal Commission began to take evidence in November 1913. It was instructed:

> "to inquire into the prevalence of Venereal Diseases in the United Kingdom, their effects upon the health of the community, and the means by which those effects can be alleviated or prevented, it being understood that no return to the policy or provisions of the Contagious Diseases Acts of 1864, 1866, or 1869 is to be regarded as falling within the scope of the inquiry[12]."

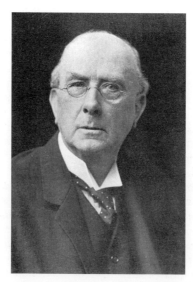

Figure 13.3. Sir Malcolm Morris (1849–1924).

Clearly the Government had no desire to be engulfed again by the trouble which had followed the earlier legislation. The chairman of the Commission was Lord Sydenham, an ex-soldier, colonial governor and businessman, and there were 14 other members. Sir Almeric Fitzroy and Sir Kenelm Digby were Whitehall mandarins, Canon J W Horsley and the Rev J Scott Lidget were clergymen with a special interest in social problems and Philip Snowden and Sir David Brynmore Jones were Members of Parliament. Mrs Louise Creighton was the widow of a former Bishop of London, and Mrs E. M. Burgwin an expert on mentally handicapped children; both were social purity campaigners with deep moral convictions. There were six members of the medical profession: James Ernest Lane was (like his father James) a surgeon on the staff at St Mary's and the London Lock Hospitals, Sir Arthur Newson had a background in public health and was principal medical officer to the Local Government Board and Sir John Collie was medical examiner to various insurance societies, with a special interest in workmens' compensation; Sir Frederick Mott, Sir Malcolm Morris and Dame Mary Scharlieb we have already met.

The Commissioners took evidence from many people concerned with the subject: surgeons, physicians, paediatricians, eye specialists, pathologists (including Major Harrison, as he then was), clergymen and welfare workers, and published their report in 1916; it became law as the Public Health (Venereal Diseases) Regulations, 1916.

It is remarkable that this disparate group of people who no doubt, like the rest of us, had personal problems and prejudices, produced such an enlightened document. It began by confirming the very high prevalence of venereal infection in Britain. It rejected the old idea that the detention or regulation of prostitutes, or any other group, had any significant effect against venereal disease. Instead, its most important recommendation was that local authorities should provide a free service for the early diagnosis and prompt treatment of venereal diseases, three-quarters of the cost to come from central funds and the remainder from local taxes. The service would be strictly confidential, and available on demand. This proposal was the cornerstone of future policy towards patients with venereal diseases in the UK, and was widely followed throughout the British Empire. The Royal Commission also recommended the arrangement of supporting laboratory facilities for the performance of the Wassermann and other tests, the prohibition of advertisements for remedies, and practical instruction in venereology for every medical student (with questions on the subject regularly set in medical and surgical examinations). These proposals were straightforward, but the commissioners also had to consider some more difficult issues relating to control: notification, health education and personal prophylaxis. They concluded that any possible advantages of notification by name were far outweighed by the need for complete confidentiality in the relationship between a patient and the clinic staff and concluded that this could not be recommended. They proposed that the *numbers* of patients with each disease should be reported, this system receiving the delightful alliteration "non-nominative notification". An exception to this had already been made in 1914, when ophthalmia neonatorum became notifiable by name.

Education of the public about the diseases was an even more difficult problem. While the commissioners recognised in principle the need for health education in this field, they were nervous about being accused of encouraging promiscuity by indicating how infections could be avoided. They stated that "such instruction should be based on moral principles and spiritual considerations, and should not be based on the physical consequences of immoral conduct", and they emphasised that private voluntary agencies, notably the National Council for Combating Venereal Diseases (NCCVD) should take the lead. They hoped that the NCCVD would "become a permanent and authoritative body, well capable of spreading knowledge and giving advice in regard to this question in its varied aspects and that it will be recognised as such by the Government". No educational literature on venereal disease should appear without its imprimatur.

The NCCVD had been founded in 1914, its first chairman being Sir Thomas Barlow, President of the Royal College of Physicians. From the outset the main thrust of its campaign was moral and social rather than medical. After the report of the Royal Commission had been accepted by the Local Government Board, from 1917 onwards the NCCVD received substantial treasury grants for its work. Lord Sydenham himself became Chairman and most of the commissioners, including Morris and Mary Scharlieb (but not Mott) joined its executive committee. The council was thus in a position of considerable power and influence. In taking a firm moral line it was later accused of being "an appendage of the Church, and more especially of the See of Canterbury", and its members "a little knot of intensely prejudiced and incapable private people"[13]. The remark of one of its founders, Sir Francis Champneys (1848–1930), is often quoted; he wrote that "it is better for venereal disease to be imperfectly controlled than that, in an attempt to prevent them, young men should be enticed into mortal sin"[14]. Champneys was an obstetrician on the staff of St Bartholomew's Hospital. He had a distinguished career as a consultant and teacher and strongly advocated, with eventual success, the legal recognition and registration of midwives; he was said to be the finest medical musician in London. Then as now, many eminent physicians and surgeons had a blind spot of prejudice about venereal disease.

The Royal Commission delegated health education to the NCCVD, but its approach to personal prophylaxis was timid. Eighty years after the event it is easy to smile at this but in the moral climate of the time it was understandable. Condoms, originally made from animal intestines but later of rubber or latex, had been used for centuries by those who could afford them to protect the user against infection. Nobody liked them – Madame de Sevigny called a condom "a cuirass against pleasure but a cobweb against danger" – but they were fairly effective if properly used. A different type of prophylaxis became possible when in 1905 Metchnikoff and Roux showed that calomel (mercurous chloride) ointment applied up to an hour after the inoculation of syphilitic material into a chimpanzee would prevent the development of a chancre. A similar inoculation of Paul Massouneuve, which was also – fortunately for him – unsuccessful has been mentioned in Chapter 6. Experiments on three monkeys and one human provided a slender scientific basis for a method of prophylaxis, but great hopes were pinned on it. It was thought that the application of calomel ointment to the genitals after coitus might be an effective prophylaxis against infection and be particularly useful for the armed forces. It was tried in some European armies and navies with encouraging results, and subsequently adopted by both the French and German armies. To the commissioners, personal prophylaxis raised some awkward moral issues: if it was available, might not a man deliberately fornicate in the knowledge that he would be protected from the consequences of his action? Therefore, although some individuals – notably Mott – wanted to mention prophylaxis, collectively the commissioners sat on their hands, and did not discuss the subject in their final report.

The First World War, 1914–1918

The First World War began in August 1914. Servicemen had always been at risk of contracting venereal diseases, and the British army had developed facilities for treating them. Control was attempted by lectures on personal hygiene and, in overseas stations, the medical examination of prostitutes. The lectures sometimes had unexpected results:

> "One English doctor, asked to lecture on venereal diseases to a group of soldiers, had just begun his talk when he saw the commander hand a note to the battalion chaplain. The clergyman got up, left the hall and did not return until the lecture's end. Curious, the doctor asked why he had left. The chaplain had replied that the colonel had asked him to go 'because he did not consider the subject a proper one' for clerical ears[15]."

The examination of prostitutes near military bases in England had been abandoned after the repeal of the Contagious Diseases Acts, but it continued overseas; Harrison related that he regularly checked enclaves of women near army stations in India[16]. The system of management of venereal disease in the British army was adequate in peacetime, but the army was unprepared for the problems which it met in France. A leaflet signed by Lord Kitchener, the Secretary of State for War, was issued to all troops. In part, it read:

> "Your duty cannot be done unless your health is sound, so keep constantly on your guard against any excesses. In this new experience you may find temptations in both wine and women. You should entirely resist both temptations and, while treating all women with perfect courtesy, you should avoid any intimacy[17]."

Not surprisingly, this exhortation had little effect. Soldiers in the British Expeditionary Force were free to patronise French regulated brothels, the *maisons tolerées*; there were said to be forty of these in Paris alone. The women were inspected weekly, but the examination was cursory, without laboratory tests, and therefore of limited value. There were soon high levels of infection. Facilities for treatment were inadequate – in France there was no irrigation equipment for the treatment of gonorrhoea, and no arsenic or mercury for syphilis[16]. After a period of improvisation (Figure 13.4) dedicated hospitals were opened in France and Britain, and adequately equipped.

The report of the Royal Commission appeared in March 1916, three months before the battle of the Somme. By this time venereal disease had become so common among British troops at home, in France and in the colonies that action by the authorities was urgently needed. In 1916 "venereal ablution rooms" were established in all barracks. An Army order directed that soldiers who had risked infection should attend for treatment within 24 hours. The standard regimen, which was self-administered, was to wash the genitals with soap and water, irrigate the urethra with potassium permanganate solution (known by the troops as "pinky panky"), and then apply calomel ointment to the whole area. The treatment was very effective if applied sufficiently soon after intercourse. Although the ablution rooms were sometimes called early treatment centres their purpose was not therapeutic but prophylactic; nevertheless, they were reluctantly accepted by the moralists.

The provision of prophylactic "packets" was seen quite differently. The author of a leading article in *The Lancet*, having observed that "young men, stirred by an unwonted spirit of adventure, must be exceedingly easy game for the temptress", went on to oppose "apparatus and instructions for use" as being "a recognition of vice"[18]. To others this moral approach had no place in a public health programme, and they favoured the issue of "packets". These usually contained calomel ointment to apply to the genitals and a tube of argyrol for the urethra, to be applied after coitus; sometimes a condom was included. The "packets" were anathema to the moralists, because a man setting out with one in his pocket had the *intention* to sin; the provision of early treatment centres was a different matter altogether. These differences, which may seem like hair-splitting today, were at the time deeply divisive and in the end irreconcilable. The Army Council at first stated that prophylaxis which would allow "unrestrained vice" was unacceptable – this at a time when easy access to maisons tolerées was permitted – but in 1917 it stopped pussyfooting, and authorised the issue of "packets" to British troops.

Although there was a marked reduction of infection among those who used the "packets" properly, they were not a panacea. They were not available everywhere, soldiers forgot to carry them, or were too drunk to use them until it was too late. Worse, they were sometimes used, by men who had not been properly instructed, for the self-treatment of established infections. In 1917 at a meeting of the Imperial War Conference it was acknowledged that venereal

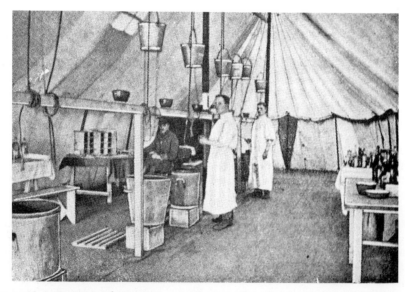

Figure 13.4. Improvised irrigation equipment for the treatment of soldiers with gonorrhoea in France (1914–1918). (From Harrison (1949) Half a lifetime in the management of venereal diseases.)

diseases were not being contained either in France or in England, and that they were seriously impeding the fighting capacity of the forces. In that year 23 000 British soldiers were hospitalised for treatment, and the French government reported that over a million cases of syphilis or gonorrhoea had been reported since the beginning of the war. Visits to the *maisons tolerées* were still allowed, and it was rumoured that the British authorities were operating a few houses of pleasure themselves at the Channel ports. In England there was no regulation of prostitutes, who were therefore free to solicit; Canadian, Australian and New Zealand troops, who were paid more than the British, were a particular target. A medical officer wrote:

> "The scenes were disgraceful. One saw thousands of men covered in mud, and although their clothing was muddy they could hardly get through the streets from Victoria station on account of the women crowding about them[19]."

Voluntary women's patrols and local vigilance committees had appeared quite early in the War. It was hoped that they might be able to curb some importuning and public displays of sexuality by young girls, but the size of the problem was too great for them to have much effect. Although by 1917 nearly half the final total of 230 civilian clinics recommended by the Royal Commission had been established, facilities for the treatment of servicemen infected in England were poor. The Dominion governments – Canada in particular – were insistent that steps were taken to protect their men. In March 1918 the British cabinet took draconian action. The *maisons tolerées* were placed out of bounds to Crown forces, and a regulation was issued (No 40D of the Defence of the Realm Act) that made it a criminal offence for a woman with a venereal infection to solicit or have sex with any member of His Majesty's forces. Predictably, these measures roused indignant protests. The army thought that denying soldiers access to brothels (which after all were a traditional part of army life) would mean that they would patronise street prostitutes and increase the risk of infection; even Sir Douglas Haig, the Commander-in-Chief, objected. Female campaigners complained that Regulation 40D discriminated against women and opened the door to persecution and blackmail. Although the Regulation was largely unenforceable and was regarded as naive by many doctors the government refused to give way, and was still embroiled in this controversy when the war ended in November 1918.

The United States entered the war in April 1917. Venereal disease had been a problem for the US army in peacetime, and a policy had been developed which was was based on encouraging temperance, suppressing prostitution near army camps, the provision of facilities for "healthy" recreation, and health education. The developing social hygiene movement, which favoured morality and sexual restraint and stressed the "loathsome" aspects of venereal disease, endorsed all these measures. But they were clearly not adequate for France. The US Army Medical Department was impressed by the aggressive control policy of the New Zealand Expeditionary Force, which had a programme of frequent medical examination of soliders for signs of infection – so-called "dangle parades" – the issue of condoms and the provision of post-coital prophylaxis. The policy of the US army thus had both moral and medical aspects[20]. Prophylactic stations were established in army camps and soldiers required to attend not more than three hours after exposure. The treatment was similar to that provided in British centres – thorough washing of the genitals, the instillation of an antiseptic into the urethra, and application of calomel ointment – but it was administered not by the soldiers themselves but by medical orderlies, who were sometimes accused of deriding their patients and thereby deterring them from attending again. If properly performed chemical prophylaxis was effective. Men who developed an infection despite prophylaxis suffered loss of pay while their illness lasted, but no other punishment. Personal prophylaxis with "packets" was not favoured, except for troops in outlying stations, besides being (as in the British army) opposed on moral grounds. The Secretary of the Navy said: "I could not look a boy . . . straight in the face . . . if I were approving the policy and use of a measure of this kind"[15].

When the US army arrived in France the French *maisons tolerées* were made available to servicemen. They were enthusiastically patronised – a journalist remembered seeing the men lined up eight deep at the entrance to one establishment – and the inevitable result was an escalation of infection, and a breakdown of the system of prophylaxis. Appeals for temperance and morality fell on deaf ears, and prophylactic stations were often not used. Soldiers on leave, frequently drunk, would return to their camp to find the queue outside the station was longer than the one outside the brothel they had just left, and did not bother to wait. General Pershing, the Commander of American forces in Europe, had to act quickly, and he issued a series of orders. Although in the past he had favoured regulated prostitution, he now changed his mind. US soldiers were prohibited from visiting the *maisons tolerées*, an edict which was greeted by the French authorities with derision; they simply could not understand how it was hoped that young men on active service could be made chaste by decree. This disagreement was to open a gulf between the American and French authorities' conception of venereal disease control. General Pershing also ordered that in future contracting a venereal disease would be a court-martial offence. Post-coital prophylaxis was to be strictly enforced. In some units men taking leave were medically examined before they left and on their return, and chemical prophylaxis was compulsory, whether they admitted to having intercourse or not. The emphasis on prophylaxis upset the social hygiene protagonists in the United States, as it had the NCCVD in Britain, but during the war social hygiene was a lost cause. US army doctors were sure that prophylactic stations had materially helped to control venereal disease, and the British authorities were impressed by the apparent success of the policy. In May 1918 an Anglo-American conference on venereal diseases was convened to discuss and compare methods of control, but the war ended before any significant progress had been made.

Other nations had their own procedures to try to control the escalation of venereal disease. The French were confident that their system of controlling infection in the *maisons tolerées* by the regular examination of the prostitutes was effective, but personal prophylaxis was also considered important; the use of condoms and the application of calomel ointment *before* intercourse were encouraged. Men underwent a medical inspection for signs of infection on enlistment, and when taking or returning from leave; inspection of officers, however, proved to be "difficult"[21]. Hospitals, polyclinics and dispensaries for the treatment of soldiers on leave and civilians were available in most French towns. In Germany Albert Neisser, who advised the army on venereal disease control until his death in 1916, thought that personal prophylaxis was essential, and condoms and calomel ointment were issued to all troops. Soldiers had access to approved military brothels – red light ones for NCOs and private soldiers, blue light ones for officers. There was a compulsory medical examination and Wassermann test for soldiers leaving the army, and those found to be infected were detained for treatment.

While they recognised its importance, none of the combatant nations in the First World War was able to solve the complex problems of venereal disease control. The need to return men to the front line meant that the duration of therapy was reduced to the minimum, and the careful prolonged follow-up practised in peacetime was not possible. In the pre-antibiotic era many patients remained infectious after apparently successful treatment and a large number of servicemen, and their wives, finished the war with chronic infections. Chemical prophylaxis, either by early treatment centres or the provision of "packets", was adopted by most of the belligerents. Prompt post-coital disinfection in a medical facility was effective, but some experienced observers were unconvinced that the efficacy of self-applied chemical prophylaxis had been proved[22]. Coercive legislation against prostitutes had, once again, been unsuccessful. *In toto*, there was a need for fresh thinking about venereal disease control in the armed forces.

Europe, 1918–1925

After the Armistice most European countries experienced a sharp decline in the incidence of venereal diseases, whose most important cause was the return of the more settled conditions of peacetime. Thereafter, improvements in the public health aspects of the infections was disappointingly slow in most countries. France continued to rely on the supervision of prostitutes and personal prophylaxis for men. In Germany, legislation in 1927 made the notification and treatment of defaulters compulsory, but the scheme was a failure because it was too costly and because many doctors refused to cooperate. Under fascist regimes the rules became stricter: state regulation of venereal diseases was reintroduced in Italy in 1931 and in Germany in 1933. Sweden adopted a rigorous system. Under an Act of 1918 the name and address of each patient, and the patient's source contact, were reported to local medical officers of health, there were penalties for not completing treatment, and doctors who did not fulfil their obligations in these matters were punished. These measures were strict, but the venereal rates in Sweden were the lowest in Europe[23]. Denmark had a similar programme. In 1923 the International Union against Venereal Diseases and the Treponematoses was formed, whose object was to encourage member nations to collaborate in the study and control of venereal diseases. It played a large part in the Brussels agreement of 1924 under which treatment facilities for seamen were made available at major ports.

Britain, 1918–1939

In Britain after the end of the First World War, the main responsibility of the developing network of venereal disease clinics was the diagnosis, treatment and post-treatment surveillance of patients. The physicians in charge were too preoccupied with establishing high standards in these matters to become involved in the debate about personal prophylaxis which erupted in the early 1920s. This had been so successful during the War that it was suggested in some quarters that it should be made available for civilians. Harrison knew more about its efficacy than anyone[22]. He held that while under service conditions, where adequate and repeated instruction was possible, the provision of "packets" was often followed by a sharp fall in infection, even then they would fail to protect men who were too drunk or stupid to use them properly. He did not favour personal prophylaxis for civilians because of the difficulty of arranging adequate instruction. Some individuals, too embarrassed or frightened to go to a public clinic, might use the "packets" for self-treatment; this had happened in the army, and in some cases the delay in getting proper advice had led to disaster. Harrison commented that prophylaxis for women had hardly been considered, and might not be practicable. This important matter had been neglected because of a mistaken belief that the elimination of infection from men would automatically be followed by its elimination from women. An alternative to self-disinfection was the provision of early treatment centres along Army lines which could be attended by anyone who had "run a risk." One was opened in Manchester and another in Portsmouth, but there were protests from local authorities who did not see why they should have to shoulder the cost of these as well as the cost of venereal disease clinics.

During the 1920s more clinics were opened. From the beginning they had been well patronised, and only a minority of patients were treated privately – an obvious advantage in preparing national statistics. The directors of clinics knew the importance of examining potentially infected sexual contacts of their patients. Harrison himself favoured finding contacts "through the patient's own efforts", and this approach often worked quite well. In some UK clinics during the 1920s and 1930s medical social workers, then called almoners, were employed to help people with financial, domestic and marital problems, and they often tried to persuade them to bring their partners to the clinic.

A more formal system of "contact epidemiology" was introduced during the Second World War. There had been an alarming escalation of infection in North-East England and the local authorities inaugurated a "Tyneside scheme" in 1943[24]. Infected patients were interviewed by specially trained staff, their contacts were identified and, if necessary, visited at home and persuaded to go to a clinic. These arrangements were so successful that they were adopted by other local authorities, and eventually virtually all the larger clinics had one or more staff members, paid by local authorities, to undertake the work.

In principle, health education is an important part of a venereal disease control programme, but its history in Britain between the wars was unhappy. Although much counselling on a one-to-one basis was given by the staff in clinics, the main educational programme in the UK had been delegated by the Royal Commission to the NCCVD. It provided books and pamphlets, supplied lecturers for public meetings, and arranged public performances of films, and plays such as "Damaged Goods". These events were very well attended at the time, but how much good they did is hard to assess. Publicising the subject was certainly desirable, but the implication of much of the educational material was that people with venereal diseases were immoral and lacking in self-control, and this may have enhanced the stigma attached to the diseases. The lectures, films and so on did not attract the young people who were most at risk of infection, and they were often followed by a flow of the "worried well" to clinics – as was to happen 60 years later after television programmes about AIDS. Unfortunately, the long-running obsession of the

NCCVD with prophylaxis continued, and more committees were convened to go over the old ground yet again[25]. Did sexual continence adversely affect health? Was post-coital disinfection morally permissible, or did it encourage vice? Was it effective, or did it engender a false sense of security? Some of the discussions lost sight of the problem of controlling venereal disease and became entangled in eugenics, contraception and feminist issues, and accusations of time-serving, dishonesty and humbug were bandied about.

In 1919 discontent with the "preach and teach" policy of the NCCVD had led some of its members to resign and form the Society for the Prevention of Venereal Disease (SPVD). Its president was Lord Willoughby de Broke, a scion of an old aristocratic family. He owned 6000 acres of land in Warwickshire and had written books on fox-hunting. Somehow he had become interested in venereal diseases, and had spoken on the subject of immediate self-disinfection in the House of Lords. The secretary was Hugh Wansey Bayly who, after spending some time as a ship's surgeon and serving in the army, developed an interest in venereology and obtained appointments at St George's and the London Lock Hospitals; he wrote a book on the subject which went through several editions. There were some very well-known figures on the council: Sir Alfred Fripp, Sir Arbuthnot Lane, Sir Berkely Moynihan, Sir D'Arcy Power, Sir Frederick Treves and Mr Wilfred Trotter were surgeons, Mr Aleck Bourne and Mr Eardley Holland were gynaecologists, and Sir Frederick Mott had resigned from the NCCVD to become a council member. Sir Bryan Donkin and Sir Archbald Reid were tireless and outspoken propagandists for the society. Donkin had been a physician at Westminster Hospital, but after being appointed a commissioner of prisons he abandoned clinical medicine and devoted the rest of his career to criminology and mental disease. Reid spent most of his professional life as a general practitioner, but during the First World War he had been medical officer at the Victoria Barracks at Portsmouth, where he had become a firm believer in the value of post-coital prophylactic treatment. The NCCVD too had some new recruits, among them William Inge, the Dean of St Paul's, London; he was a well-known Anglican divine and publicist, who later became known as "the gloomy Dean" because of his pessimistic views on progress, education and democracy. It is strange that with the exception of Mott none of these eminent people had any special knowledge, or indeed experience, of venereology.

There was a rancorous public debate between the NCCVD and the SPVD. The central issue was whether control of venereal disease should depend on sexual continence, public health education and good treatment facilities, as recommended by the NCCVD, or on personal prophylaxis, as advocated by the SPVD. The SPVD was quite explicit. It wanted notices placed in public lavatories stating:

> "Every time you have sexual intercourse with a woman who is not your wife you run the risk of venereal disease. You can avoid disease in one way. In every public water closet is an automatic machine. By putting a penny in the slot you will obtain a packet with the necessary material. Apply this according to the instructions and you will be safe[26]."

This was totally opposed to the policy of the NCCVD, and feelings between the two factions ran high. Efforts to resolve the dispute – referred to by *The Times* as "an unedifying wrangle" – failed. Eventually, as public interest in the subject declined, the argument died down.

In 1925 the NCCVD changed its name to the British Social Hygiene Council, and it diversified into other areas of health education. During the 1930s it continued to issue books and pamphlets about venereal disease – at one time there were more than 100 on its recommended reading list – but there was now little demand for them. The council slowly faded away, and was absorbed into the Health Education Council in 1943. The SPVD, which was never an effective pressure group and was handicapped by the opposition of the Ministry of Health, succumbed at about the same time. It is sad that so many committees, meetings, publications, speeches and reports seemed to have had so little effect on the control of venereal disease in Britain. Today, the details of the anguished debates seem hardly more relevant than those of previous disputes about syphilisation or the use of mercury. The local authorities, who in principle should have been concerned about health education in this field, in practice spent next to nothing on it, the only overt evidence of their activity being the notices about the times of local venereal disease clinics erected in public lavatories.

Health education in sexually transmitted diseases remains an important part of any control programme. Mistakes were undoubtedly made in the past, and today the goals of such education, and the methods to achieve them, are better understood. Whether the programmes will be more effective remains to be seen.

USA, 1918–1939

In the United States there was a marked decline of interest in venereal diseases after the First World War, and federal control programmes virtually halted. Throughout history older people have been dismayed by the behaviour of the young, and in the USA in the 1920s this dismay was focused on illicit intercourse; this was now less often with prostitutes, and more often between men and women who had rejected earlier ideas of premarital chastity, the automobile providing a convenient venue for their encounters.

It was paradoxical that while sex was now freely discussed, venereal disease was not. Social hygienists emphasised moral uplift, the authorities were uncommitted, and the escalating levels of venereal disease seem to have been simply ignored. Throughout the 1920s and 1930s there were some clinicians and public health workers who, alarmed by the size of the problem, pressed for new federal and state control programmes, pointing out the poor quality of US services compared with those in many European countries. One of the most influential leaders of this agitation was Thomas Parran (1892–1968; Figure 13.5). He was born in Maryland and received his medical education at Georgetown University[27]. He joined the US Public Health Service in 1917, and was appointed chief of the Venereal Disease Division in 1926. Unfortunately it had become, in his words, "a dying operation", and funds became even scarcer after the slump began in 1930. Between 1930 and 1936 he was health commissioner of New York State, and from 1936 to 1948 surgeon-general of the US Public Health Service. In later life he became dean of the Graduate School of Public Health at Pittsburg and was involved in many international health issues, including the foundation of the World Health Organisation in 1946. Parran and his collaborators were determined to bring the venereal disease problem to national attention. They were resourceful in their use of the media. In 1934 Parran himself had a furious dispute with the Columbia Broadcasting Company who had told him, minutes before he was due to broadcast a talk on public health issues, that he could not mention syphilis or gonorrhoea by name. He refused to give the talk and publicly accused the company of hypocrisy and double standards. He had an article, "The Next Great Plague to go" in the *Reader's Digest* in 1936, and his book *Shadow on the land: syphilis*, published in 1937, became a best-seller. He wrote:

> "a symbolic picture of syphilis control ... would show a few green islands of intelligent activity, a good many sand bars of effort, and the whole surrounded by the vast grey waters of apathy, futility and ignorance."

Parran was an epidemiologist. His programme for controlling syphilis was based on case-finding by the free provision of serology, prompt treatment, tracing and examining contacts, compulsory blood tests before marriage and during pregnancy, and health education. He made no appeal to morality, admitting that in the twentieth century "continence was perhaps an unrealistic solution to the problem of venereal disease control". Like Harrison, he was unenthusiastic about chemical prophylaxis for civilian populations. He avoided the discussion of condoms in this context; he was a Roman Catholic, and may have felt that he had already gone as far as he could. Slowly, his efforts bore fruit. The mid-1930s saw the introduction of mandatory syphilis serology before marriage and during pregnancy which soon became general throughout the country. Clinical services began to improve, and some states required the reporting of cases of syphilis and gonorrhoea. Finally, in 1938 Franklin D. Roosevelt signed the National Venereal Disease Control Act, which authorised the provision of federal funds for a comprehensive control programme. Money became available for improving public clinics, making laboratory tests for syphilis generally available, and

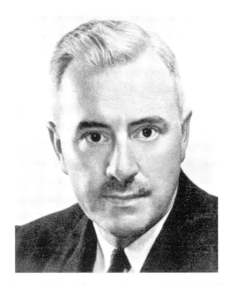

Figure 13.5. Thomas Parran (1892–1968).

207

providing services for private practitioners. Like the publication of the report of the Royal Commission on Venereal Diseases in Britain, this was the beginning of a new era for US venereology, and Parran had done more than anyone to make it possible.

Health education about venereal diseases in the US between the two World Wars was influenced by the American Social Hygiene Association, a voluntary body founded in 1913. Unfortunately its attitude to the problem was prudish and moralistic; it regarded public health approaches with suspicion and, like the NCCVD in Britain, was completely opposed to prophylaxis. Parran favoured a much more open style of health education, emphasising the need for diagnosis and treatment rather than behavioural reform. He published books and articles himself, and persuaded the popular press to do the same. The public responded. In one of the first Gallup polls, in 1936, 90 per cent of respondents favoured the distribution of educational material about venereal diseases by a government agency[28]. The American Social Hygiene Association, while continuing to emphasise the importance of family values, as they are called nowadays, moderated some of its puritanical views; but in 1940 it was still failing to promote, or even mention, the possible value of condoms as a protection against infection.

The Second World War, 1939–1945

By the late 1930s it was clear that war was coming, and contingency planning for a probable escalation of venereal disease began. In Britain, civilian clinics were now well established. Service medical officers and ancillary staff were instructed in venereology, and there was none of the shortage of equipment which had occurred in the First World War. After its past experiences the British army attached great importance to preventing infection. The dispute about personal prophylaxis was over. There were now ablution centres in most units, and "packets" were available everywhere. Free condoms were provided for troops overseas, although the army fought shy of providing them at home[29].

The American authorities embarked on a programme which comprised a good clinical service, the suppression of prostitution, personal prophylaxis and health education. Additional rapid treatment centres were built for the intensive arsenotherapy of syphilis in civilians and the 5 per cent of service recruits who were found to be infected. Hundreds of post-coital prophylactic stations were opened at home and overseas (Figure 13.6) and there was an abundant supply of condoms – fifty million a month according to one account. In 1943, after a bitter debate, the law by which servicemen did not receive pay during the treatment of venereal infections was repealed.

Nevertheless, control was as difficult as ever. Between 1939 and 1941 the number of new cases of venereal disease reported from clinics in England nearly doubled, and a further massive increase followed the arrival of American troops in 1942. The centres for chemical prophylaxis were not much used because most of the sexual exposures were "friendly" rather than commercial, and servicemen did not think prophylaxis was necessary. The epidemiology of sexually transmitted diseases was changing. In the First World War the majority of infections came from prostitutes but this was no longer the case. Some doctors implied that men's partners – "pickups", "good time girls" and so on

– were little more than amateur prostitutes. The American venereologist John Stokes wrote:

> "The old type of prostitute in a house or on the street is sinking into second place. The new type is the young girl in her late teens and early twenties, the young woman in every field of life who is determined to have one fling or better[30]."

For centuries it had been habitual to blame women for venereal disease. The people castigated by Stokes were not paid by their partners, so were not prostitutes. In truth, their motives were little different from those of the men – a desire for companionship and sex amid the uncertainties of wartime. The women's services were important to all combatant nations in the Second World War. Predictably, there were covert charges of immorality which in Britain were even investigated by a parliamentary committee, which found the level of infection to be actually less than in corresponding civilian groups. At least in some units periodic examinations for evidence of infection were performed; surprisingly, nobody seems to have objected.

In England the increase in the number of cases imposed a severe strain on the venereal disease services. The American forces operated a very successful system of contact tracing, and the Tyneside scheme began in 1943, but the epidemic was not contained. The British government, alarmed by the deteriorating situation, once again decided to introduce compulsion. Defence Regulation 33B required specialists in venereal disease to supply to medical officers of health details of sexual contacts named by patients on two occasions as the likely source of

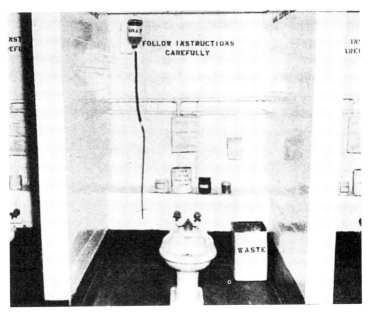

Figure 13.6. Interior of prophylactic station at Staging Area No 1, Naples, April 1944. From Holmes et al. (eds) (1984) Sexually transmitted diseases. (Courtesy of McGraw Hill Inc.)

their infections; treatment was then obligatory. Two accusations were required to comply with the law, and to guard against mistakes, malice or blackmail but the number of these which were actually made was "woefully small"[31]. Some unofficial attempts were made to approach contacts after a single report, and these were much more successful. The regulation was abandoned in 1947.

In 1943 the Ministry of Health introduced a large-scale programme of health education involving posters, films and radio broadcasts. At first these were so mealy-mouthed and cautious that they were difficult for the average person to understand, but later in the war they became more explicit. Fears that the public would be upset by hearing about sex organs, syphilis and gonorrhoea proved to be groundless; times were changing. Whether the campaign achieved anything is impossible to say.

The Second World War was a world-wide conflict in a way that the First World War had never been. From the outset servicemen were seeking sex not only in Europe but in the Middle East, the Far East, North Africa and elsewhere. The incidence of venereal disease was very high and control very difficult. The problem became even worse during the Allied invasion of Europe. In Italy – particularly in Naples – the British and American medical authorities later admitted that they had lost the battle and that the situation was for a time out of control. The courageous decision was made to make some of the scarce supplies of penicillin available for the treatment of servicemen with venereal disease, and the effect on this epidemic was immediate and spectacular.

In France, troops were exposed to the *maisons tolerées* which had been the undoing of many of their predecessors in 1914–1918, but the liberation gave many other opportunities for casual sex. There had been an escalation of venereal disease in Germany during the war, which duly affected the armies of occupation. The distinguished venereologist Robert Morton recalls that in one centre in West Germany at this time three medical officers each treated an average of 30 cases of gonorrhoea and six cases of early syphilis every day, six days a week, for six months. However, although the levels of infection were very high, treatment of both gonorrhoea and syphilis were revolutionised once penicillin was available. Its major advantage for the public health worker was the rapidity with which it rendered a patient non-infectious, and for the clinician the prospect of achieving a complete cure, without complications, with a drug that was remarkably free from side effects. The post-war period therefore began in an atmosphere of therapeutic optimism.

The Post-War Period, 1945–1955

Some commentators were concerned that simple and effective treatment would promote promiscuity by removing the supposed deterrent effect of a fear of infection. The old dread of any sort of control which was not based on morality re-emerged, and there was apocalyptic talk of "subsidising venery" and "bringing mankind to its fall". In fact, from 1946 onwards there was a marked reduction in the number of infections in most developed countries. This had also happened after the First World War; although it was now attributed to penicillin, a major contributory factor was probably the ending of the social upheaval and emotional stresses of the war. Nevertheless, the fall in the number of new cases of syphilis was maintained into the 1950s, and this may well have been due to the use of antibiotics for the treatment not only of syphilis but more generally for a multitude of other infections. In Britain the fall in the number of new cases of syphilis, and to a lesser extent gonorrhoea, made the authorities reluctant to spend any more public money on venereal disease services once the worst damage and dilapidation caused by the war had been corrected, and the speciality steered into the National Health Service in 1948.

In the United States, a policy of mass testing for syphilis was inaugurated in 1945, and by the early 1950s more than two million people had been treated; it was then ended as being no longer cost-effective. With the decline in the number of cases of early syphilis and gonorrhoea the venereal diseases appeared to be of diminishing public health importance, and this was reflected in a reduction in federal funding. Two important publications, *The American Journal of Syphilis* and the *Journal of Social Hygiene* disappeared. The great American syphilologists concluded, not without some personal sadness, that the subject of their life work was now finished. Earle Moore wrote in 1956:

"One might anticipate the nearly complete disappearance of syphilis as a public health problem within the next 5 or 10 years[32]."

Earle Moore himself turned his department of syphilis over to the study of chronic diseases. By the mid 1950s, therefore, it seemed that the venereal diseases, like many other conditions which had plagued humanity for centuries, had yielded to the power of modern medicine. How wrong this was will be seen in the following chapter.

Chapter 14
No Happy Ending

I tell you naught for your comfort,
Yea, naught for your desire,
Save that the sky grows darker yet
And the sea rises higher.

G.K. Chesterton, *Ballad of the White Horse*

By 1950 there were reasons for optimism about the venereal diseases. The natural history of syphilis and gonorrhoea were well understood, reliable laboratory tests were available for diagnosis and post-treatment surveillance and good methods of control by case finding and contact epidemiology had been established; above all, penicillin now provided safe and rapidly effective treatment. The results were there for all to see. In Britain and the USA the mortality from late syphilis, the number of patients admitted to mental hospitals with syphilitic psychoses and the number of congenital infections were all declining; furthermore, since 1946 the incidence of early syphilis was falling as well. The number of new cases of gonorrhoea reported from most developed countries had steadily fallen to a stable, relatively low level. Non-gonococcal urethritis was less common than gonorrhoea. Its causes were largely unknown, but it was not thought to be a serious infection and its treatment was much improved by the introduction of the tetracyclines in the early 1950s. There was believed to be an analogous condition in women, but this could not be defined clinically as there were no laboratory tests for causal organisms. Chancroid, lymphogranuloma venereum and donovanosis were hardly seen outside developing countries. The effectiveness of penicillin induced a state of euphoria in many workers; in 1958 the British venereologist Ambrose King was told by the chairman of a regional hospital board: "We don't want to spend any more money on these dying diseases"[1]. In some countries, for example the USA, public health administrators reduced the funds available for laboratory tests, venereal disease clinics and contact tracing. These optimists had forgotten that in the long history of venereal diseases there had been periods, particularly after major wars, when their incidence had fallen to a low level, only to rise again later. Moreover, infectious diseases have never been controlled by improved treatment alone. The warnings from some physicians that the current happy state of affairs might not last for long went largely unheeded.

In the event, the decline in the incidence of these infections proved to be short-lived. Although it had been thought that penicillin mitigated gonorrhoea as a public health problem, from the mid 1950s onwards its incidence rapidly rose; in Britain the number of new infections in men doubled between 1951 and 1960, and similar increases were reported from many other countries[2]. Non-gonococcal urethritis was also escalating. The incidence of syphilis varied between countries. The arrival of penicillin had led to a rapid fall in the number of early infections throughout the world. In Britain this decline was maintained, apart from a small increase, mostly in homosexual men, in the 1970s. In the USA, on the other hand, there had been a continuous increase in early infectious syphilis since the 1950s, and it quadrupled in the following 20 years. It was obvious that, despite the general availability of effective treatment, venereal diseases were becoming a problem again. The reasons for this were much discussed, although poorly understood. A complex of demographic and social variables was involved which included population movements, increasing affluence, more holiday travel, oral contraception, the promulgation of sex in popular culture and some relaxation in the laws affecting male homosexuals.

The result was a revolution in attitudes to sexuality, particularly among young people – the so-called sexual revolution – but more sex partners and more casual affairs meant more unwanted pregnancies and more venereal diseases. Doctors and health administrators cannot escape some responsibility for the renewed epidemics of the 1960s and 1970s. Health education in this field, although active during the recent war, was now desultory. Because of confidence in the power of antibiotics the subject of prophylaxis, which had formerly received so much attention, was forgotten; the use of condoms to prevent the transmission of infection was not advocated until the HIV epidemic 30 years later. Doctors in family planning clinics were of course right to stress the need to avoid unwanted pregnancies, but they often failed to add that sexual freedom combined with non-barrier contraception brought with it a risk of sexually transmitted diseases.

The rising levels of infection were not the only problem to confront venereologists. Bacterial resistance had already destroyed the value of sulphonamides for the treatment of gonorrhoea, so there was little surprise when strains of N. gonorrhoeae appeared in the early 1950s which showed an increased resistance to penicillin. It was still possible to use penicillin for treating gonorrhoea by increasing its dosage, but in 1976 there was a more serious development; strains appeared in Africa and the Far East which showed a very high level of resistance because of the plasmid-mediated production of β-lactamase[3]. In due course these organisms became widespread, so that in some parts of the world penicillin could no longer be used for the treatment of gonorrhoea. Fortunately, Treponema pallidum has not become resistant to penicillin, but the problem with gonorrhoea was a blow; venereologists may well have murmured "Never glad confident morning again!" Since its foundation in 1948 the World Health Organisation had emphasised the size of the venereal disease problem in developing countries, which was aggravated by a serious lack of resources. Syphilis remained common, and many of the complications and sequels of sexually transmitted infections – salpingitis, epididymitis, infertility, neonatal disease and so on – were widespread. Resistance to antibiotics was extensive, and consequently there were difficulties in treating not only gonorrhoea but chancroid; this disease had become uncommon in the West, but was still a major cause of genital ulceration in developing countries.

The "Second Generation" Infections

The escalation of the classical venereal diseases was compounded by the increased occurrence of many less familiar infections, the so-called "second generation" diseases. These were not new, but their importance had become recognised through study and research. Sexually transmitted diseases were no longer taboo; they were fully (and sometimes inaccurately) discussed in the media amid public concern at their increasing incidence. *Chlamydia trachomatis* attracted much attention. During the 1960s and 1970s it became accepted as a major cause of non-gonococcal and post-gonococcal urethritis in men and cervicitis in women. An association with pelvic inflammatory disease had been mentioned in the 1930s, and this was now confirmed when new laparoscopic techniques and better laboratory tests became available[4]. Neonatal ocular chlamydial infection was already well known, but in 1977 a neonatal pneumonia syndrome was described for the first time[5]. These discoveries were to make genital chlamydial infection as important a subject as gonorrhoea.

Genital herpes became prominent during the 1970s, probably because of an increase in incidence. The public knew that it was incurable, that many patients had frequent recurrences and that newborn babies could be at risk of serious or even fatal disease. Worse still, there was some evidence (now discounted) that the virus might be involved in cervical cancer[6]. These anxieties were fuelled by alarmist reports in sections of the media, and as a result, the diagnosis was often greeted with something like panic. Genital warts were another old disease; although patients disliked having them, doctors regarded them as little more than a nuisance. An association of some papillomavirus types with cervical dysplasia and invasive cancer was shown in the late 1970s, and within a few years these types were associated with dysplasias and malignancies throughout the lower genital tract. Since papillomavirus infections are common, these discoveries posed a series of management problems which have not yet been resolved. The prevalence of these incurable sexually transmitted viral infections cast a shadow over the therapeutic optimism which had followed the discovery of antibiotics.

The need to diagnose this expanding range of sexually transmitted infections increased the workload of microbiology departments. New and more sophisticated diagnostic tests became available, but their use was often constrained by their expense. The increasing number of patients attending venereal disease clinics necessitated an increase in staff. In countries where venereology was a recognised speciality a patient attending a clinic could expect to see a doctor with experience of the subject but this was not possible in some places, where paramedical "physician's assistants" dealt with the routine work under the supervision of a consultant. Throughout the years following the Second World War there was an increased emphasis on case finding. In the larger clinics and departments the tracing of sexual contacts was actively pursued by trained health workers. "Cluster testing", the examination of social as well as sexual contacts of infected individuals, was sometimes arranged. Epidemiological treatment – when the diagnosis was likely on clinical or behavioural grounds but the results of laboratory tests, if any, were not known – was adopted in some areas where the prevalence of infection was high.

Infections in Male Homosexuals

From the early 1950s onwards venereologists became aware that they were seeing more men with homosexually acquired infections. Again, these were not new. They had been described, particularly in the European literature, for many years; in a review published in 1926, 262 cases of anal primary syphilis, mostly in homosexual men, were reported[7]. The incidence may have been far higher than this, because at that time doctors were evidently reluctant to examine the anorectal region of their patients. There were problems facing homosexual men seeking medical advice. In many countries buggery had been a criminal offence for centuries, and in England *any* sexual acts between men were made illegal by the Criminal Law Amendment Act of 1885; Oscar Wilde was imprisoned for two years under this Act. In the United States the penalties were even more severe, and in some states men convicted of buggery could receive life imprisonment. Quite apart from its legal aspects male homosexual behaviour was regarded as abnormal, deviant or worse. To many doctors it was a disgusting offence, and their disapproval is apparent in many writings on the subject. Thus the American venereologist Robert Taylor wrote in 1890:

> "There is a class of men, chiefly young (but there are some older ones among their number), who are the victims of sexual perversion and who grant to and receive from men libidinous favours in revolting and unnatural practices. By the laity they are called Charleys and Sissies, and obscene epithets are often applied to them. They circulate in our midst and patrol dark and unfrequented streets, and prove a constant source of annoyance to the police after dark by "hanging around" our public parks and haunting the public places of urination, and also water closets in hotels. They are rarely, I am told, of a mercenary turn like their sister colleagues in prostitution, but seem impelled by an irresistible impulse to toy with and fondle the genitals of their fellow men."

Taylor went on to describe a homosexual man with a chancre of the tonsil, and concluded:

> "The members of this promising fraternity are well known to the police who, having an antipathy to them as a rule, keep a sharp eye upon them, cause them to keep moving, and in every possible way interfere with their beastly pursuits[8]."

Fifty years later Josephine Hinrichsen, of the Division of Venereal Diseases of the US Public Health Service, began a long review article by stating:

> "Human sexual habits, particularly if they come under the classification of 'perversions', do not interest most physicians, not even those who specialise in venereal diseases. They have a healthy aversion to abnormal sexual behaviour[9]."

This hearty, "I'm glad I'm normal" stance was bound to affect doctor – patient relationships. Fear of moral condemnation led some men to say that they had consorted with women (thereby making contact tracing impossible), and others were deterred from seeking medical advice at all if it could possibly be avoided.

Homosexuality has existed in all civilisations without exception, and the reaction of society has not always been one of condemnation – in some cultures sexual relations between men were tolerated or approved. During the Second World War such liaisons were not at all unusual, so there should have been no surprise – although there was – when in his *Report on Sexual Behaviour in the Human Male*, published in 1948, Alfred Kinsey wrote that over one third of North American men had had homosexual experience to the point of orgasm at some time in their lives. However, the legal situation marred the sex life of men who were predominantly homosexual. In many cases, their only possible outlet was intercourse with strangers, and this encouraged the spread of venereal disease. This was pointed out by the British venereologist James Jefferiss in a paper published in 1956[10]; he had observed that in London a significant proportion of men with venereal diseases were now homosexual.

Review of the repressive laws against homosexuals was overdue, but it took a long time. It began in 1957 with the report of the Wolfenden Committee on Homosexual Offences and Prostitution, which recommended that sexual acts performed in private between men over the age of 21 should no longer be criminal offences. This proposal was greeted with expressions of outrage by the popular press and, sadly, by many doctors. Even the comment in the British Journal of Venereal Diseases was chilly:

> "The Committee's analysis of homosexuality, homosexual behaviour and homosexual offences has led to recommendations that are unacceptable to many[11]."

Those who could think rationally about the subject often saw homosexuality as a pathological state, perhaps requiring treatment with the object of achieving "cure". This was brought out in a leading article on the Wolfenden report in *The Lancet*:

> "The claim of doctors to be heard on homosexuality is weakened by deep divisions of opinion within the profession. To the psychiatric wing homosexuality is a medical disorder, but at the opposite extreme there are doctors to whom homosexual behaviour is the abominable offence – in the realm of morals, not medicine[12]."

Nevertheless, the recommendations became law in the Sexual Offences Act of 1967. Ten years later a proposal that the age of consent should be reduced from 21 to 18 excited so much opposition that it was dropped.

Despite these legal reforms, prejudice against homosexuals persisted, and in defence a "gay rights" movement developed, first in the USA and later in many other countries. Its members publicly expressed anger at the stigmas of "illness" and "perversion" often directed at them by the medical profession. At the same time, sexual activity within the group increased. While some homosexual men lived in stable single-partner relationships, many did not and some were very promiscuous. It would be a mistake to regard this as a new phenomenon – in 1922 a German physician reported the case of a homosexual man who admitted sex with 965 men[13] – but from the 1960s onwards the number of new infections in homosexual men steadily increased. For example, in London at this time 20 per cent of gonorrhoea and 70 per cent of early syphilis was acquired homosexually. As well as syphilis and gonorrhoea, viral infections such as hepatitis B and a variety of bowel pathogens, including *Entamoeba histolytica*, *Giardia lamblia*, *Salmonella* and *Shigella* spp, transmitted through oral – anal contact, were present. The diagnosis and treatment of these varied conditions presented a challenge to physicians working in this field. Doctors learned new approaches to patients who had adopted a sexual life-style with which they were for the most part unfamiliar, and as they did so earlier concepts of homosexuality as a disease requiring treatment were abandoned.

The scope of venereology was increasing. The speciality had been built on a major disease of outstanding interest and importance – syphilis – and to a lesser extent on other sexually transmitted infections: gonorrhoea, chancroid, herpes and so on. In the 1970s there were some physicians, particularly in Britain, who argued that this viewpoint had become too narrow. Sexual activities promoted a range of genito-urinary ailments, both infective and non-infective in nature. Patients would benefit if they could receive at the same clinic advice on not only venereal infections but problems like vaginal discharge, genital dermatoses and psychosexual difficulties. In Britain a new name for the speciality, genito-urinary medicine, was proposed which, it was hoped, would reflect these ideas and carry less social stigma. This proposal triggered another vituperative debate between venereologists of different persuasions; some feared that attention would be diverted from the prime purpose of a clinic, i.e. the diagnosis and treatment of venereal diseases, towards problems which were the proper concern of other specialities. Eventually the name "genito-urinary medicine" was adopted in Britain, and the concept of total patient care for sexually associated conditions was gradually put into practice. Most European countries, however, adhered to the traditional "dermato-venereology".

HIV Infection

In 1981 there was a new and unexpected event which was to transform the practice of venereology: the first cases of an apparently new illness in American homosexuals were described[14]. It spread rapidly, and received the acronym AIDS in 1982. Although homosexuals were predominantly affected, the disease was not confined to them, as cases were soon identified in haemophiliacs, recipients of blood transfusions, intravenous drug abusers and a few heterosexuals. This distribution made it probable that AIDS was due to a sexually transmissible infectious agent and the first of these, a retrovirus called HIV-1, was identified by the virologist Luc Montagnier in Paris in 1983. A second virus, HIV-2, was identified in some patients with AIDS in West Africa in 1986. In some ways the debate about the origin of HIV paralleled nineteenth century discussions of the origin of syphilis. Some commentators suggested that the viruses might have existed for centuries, causing sporadic cases and minor epidemics which remained undiagnosed until in recent times more virulent strains appeared. Others suggested that a mutant of an existing simian retrovirus, pathogenic to man, appeared in Africa and later reached first North American homosexual men and subsequently other homosexual groups before fanning out into the general population. It was soon realised that there was a major epidemic of AIDS in central Africa, and that in that area heterosexual transmission was the commonest route of infection; this was to be the pattern in other developing countries as the epidemic progressed.

Many commentators have been tempted to compare the initial outbreak of HIV infection with that of syphilis. Both infections appeared suddenly and spread rapidly, are sexually transmitted, involve adults and babies and often end fatally. There the comparisons end, because the social, cultural and medical milieux in which they occurred are totally different. But there are similarities between *reactions* to the two great epidemics. Just as syphilis had been regarded as a punishment for sin, AIDS was now seen as a result of sexual deviance and promiscuity, and just as prostitutes were held responsible for the epidemic of syphilis homosexual men were held responsible for AIDS – the "gay plague". In both cases there were atavistic proposals that infected subjects should be banished to a remote place, or locked up. Historians of the social aspects of medicine have pointed out that the control of these infections by compulsion has never been successful[15]. In Britain the Contagious Diseases Acts of the 1860s, directed against prostitutes, did not reduce the spread of infection and caused endless trouble from pressure groups; they had to be repealed. In both the World Wars of this century legal regulations directed at women with the object of protecting soldiers from infection were likewise unsuccessful. They were aberrations. The Royal Commission laid down that while control by a voluntary and collaborative effort might be possible, it would never be achieved by compulsion. Unfortunately, as the German philosopher Georg Hegel (1770–1831) remarked:

> "What experience and history teach is this – that nations and govern-
> ments have never learned anything from history, or acted upon any
> lessons they might have drawn from it[16]."

Governments and individuals have to accept that coercive measures have never been effective in the control of sexually transmitted diseases. Moreover, in the (unlikely) event of a cure for HIV infection being discovered it should not be assumed that this would end the epidemic; gonorrhoea has continued to flourish despite half a century of effective antimicrobials. A prophylactic HIV vaccine is a chimera. There remains only health education, with its goal of "behaviour modification". Experience between the two World Wars showed many such efforts simply added to the fear of infection and to discrimination against its victims[17]. Other programmes – for example those directed at soldiers in the First World War, which had a particular emphasis on prophylaxis – were somewhat more successful. A too broadly conceived health education programme has little hope of changing people's sexual habits, but "behaviour modification" may be achieved by messages which are accurately directed at people most at risk, explicit and easily understood. It will be for future historians of medicine to decide whether these approaches have been successful.

HIV infection presents medical and social problems of daunting complexity, and it has had a profound effect on venereology. It is providing the same human, clinical and scientific challenges as were at one time provided by syphilis. Earle Moore's valedictory remarks about the old infection apply exactly to the new one:

"But syphilis! . . . Here was an infectious disease of the most fascinating interest . . . It demanded a broad knowledge of internal medicine and more than a bowing acquaintance with dermatology, ophthalmology, neuropsychiatry, pathology, immunology, chemotherapy, epidemiology and public health . . . This infectious disease offered avenues of investigation and research interest unmatched by any other infection[18]."

Because of the public health importance of HIV infection, funds have been provided by many health care authorities for clinical and supportive services. The importance of not allowing attention to be diverted from other sexually transmitted diseases has been shown recently by an unexpected marked increase in both adult and congenital syphilis in many parts of the USA[19]. In developing countries the control of venereal diseases, particularly those which cause genital ulceration, is an important part of AIDS prevention programmes. The capacity of these infections to cause trouble has been shown again and again over the centuries, and must never be forgotten.

Envoi

Twentieth century venereology began well. In 1903 Metchnikoff and Roux succeeded in inoculating monkeys with syphilis, in 1905 Schaudinn and Hoffmann discovered *T. pallidum*, in 1906 Wassermann, Neisser and Bruck developed the first blood test for syphilis, and in 1910 Ehrlich and Hata introduced arsphenamine. Many further clinical, scientific and therapeutic advances followed, culminating in the appearance of penicillin in 1943. Recently, as has been shown in this chapter, things have gone badly wrong and the century is ending with HIV infection casting a dark shadow of uncertainty over doctors and fear over the general public.

It is impossible to predict the future, but can we learn anything from studying the past? For good medical practice it is the recent literature which matters. Henry Ford made this point in another context with his famous remark: "History is more or less bunk. It's tradition. We don't want tradition, we want to live in the present". Yet to read the history of venereology – the successes and failures, the slow growth of ideas, the emergence of the truth, the occasional flashes of inspiration – helps in the development of that "scepticism, supported by a healthy philosophy" (the expression is Swediaur's) which is a virtue in any medical worker. Furthermore, reading about our predecessors engenders hope. They struggled with problems, no less intractable at their time than ours are today, which eventually yielded to human ingenuity, knowledge and organisation. So will ours, but we must also hope that future practitioners in this old and rewarding speciality will retain the breadth of clinical experience of Jonathan Hutchinson, the wit and panache of Philippe Ricord and the insight and human understanding of Benjamin Bell.

Chronology of Events

Venereology		World Events	
1493	First cases of syphilis		
		1517	Luther at Wittenberg
1530	Fracastoro: *Syphilis sive morbus Gallicus*		
1553	Paracelsus: oral mercury		
		1642	English Civil War
1736	Astruc: *De morbis veneris*		
		1776	American Declaration of Independence
1786	Hunter: *A treatise on the venereal disease*		
		1789	French Revolution
1793	Bell: *Treatise on gonorrhoea virulenta and lues venerea*		
		1814	Battle of Waterloo
1831	Ricord appointed to l'Hôpital du Midi		
1836	Donné discovers *T. vaginalis*		
1836	Wallace introduces iodides for syphilis		
1852	Bassereau separates chancroid from syphilis		

(*continued*)

Venereology	World Events
	1854–
	1856 Crimean War
1857–	
1860 Hutchinson's triad	
	1861–
	1865 American Civil War
	1870–
	1871 Franco-Prussian War
1876 Fournier appointed to l'Hôpital St Louis	
1876 Noeggerath: *Latent gonorrhoea*	
1879 Neisser discovers gonococcus	
1889 Ducrey discovers *H. ducreyi*	
	1899–
	1902 Second Anglo-Boer War
1905 Schaudinn and Hoffmann discover *T. pallidum*	
1906 Wassermann reaction	
1907 Halberstaedter and von Prowazek discover *C. trachomatis*	
1910 Ehrlich and Hata introduce arsphenamine	
1913–	
1916 Royal Commission on Venereal Diseases	
	1914–
	1918 First World War
1917 Von Jauregg introduces malaria treatment of general paresis	

(*continued*)

Venereology	*World Events*
	1917 Russian Revolution
1921 Sazerac and Levaditi introduce bismuth	
1937 Domagk introduces sulphon-amides	
	1939–1945 Second World War
1943 Fleming, Florey and Chain introduce penicillin	
1948 Introduction of tetracyclines	
	1950–1953 Korean War
	1964–1973 Vietnam War
1981 First cases of AIDS reported	

References and Recommended Further Reading

Chapter 1. Origins

1. Burnet FM, White DO (1982) Natural history of infectious disease, 4th edn. Cambridge University Press, Cambridge pp 22–31
2. Oriel JD, Hayward AHS (1974) Sexually transmitted diseases in animals. Br J Vener Dis 50: 412–420
3. Fribourg-Blanc A, Niel G., Mollaret MH (1966) Confirmation sérologique et microscopique de la tréponémose du cynocéphale de Guinée. Bull Soc Pathol Exot 59: 54–59
4. Lancereaux E (1868) A treatise on syphilis, vol.1, translated by G. Whitley. New Sydenham Society, London, pp 8–22
5. Willcox RR (1949) Venereal disease in the Bible. Br J Vener Dis 25: 28–33
6. Luys G (1913) Gonorrhoea and its complications, translated by A. Foerster. Baillière Tindall and Cox, London, pp 1–5
7. Rolleston JD (1935) Venereal disease in literature. Br J Vener Dis 11: 147–174
8. Vertue H St H (1953) An enquiry into venereal disease in Greece and Rome. Guys Hosp Rep 102: 277–302
9. Hirsch EW (1930) A historical survey of gonorrhoea. Ann Med Hist 2: 414–423
10. Sudhoff K (1917) The origin of syphilis. Bull Soc Med Hist 2: 1–14
11. Mettler CC (1947) History of medicine. Blakiston, Philadelphia, pp 612–616
12. Roucayrol (1909) Considérations historiques sur la blennorragie. Steinheil, Paris (Quoted Luys G, *op. cit.* (6) p.1)
13. Mesue Junior (Pseudo-Mesue) (Tenth Century; quoted Luys G, *op. cit.* (6) p 3)
14. Anon (1895) John Freind MD. Dictionary of national biography 20: 241–243
15. Power, d'A (1934) Clap and the pox in English literature. Br J Vener Dis 10: 105–113
16. Lanfranchi of Milan (1306) Quoted Mettler CC, *op. cit.* (11) p 617

Recommended Further Reading
Cockburn A (1963) The evolution and eradication of infectious diseases. Johns Hopkins University Press, Baltimore
Bäfverstedt B (1966) How old are the venereal diseases? Acta Derm Venereol Sven Hellerstrom 65 years: 23–25

Chapter 2. The French Disease

1. Cumston CG (1923) Syphilis in the fifteenth and sixteenth centuries, especially at Paris. Br J Dermatol 35: 351–363
2. Creighton C (1891) A history of epidemics in Britain. Cambridge University Press, Cambridge pp 414–438

3. Mettler CC (1947) History of medicine. Blakiston, Philadelphia, pp 618–621
4. Friedenwald H (1939) Francisco Lopez de Villalobos: Spanish court physician and poet. Bull Hist Med 7: 1129–1135
5. Sudhoff K (1917) The origin of syphilis. Bull Soc Med Hist 2: 1–14
6. Moore M, Solomon HC (1935) Joseph Grünpeck and his neat treatise (1496) on the French evil. Br J Vener Dis 11: 1–27
7. Bechet PE (1932) Hieronymus Fracastorius. A brief survey of his life and work on syphilis. Arch Dermatol Syph 26: 888–893
8. Fracastoro G (1546) De morbis contagiosis. Venice. In Lancereaux E (1868) A treatise on syphilis, vol. 1, translated by G. Whitley. New Sydenham Society, London, pp 25–26
9. McNeill WH (1976) Plagues and peoples. Doubleday, New York, p 201
10. Burnett M, White DO (1972) Natural history of infectious disease, 4th edn. Cambridge University Press, Cambridge, pp 16–17
11. Beeson BB (1926) The treatment of syphilis according to Jacques de Bethencourt. Arch Dermatol Syph 14: 427–433
12. Garrison FH (1929) An introduction to the history of medicine, 4th edn. Saunders, Philadelphia and London, pp 196–197
13. Lancereaux E (1868) Op. cit. (8), pp 29–30
14. Goodman H (1944) Notable contributors to the knowledge of syphilis. Froben Press, New York, p 45
15. Paré A (1560) Livre 19, chap 4. Quoted Lancereaux E (1868) Op. cit. (8), pp 125–126
16. Waugh MA (1973) Venereal diseases in sixteenth-century England. Med Hist 17: 192–199
17. Lancereaux E (1868) Op. cit. (8), pp 123–126
18. Oviedo y Valdes, Fernandez de (1535) La general y natural historia de las – Indias, translated by V. Robinson (1938). Br J Dermatol 50: 593–605
19. Las Casas, Fray Bartolome de (1875) Historia de las Indias, translated by V. Robinson (1938). Br J Dermatol 50: 593–605
20. De Isla, Rodrigo Ruiz Diaz (1539) Tractado contra el mal serpentino, translated by V. Robinson (1938). Br J Dermatol 50: 593–605
21. Cole NH, Harkin JC, Kraus BS, Moritz AR (1955) Pre-Columbian osseous syphilis. Arch Dermatol 71: 231–238
22. Harrison LW (1959) The origin of syphilis. Br J Vener Dis 35: 1–7
23. Holcomb RC (1936) Ruiz Diaz de Isla and the Haitian myth of European origin of syphilis. Med Life 41: 535–541
24. Pusey WA (1933) The history and epidemiology of syphilis. Thomas, Springfield, Ill. p 22
25. Robinson V (1938) Did Columbus discover syphilis? Br J Dermatol 50: 593–605
26. Petronius, Alexander Trajanus (1565) Quoted Melville CH (1906). In: Power d'A, Murphy JK (eds) A system of syphilis, vol 6. Oxford University Press, London, p 8
27. Gaddesden, John of (1492) Rosa anglica, quatuor libris distincta, Pavia. Translated by C.C. Mettler (1947) History of medicine. Blakiston, Philadelphia, p 615
28. Gordon, Bernard de (1496) Quoted Lancereaux E (1868) Op. cit. (8), p 20
29. Hudson EH (1958) Non-venereal syphilis, a sociological and medical study of bejel. Livingstone, Edinburgh
30. Hollander DH (1981) Treponematosis from pinta to venereal syphilis: hypothesis for temperature determination of disease patterns. Sex Transm Dis 8: 34–37

Recommended Further Reading

Bloch I (1908) The history of syphilis. In: Power d'A, Murphy JK (eds) A system of syphilis, Oxford University Press, London, pp 3–25
Sudhoff K (1917) The origin of syphilis. Bull Soc Med Hist 119: 1–14

Cripps DJ, Curtis AC (1967) Syphilis maligna praecox. Arch Intern Med 119: 411–418
Morton RS (1968) A new look at the Morbus Gallicus. Br J Vener Dis 44: 174–177

Chapter 3. "Mr Hunter's singular opinions": Early and Experimental Syphilis

1. Astruc J (1737) A treatise on the venereal disease, 2 vols, translated by W Barrowby. London
2. Kemp JE (1940) Outline of the history of syphilis. Am J Syph 24: 759–799
3. Shorter Oxford dictionary (1973) 3rd edn. Oxford University Press, Oxford
4. Boerhaave H (1751) Praelectiones academicae de lue venerea. Leyden
5. Mettler CC (1947) History of medicine. Blakiston, Philadelphia, p 641
6. Qvist G (1981) John Hunter 1728–1793. Heinemann, London, pp 29–41
7. Hunter J (1786) A treatise on the venereal disease. For the Author, London
8. Power d'A (1931) Hunterian oration 1925. John Hunter: a martyr to science. In: Selected writings 1877–1930. Clarendon Press, Oxford, pp 1–28
9. Lancereaux E (1868) A treatise on syphilis, vol 1, translated by G. Whitley. New Sydenham Society, London, pp 77–78
10. Ibid., vol 2 p 219
11. Proksch JK (1908) Quoted Bloch I. In: Power d'A, Murphy JK (eds) A system of syphilis, vol 1. Oxford University Press, London, p 32
12. Paget S (1897) John Hunter, man of science and surgeon. Fisher Unwin, London, p 126
13. Bell B jr (1868) The life, character and writings of Benjamin Bell, FRCSE, FRSE. Edmonston and Douglas, Edinburgh, pp 31–32
14. Ibid., p 104
15. Bell B (sr) (1793) A treatise on gonorrhoea virulenta and lues venerea, 2 vols. James Watson and Company, Edinburgh
16. Bell B jr (1868) Op. cit. (13), pp 114–115
17. Hernandez JL (1812) Essai analytique sur la non-identité des virus gonorrhéique et syphilitique. JJ Paschoud, Toulon
18. Lane JE (1934) Francois-Xavier Swediaur 1748–1824. Arch Dermatol Syph 29: 80–91
19. Kelly M (1967) Swediaur: the vicious anti-Hunter rheumatovenereologist. Med Hist 11: 170–174
20. Colles A (1837) Practical observations on the venereal disease and the use of mercury. Sherwood, Gilbert and Piper, London
21. Anon (1836) Colles on the venereal disease. Lancet ii: 23
22. Wallace W (1837) Clinical lectures and remarks delivered on diseases of the skin, venereal diseases and surgical cases at the Skin Infirmary and at the Jervis Street Hospital, Dublin. Lancet ii: 534–540
23. Widdess JDH (1965) William Wallace (1791–1837). Br J Vener Dis 41: 9–14
24. Oriel JD (1989) Eminent venereologists 3. Philippe Ricord. Genitourin Med 65: 388–393
25. Ricord P (1838) Traité pratique des maladies vénériennes ou recherches critiques et experimentales sur l'inoculation appliquée à l'étude de ces maladies. Rouvier et le Bouvrier, Paris, pp 5–198
26. Proksch JK (1928) Quoted Jacobi A, Lessons of medical history. Med Life 35: 404
27. Lancereaux E (1868) Op. cit. (9), vol 2, p 219
28. Beeson BB (1930) Philippe Ricord MD 1800–1889. Arch Dermatol Syph 22: 1061–1068
29. Stillians AW (1938) Syphilisation. An episode in the evolution of syphilology. Arch Dermatol Syph 37: 272–278
30. Ricord P (1856) Lettres sur la syphilis, 2nd edn. Paris, p 348

31. Lancereaux E (1868) Op. cit. (9), vol 2, p 245
32. Anon (1889) Death of M. Ricord. Br Med J ii: 939
33. Ricord P (1856) Quoted Crissey JT, Parish LC (1981) The dermatology and syphilology of the nineteenth century. Praeger, New York, p 141
34. Gousselin L (1843) De la valeur symptomatique des ulcerations du col utérin. Arch Gen de Méd 2: 129–146
35. Anwyl Davis T (1931) Primary syphilis in the female. Oxford University Press, London, p 46
36. Lancereaux E (1868) Op. cit. (9), vol 2, pp 238–243
37. Zimmermann EL (1938) Extragenital syphilis as described in the early literature (1497–1524) with special reference to focal epidemics. Am J Syph Gonorrhea Vener Dis 22: 757–780
38. Hutchinson J (1877) Illustrations of clinical surgery, vol l. Churchill, London, pp 113–140
39. Gray H (1921) History of lumbar puncture (rachicentesis). Arch Neurol Psychiat 6: 61–69
40. Lawrence WS (1830) On the venereal diseases of the eye. London
41. Hutchinson J (1896) Syphilis. Cassell, London, p 31
42. Willcox RR, Goodwin PG (1971) Nerve deafness in early syphilis. Br J Vener Dis 47: 401–405
43. Metchnikoff E, Roux E (1903–5) Études experimentales sur la syphilis. Ann Inst Pasteur 17: 809–821; 19: 673 (English translation in Selected essays (1906), New Sydenham Society, London, pp 85–95)
44. Neisser A (1911) Beiträge zur Pathologie und Therapie der Syphilis. Springer, Berlin
45. Crissey JT, Parish LC (1981) The dermatology and syphilology of the nineteenth century. Praeger, New York, p 355

Recommended Further Reading

Hutchinson J (1886) Syphilis. Cassell, London
Metchnikoff E (1908) Discovery of the spirillum of syphilis. In: Power d'A, Murphy JK (eds) A system of syphilis, vol 1. Oxford University Press, London, pp 52–59
Crissey JT, Parish LC (1981) The dermatology and syphilology of the nineteenth century. Praeger, New York

Chapter 4. "He sees syphilis everywhere": Late Syphilis

1. Lancereaux E (1868) A treatise on syphilis, 2 vols. translated by G. Whitley. New Sydenham Society, London, p 210
2. Lambert M (1983) Jan Fryderyk Knolle's forgotten dissertation on osseous syphilis. Sex Transm Dis 10: 36–40
3. Rolleston JD (1934) Venereal disease in literature. Br J Vener Dis 10: 147–174
4. Bell B (1793) A treatise on gonorrhoea virulenta and lues venerea, vol 2. James Watson, Edinburgh, p 128
5. Hunter J (1786) A treatise on the venereal disease. London
6. Ricord P (1838) Traité pratique des maladies vénériennes. de Just, Rouvier et le Bouvier, Paris
7. Virchow R (1858) Über die Natur der constitutionell syphilitischen Affectionen. Virchows Arch Pathol Anat 15: 217–336
8. Kampmeier R (1981) Clarification of the systemic manifestations of syphilis, especially in the tertiary stage. Sex Transm Dis 8: 82–84
9. Schonfeld W (1939) Friedrich Wilhelm Felix von Baerensprung (1822–1864). Urol Cutan Rev 43: 470–475
10. Wilks S (1863) On the syphilitic affections of internal organs. Guys Hosp Rep 9: 1–64

11. Paré A (1564) Treatise on surgery. Quoted Osler W (1909) Syphilis and aneurysm. Br Med J ii: 1509–1513
12. Lancisi GM (1728) De motu cordis et aneurysmatibus. Naples. Quoted Osler W, op. cit. (11)
13. Welch FH (1876) On aortic aneurysm in the army and conditions associated with it. Med-Chir Trans 41: 59–77
14. Bloomfield AL (1958) A bibliography of internal medicine: communicable diseases. University of Chicago Press, Chicago, p 318
15. Conner LA (1934) Development of knowledge concerning role of syphilis in cardiovascular disease. JAMA 102: 575–581
16. Heubner O (1874) Die luetische Erkrantung der Hinarterien. Leipzig
17. Beeson BB (1924) Alfred Fournier, his life and works. Arch Dermatol Syph 10: 297–303
18. Crissey JT, Parish LC (1981) The dermatology and syphilology of the nineteenth century. Praeger, New York, p 261
19. Romberg MH (1846) Lehrbuch der Neurokrankheiten des Menschen. A Drucker, Berlin. Translated by E.H. Sieveking, New Sydenham Society, London
20. Argyll Robertson, D (1869) On an interesting series of eye symptoms in a case of spinal disease. Edinb Med J 14: 696
21. Garrison FH (1929) An introduction to the history of medicine, 4th edn. Saunders, Philadelphia, pp 637–639
22. Bloomfield AL (1958) Op. cit. (14), pp 314–315
23. Moore M, Solomon HC (1934) Contributions of Haslam, Bayle and Esmarch and Jessen to the history of neurosyphilis. Arch Neurol Psychiat 32: 804–839
24. Mettler CC (1947) History of medicine. Blakiston, Philadelphia, p 574
25. Fournier A (1897) Syphilis and general paralysis. In: Selected essays and monographs. New Sydenham Society, London, pp 375–392
26. Mott FW (1899) Observations upon the aetiology and pathology of general paralysis. Arch Neurol 1: 166–203
27. Anon (1926) Obituary, Frederick Mott KBE, MD, FRCP, LlD, FRS. Lancet i: 1228–1230
28. Noguchi H, Moore JW (1913) A demonstration of *Treponema pallidum* in the brain in cases of general paresis. J Exp Med 17: 232–238
29. Oriel JD (1990) Eminent venereologists 4: Jonathan Hutchinson. Genitourin Med 66: 401–406
30. Hutchinson J (1879) An address on syphilis as an imitator. Br Med J i: 499–501, 541–542
31. Hutchinson J (1909) Syphilis, new edn. Introduction.
32. Godlee R (1925) Sir Jonathan Hutchinson FRS, 1828–1913. Br J Ophthalmol 9: 257–281

Recommended Further Reading

Lancereaux E (1868) A treatise on syphilis, 2 vols. Translated by G. Whitley. New Sydenham Society, London
Mott FW (1910) Neurosyphilis. In: Power D'A, Murphy JK (eds) A system of syphilis, vol 2. Oxford University Press, London
Dickson Wright A (1971) Venereal disease and the great. Br J Vener Dis 47: 295–306

Chapter 5. "The sins of the fathers": Congenital Syphilis

1. Hunter J (1786) A treatise on the venereal disease. London, pp 291–292
2. Bell B (1793) A treatise on gonorrhoea virulenta and lues venerea, vol 2. Watson, Mudie and Murray, Edinburgh, p 416

3. Doyon A (1894) Notice nécrologique sur P Diday. Ann Dermatol Syph 5: 53–57
4. Diday P (1859) A treatise on syphilis in new-born children and infants at the breast, translated by G. Whitley. New Sydenham Society, London
5. Barlow T (1877) Enlargement of the spleen and heart in a case of congenital syphilis. Trans Pathol Soc Lond 28: 353
6. Lawrence W (1830) Quoted by Chance B (1926) Sir William Lawrence. Ann Med Hist 8: 270
7. Hutchinson J (1861) Clinical lecture on heredito- syphilitic struma and on the teeth as a means of diagnosis. Br Med J i: 515–517
8. Hutchinson J (1859) On the different forms of inflammation of the eye consequent on inherited syphilis. Ophth Hosp Rep and J Royal Lond Ophth Hosp 1: 244; 2: 54–105, 258–283
9. Hutchinson J, Hughlings Jackson J (1861) Cases of deafness associated with syphilis. Med Times Gaz 2: 530–531
10. Hutchinson J (1863) A clinical memoir on certain diseases of the eye and ear consequent on inherited syphilis. Churchill, London, p 174–177
11. Moon H (1876) On irregular and defective tooth development. Trans Odont Soc Gr Br (new series) 9: 223–243
12. Hutchinson J (1958) On the means of recognising the subjects of inherited syphilis in adult life. Med Times Gaz, Sept 11: 264–265
13. Lancereaux É (1869) A treatise on syphilis: historical and practical, 2 vols, translated by G. Whitley. New Sydenham Society, London, pp 139–178
14. Colles A (1951) Practical observations on the venereal disease and on the use of mercury. Sherwood, London
15. Profeto G (1865) Sulla sifilide per Allattamento. Lo sperimentale 15: 328, 339–418
16. Kassowitz M (1875) Die Vererbung der Syphilis. Med Jb Wien, pp 359–495
17. Wegner FRG (1870) Ueber hereditare knochensyphilis bei jungen Kindern. Virchows Arch Pathol Anat 50: 305–322
18. Parrot J (1872) Sur une pseudo-paralysie causée par une alteration du système osseux chez les nouveau-nés atteints de syphilis héréditaire. Arch de Physiol Norm et Pathol 4: 319
19. Parrot JM (1879) The osseous lesions of congenital syphilis. Lancet i: 696–698
20. Taylor RW (1875) Syphilitic lesions of the osseous system in infants and young children. William Wood, New York
21. Clutton HH (1886) Symmetrical synovitis of the knee in hereditary syphilis. Lancet i: 391–393
22. Hutchinson J (1896) Syphilis. Cassell, London, p 76
23. Hochsinger C (1904) Studien über hereditare Syphilis, 2 vols. Franz Deuticke, Vienna
24. Thomsen O (1907) Abstract from Danish in Jb Kinderheilk 66: 125
25. Levaditi C, Sauvage (1905) Sur un cas de syphilis héréditaire. C R Soc Biol 59: 374
26. Dressler W (1854) Quoted Nabarro D (1954) Congenital syphilis, Edward Arnold, London, p 247
27. Donath J, Landsteiner K (1904) Ueber paroxysmale Hämoglobinuria. Münch Med Wochenschr 51: 1590–1593
28. Clouston TS (1877) A case of general paralysis at the age of sixteen years. J Ment Sci 23: 419
29. Mott FW (1899) Notes of 22 cases of juvenile general paresis with 16 post-mortem examinations. Arch Neurol 1: 250–327
30. Hutchinson J (1896) Op. cit. (22), p 223
31. Warthin AS (1911) Congenital syphilis of the heart. Am J Med Sci 141: 398–411
32. Turnbull HM (1915) Alterations in arterial structure and their relation to syphilis. Q J Med 8: 201–254
33. McDonald S (1934) Syphilitic aortitis in young adults with special reference to a congenital aetiology. Br J Vener Dis 10: 183–201

34. Hutchinson J (1906) The transmission of syphilis to the third generation. Med Press 82: 110–112
35. Golay J (1947) De l'hérédo-syphilis paternelle a la syphilis conceptionnelle (From paternal inherited syphilis to conceptional syphilis) Bull Hyg 22: 185

Recommended Further Reading

Still GF (1908) Congenital syphilis. In: Power d'A, Murphy JK (eds) A system of syphilis. Henry Frowde, Hodder and Stoughton, London, pp 281–368
Hutchinson J (1909) Syphilis (new edn). Cassell, London
Nabarro D (1954) Congenital syphilis. Edward Arnold, London

Chapter 6. *Spirochaeta Pallida*: The Microbiology of Syphilis

1. Donné MA (1836) Animalcules observés dans les matières purulentes et le produit des sécrétions des organes genitaux de l'homme et de la femme; extrait d'une lettre de MA Donné. C R Acad Sci Paris 3: 385–386
2. Trussell RE (1947) *Trichomonas vaginalis* and trichomoniasis. Blackwell, Oxford, p 103
3. Hohne O (1916) *Trichomonas vaginalis* als haufliger Erreger einer typischen Colpitis purulenta. Zentralb f Gynak 40: 4–15
4. Metchnikoff A (1906) Historical account of researches on the microbiology of syphilis. In: Power d'A, Murphy JK, A system of syphilis, vol 1. Oxford University Press, London, pp 43–51
5. Stokes JH (1931) Schaudinn: a biographical appreciation. Science 74: 502–506
6. Blumenthal FL (1959) Erich Hoffmann MD, 1868–1959. Arch Dermatol 80: 595–596
7. Schaudinn F, Hoffmann E (1905) Vorläufiger Bericht über das Vorkommen von Spirochaeten in syphilitischen Krankheitsprodukten und bei Papillomen. Arb K Gesundhamt 22: 527–534. English translation in: Selected essays on syphilis and smallpox. New Sydenham Society, London (1906), pp 3–15
8. Winkler A (1987) Dermatology in Berlin – a retrospective view. In: Herzberg JJ, Kortin GW (eds) On the history of German dermatology. Grosse Verlag, Berlin: p 139
9. Levaditi C, Manouelian Y (1906) Histologie pathologique de la syphilis expérimentale du singe dans ses rapports avec le *Spirochaeta pallida*. C R Soc Biol 60: 304–306
10. Noguchi H, Moore JW (1913) A demonstration of *Treponema pallidum* in the brain in cases of general paralysis. J Exp Med 17: 232–238
11. Castellani A (1905) On the presence of spirochaetes in two cases of ulcerated parangi (yaws). Br Med J ii: 1280, 1330–1331
12. Noguchi H (1911) Cultivation of pathogenic *Treponema pallidum*. JAMA 57: 102
13. Willcox RR, Guthe T (1966) *Treponema pallidum*. A bibliographical review of the morphology, culture and survival of T. *pallidum* and associated organisms. Bull WHO 35 (Suppl), Geneva
14. Reiter H (1960) An account of the so-called Reiter treponeme. Br J Vener Dis 36: 18–20
15. Wassermann A, Neisser A, Bruck C (1906) Eine serodiagnostische Reaktion bei Syphilis. Dtsch Med Wochenschr 32: 745–746
16. Wassermann A, Plaut F (1906) Ueber das Vorhandensein syphilitischer Antistoffe in der Cerebrospinalflussigkeit von Paralytikern. Dtsch Med Wochenschr 32: 1769
17. Neisser A (1911) On modern syphilotherapy. In: Bull Hist Med (1944) 16: 469–510
18. Gray H (1921) History of lumbar puncture. Arch Neurol Psychiat 6: 61–69
19. Ellis AWM, Swift HF (1913) The cerebrospinal fluid in syphilis. J Exp Med 18: 162

20. Gillert K-E (1981) In: Dictionary of scientific biography, vol 15. Scribner, New York, pp 521–524
21. Kampmeier RH (1983) The evolution of the flocculation screening test for syphilis. Sex Transm Dis 10: 156–159
22. Nelson RA, Mayer MM (1949) Immobilisation of *Treponema pallidum* in vitro by antibody produced in syphilitic infection. J Exp Med 89: 369–393
23. King A (1964) Recent advances in venereology. Churchill, London, pp 162–220

Recommended Further Reading

Metchnikoff A (1906) Discovery of the spirillum of syphilis. In: Power d'A, Murphy JK (eds) A system of syphilis, vol 1. Oxford University Press, London, pp 52–59
Hollander A (1955) Fiftieth anniversary of the discovery of *Spirochaeta pallidum*. Arch Dermatol 71: 289–292
Bloomfield AL (1958) A bibliography of internal medicine and communicable diseases, section 18: Syphilis part 2. University of Chicago Press, Chicago, pp 322–339

Chapter 7. "For one pleasure a thousand pains": The Treatment of Syphilis

1. Abramowitz EW (1934) Historical points of interest on mode of action and ill effects of mercury. Bull NY Acad Med 10: 695–705
2. Von Hutten U (1519) The remarkable medicine guaiacum and the cure of the Gallic disease, translated by C.W. Mendell. Arch Dermatol Syph (1931) 23: 409–428, 681–704, 1045–1063
3. Lancereaux E (1868) A treatise on syphilis, vol 1, translated by G. Whitley. New Sydenham Society, London, pp 283–302
4. Kemp JE (1940) An outline of the history of syphilis. Am J Syph Gonorrhea Vener Dis 24: 759–779
5. Zimmermann EL (1934) The early pathology of syphilis, especially as revealed by accounts of autopsies of syphilitic corpses (1497–1563). Janus 38: 37–69
6. Garrison FH (1929) An introduction to the history of medicine, 4th edn. Saunders, Philadelphia, pp 204–207
7. Boag Watson, WN (1972) The bagnio at St Thomas' Hospital. Guys Hosp Rep 121: 199–204
8. Lane JE (1934) Francois Xavier Swediaur. Arch Dermatol Syph 29: 80–91
9. Rose T (1817) Observations on the treatment of syphilis with an account of several cases of that disease in which a cure was effected without mercury. Med-Chir Trans 8: 550
10. Doyon A (1883) Karl von Sigmund. Ann Dermatol Syph 4: 121–122
11. Lang E (1887) The therapy of syphilis. J Cutan Genitourin Dis 5: 97–98
12. Gilmour AJ (1908) The hypodermic treatment of syphilis. NY State J Med 8: 535–539
13. Fournier A (1858) Leçons sur le chancre professées par le Docteur Ricord. Paris, A Delahaye. Translated by A.L. Bloomfield (1858) A bibliography of internal medicine: communicable diseases. University of Chicago, pp 310–311
14. Colles A (1837) Practical observations on the venereal disease and the use of mercury. Sherwood, Gilbert & Piper, London, p 77
15. Wallace W (1835) Treatment of the venereal disease by the hydriodate of potash, or iodide of potassium. Lancet ii: 5–11
16. Hayes R (1917) The intensive treatment of syphilis and locomotor ataxia by Aachen methods, 2nd edn. Baillière Tindall & Cox, London
17. Hutchinson J (1887) Syphilis. Cassell, London, p 57
18. Montgomery Hyde H (1986) A tangled web: sex scandals in British politics and society. Constable, London, pp 100–105

19. Nuttall GHF (1924) Paul Ehrlich. Parasitology 16: 224–229
20. Dolman CE (1981) Paul Ehrlich. In: Dictionary of scientific biography, vol 4. Scribner, New York, pp 295–305
21. Ehrlich P, Hata S (1910) Die experimentelle Chemotherapie der Spirillosen. Julius Springer, Berlin.
22. Neisser A, Kuznitsky E (1910) Ueber die Bedeutung des Ehrlich'schen Arsenobenzols fur die Syphilisbehandlung. Berlin Klin Wochenschr 47: 1485–1490
23. Kampmeier RH (1977) Introduction of Salvarsan. Sex Transm Dis 4: 66–68
24. Meltzer SJ (1910) Dioxydiaminoarsenobenzol or "606", Ehrlich's newest remedy for syphilis. NY Med J 92: 371–372
25. Schreiber E (1912) Ueber Neosalvarsan. Munch Med Wochenschr 59: 905–907
26. Jokl E (1954) Paul Ehrlich – man and scientist. Bull NY Acad Med 30: 968–975
27. Marquardt M (1949) Paul Ehrlich. Heinemann, London
28. Almkvist J (1938) Reminiscences of Paul Ehrlich. Urol Cutan Rev 42: 214–220
29. Almkvist J (1920) Re continuous treatment of syphilis instead of chronic intermittent treatment. Acta Derm-Vener (Stockh) 1: 97–108
30. Moore JE, Keitel A (1926) The treatment of early syphilis. I. A plan of treatment for routine use. Bull Johns Hopkins Hosp 39: 1–15
31. Moore JE (1947) Penicillin in syphilis. Blackwell, Oxford, p 3
32. Sazerac R, Levaditi C (1921) Traitement de la syphilis par le bismuth. C R Acad Sci Paris 173: 338–339
33. Moore JE (1941) Modern treatment of syphilis. Baillière Tindall & Cox, London, p 42
34. Wagner von Jauregg J (1921) Die Behandlung der progressiven Paralyse und Tabes. Wien Med Wochenschr 71: 1106, 1210
35. King AC, King AJ (1990) Strong medicine. Churchman Publishing, Worthing and Folkestone, p 1086
36. Moore JE (1941) Op. cit. (33), pp 581–588
37. Selwyn S (1980) The Beta-Lactam antibiotics. Hodder and Stoughton, London, pp 4–11
38. Mahoney JF, Arnold RC, Harris A (1943) Penicillin treatment of early syphilis – a preliminary report. Am J Publ Hlth 33: 1387–1391
39. Syphilis Study Section, National Institutes of Health (1947) The status of penicillin in the treatment of syphilis. JAMA 136: 873–879
40. Pillsbury DM (1945) Penicillin therapy of early syphilis. Br J Vener Dis 21: 139–147
41. Curtis AC, Kitchen DK, O'Leary PA et al. (1951) Penicillin treatment of syphilis. JAMA 145: 1223–1226
42. Jarisch A (1895) Therpeutische Versuche bei Syphilis. Wien Med Wochenschr 45: 722–724
43. Herxheimer K, Krause (1902) Ueber eine bei syphilitischen vorkommende Quecksilberreaction. Dtsch Med Wochenschr 28: 895–897
44. Gjestland T (1955) The Oslo study of untreated syphilis: an epidemiologic investigation of the natural course of syphilitic infection based on a restudy of the Boeck – Bruusgaard material. Acta Derm-Vener (Suppl 34) 35: 1–368
45. Rockwell DH (1964) The Tuskegee study of untreated syphilis. Arch Intern Med 114: 792–797

Recommended Further Reading

Lancereaux E (1868) A treatise on syphilis, vol 2, translated by G. Whitley. New Sydenham Society, London, pp 283–351
Moore JE (1941) Modern treatment of syphilis. Baillière Tindall and Cox, London
Kampmeier RH (1976) Syphilis therapy: an historical perspective. J Am Vener Dis Assoc 3: 99–108

Jones JH (1981) Bad blood: the Tuskegee syphilis experiment. The Free Press, McMillan Publishing, New York

Chapter 8. Chancroid and Donovanosis

1. Lanfranchi (Lanfranc of Milan) (1490) Chirurgia magna et parva, Venice. Translated by C.C. Mettler (1947) History of medicine, Blakiston, Philadelphia, p 617
2. Fergusson W (1813) Observations on the venereal disease in Portugal. Medico-surg Trans 4: 10
3. Hunter J (1786) A Treatise on the Venereal Disease. London, pp 215–221
4. Bell B (1793) A Treatise on Gonorrhoea Virulenta and Lues Venerea, vol 2. Watson Mudie and Murray, Edinburgh, p 13
5. Carmichael R (1825) An essay on the venereal diseases. London. Quoted Lancereaux E (1868) A treatise on syphilis, vol 1, translated by G. Whitley. New Sydenham Society, London, p 97
6. Ricord P (1838) Traité pratique des maladies vénériennes. Paris
7. Merklen P (1887) Leon Bassereau. Ann Dermatol Syph 8: 683–685
8. Bassereau L (1852) Traité des affections de la peau symptomatiques de la syphilis. J-B Baillière, Paris, p 197. Translated by A.L. Bloomfield (1958) A bibliography of internal medicine. University of Chicago Press, Chicago pp 309–310
9. Clerc F-F (1855) Considérations nouvelles sur la chancre infectant et le chancroid. Union Med 9: 509
10. Pellerat J (1947) A great figure of French syphilology; Joseph Rollet (of Lyon). Urol Cutan Rev 51: 551–556
11. Rollet J (1861) Recherches cliniques et expérimentales sur la syphilis, le chancre simple et la blennorrhagie. J-B Baillière et fils, Paris
12. Lancereaux E (1868) A treatise on syphilis. Op. cit. (5), pp 95–117
13. Bumstead FJ, Taylor RW (1883) The pathology and treatment of venereal diseases, 5th edn. Henry C. Lea's Sons, Philadelphia pp 344–345
14. Zinsser F (1870) The doctrines of unicism and dualism of the syphilitic contagion. Am J Syph Dermatol 1: 220–239
15. Bumstead FJ, Taylor RW (1883) Op. cit. (13), pp 48–49
16. Ducrey A (1889) Experimentelle Untersuchungen über der Austeckungsstoff des weichen Schenkers und über die Bubonen. Mschr Prakt Derm 9: 387
17. Unna PG (1892) Der Streptobacillus des weichen Schankers. Mschr Prakt Derm 14: 24
18. Sullivan M (1940) Chancroid. Am J Syph 24: 482–521
19. Ito T (1913) Klinische und bacteriologische Studien über Ulcus Molle und Ducreysche Streptobazillen. Arch Dermatol Syph 116: 341–374
20. Greenblatt RB, Sanderson ES (1938) The intradermal chancroid bacillary antigen test as an aid in the differential diagnosis of the venereal bubo. Am J Surg 41: 384–392
21. McEntegart MG, Hafiz S, Kinghorn GR (1982) Haemophilus ducreyi infections: time for reappraisal. J Hygiene (Camb) 89: 467–478
22. King A (1964) Recent advances in venereology. Churchill, London, pp 295–303
23. Greenblatt RB (1943) The management of chancroid, granuloma inguinale and lymphogranuloma venereum in general practice. United States Public Health Service, Washington, D.C., Venereal disease information, suppl 19
24. Anon (1922) Obituary: Kenneth MacLeod. Br Med J ii: 1246
25. MacLeod K (1882) Precis of operations performed in the wards of the First Surgeon, Medical College Hospital, during the year 1881. Indian Med Gaz 17: 113–123
26. Galloway J (1897) Ulcerating granuloma of the pudenda. Br J Dermatol 9: 133–147
27. Anon (1951) Obituary: Charles Donovan. Br Med J ii: 1158, 1286

28. Donovan C (1905) Medical cases from Madras General Hospital: ulcerating granuloma of the pudenda. Indian Med Gaz 40: 414
29. Anderson K, de Monbreun WA, Goodpasture EW (1945) An etiologic consideration of *Donovania granulomatis* cultivated from granuloma inguinale (three cases) in embryonic yolk. J Exp Med 81: 25–39
30. King A (1964) Op. cit. (22) pp 335–336
31. Goldberg J (1964) Studies on granuloma inguinale. VII. Br J Vener Dis 40: 140–145

Recommended Further Reading

Lancereaux E (1868) A treatise on syphilis, translated by G. Whitley. New Sydenham Society, London, pp 97–108
Zinsser F (1879) The doctrines of unicism and dualism of the syphilitic contagion. Am J Syph Dermatol 1: 220–239

Chapter 9. Gonorrhoea Virulenta

1. Le Monnier L (1689) Nouveau traité de la maladie vénérienne et tous les accidents qui la précedent et qui l'accompagnent; avec la plus seure et la plus facile méthode de les guerir. Amable Auroy, Paris. Translation: Readings in the history of gonorrhoea. Med Life (1932) 39: 487–504
2. Lane JE (1919) Daniel Turner and the first degree of doctor of medicine conferred in the English colonies of North America by Yale College in 1723. Ann Med Hist 2: 367–380
3. Turner D (1732) Syphilis, a practical dissertation on the venereal disease, 4th edn. Wilkin, Bonwicke et al. London
4. Hunter J (1786) A treatise on the venereal disease, 2nd edn. London, pp 32–34
5. Bell B (1793) A treatise on Gonorrhoea Virulenta and Lues Venerea, vol 1. Watson, Mudie and Murray, Edinburgh, p 100
6. Spencer FJ (1986) Byrd's "running". Bull NY Acad Med 62: 918–922
7. Turner D (1714) De morbis cutaneis. Bonwicke, Freeman, Goodwin et al. London, p 217
8. Heister L (1757) A general system of surgery, vol 2. London, pp 148–149
9. Willcox RR (1951) Views on the treatment of venereal disease in the early nineteenth century as reflected in the writings of Samuel Cooper. Br J Vener Dis 27: 179–182
10. Swediaur F (1805) Traité complet sur les symptomes, les effects, la nature et le traitement des maladies syphilitiques. Chez l'auteur, Paris. Translation: Readings in the history of gonorrhoea. Op. cit. (1) pp 487–504
11. Ricord P (1848) Lectures on venereal and other diseases arising from sexual intercourse. III. Blennorrhagia. Lancet ii: 484–485
12. Ricord P, quoted Taylor RW (1895) The pathology and treatment of venereal diseases. Lea Bros, Philadelphia, p 102
13. Norris CC (1913) Gonorrhoea in women. Saunders, Philadelphia and London, pp 29–31
14. Ricord P, quoted Wolbarst AL (1942) Gonorrhoea one hundred years ago. Med Rec 155: 134–139
15. Stark JN (1903) A retrospect and prospect in obstetrics and gynaecology. Glasgow Med J 59: 1–26
16. Ricord P (1848) Lectures on venereal and other diseases arising from sexual intercourse. XII. Vaginal blennorrhagia. Lancet i: 144–147
17. Von Bumm E (1887) Der Mikro-organismus der Gonorrhoischen Schleimhaut-Erkrankungen "Gonococcus-Neisser". Bergmann, Wiesbaden. In: Readings in the history of gonorrhoea. Op. cit. (1), pp 553–568
18. Bernutz G, Goupil E (1862) Clinique médicale sur les maladies des femmes, vol 2. F Chamerot, Paris, p 140

19. Noeggerath E (1876) Latent gonorrhoea, especially with regard to its influence on fertility in women. Trans Am Gyn Soc 1: 268–300
20. Neisser A (1879) Ueber eine der Gonorrhoe eigentümliche Micrococcusform. Centralb Med Wochensch 17: 497–500
21. Quelmaltz ST (1740) De caecitate infantum fluoris albi materni ejusque virulanti pedisseque dissertatione. Leipzig
22. Gibson B (1807) On the common cause of the puriform ophthalmia of new-born children. Edinburgh Med Surg J 3: 159–161
23. Norris CC (1913) Gonorrhoea in women. Op. cit. (12), pp 376–379
24. Pauli of Landau (1854) In: Stephenson S (1907) Ophthalmia neonatorum. George Pulman, London, pp 28–29
25. Stephenson S (1907) Op. cit. (23), pp 1–21
26. Leopold G (1891) Carl Siegmund Franz Credé, Gedachtnissende. Arch Gynaek 42: 193–212
27. Credé CSF (1883) Die Verhütung der Augenentzündung der Neugeborenen. Arch Gynaek 21: 179–195

Recommended Further Reading

Bell B (1793) A treatise on Gonorrhoea Virulenta and Lues Venerea, vol 1. Watson, Mudie and Murray, Edinburgh
Luys G (1913) A textbook on gonorrhoea and its complications. Baillière Tindall and Cox, London
Readings in the history of gonorrhoea. Med Life (1932) 39: 475–588

Chapter 10. Gonorrhoea after Neisser

1. Oriel JD (1989) Albert Neisser. Genitourin Med 65: 229–234
2. Neisser A (1879) Ueber eine der Gonorrhoe eigentümliche Micrococcusform. Centralb Med Wochenschr 17: 497–500
3. Neisser A (1882) Die Micrococcen der Gonorrhoe. Dtsch Med Wochenschr 8: 279–282
4. Leistikow (1882) Ueber Bacterien bei den venerischen Krankheiten. Charité Ann 7: 750–772
5. Bockhart M (1883) Beitrag zur Aetiologie und Pathologie des Harnröhrentrippers. Vrtlschr für Derm und Syph 10: 3–18
6. Von Bumm E (1885) Der Micro-organismus der gonorrhoischen Schleimhaut-Erkrankung, "Gonococcus-Neisser." J.E. Bergmann, Wiesbaden
7. Wertheim E (1891) Reinzüchtung des Gonococcus Neisser mittels des Platten-verfahrens. Dtsch Med Wochenschr 17: 1351–1352
8. Elser WJ, Huntoon FM (1909) Studies of meningitis. J Med Res 20: 371–541
9. Barlow R (1899) Urethritis non-gonorrhoica: eine kritische Studie. Dtsch Arch Klin Med 66: 444–469
10. Diday P, Doyon (1876) Mal vén et cutanées, p 129. Quoted Bumstead FJ, Taylor RW (1883) The pathology and treatment of venereal diseases, 5th edn. Henry C Lea's Sons, Philadelphia, p 234
11. Bumstead FJ, Taylor RW (1883) Op. cit. (10), pp 211–212
12. Oldershaw HL (1929) Outbreak of gonorrhoea in a residential boys' school. Br J Vener Dis 5: 302–303
13. Welander (1884) Pathogenen Mikro-parasiten der Gonorrhöe. Verhandlungers des Vereins der Ärzte zu Stockholm (Oct 1883). Quoted Norris CC (1913) Gonorrhoea in women. Saunders, Philadelphia, p 39
14. Arning E (1883) Ueber das Vorkommen von Gonococcen bei Bartholinitis. Vrtljschr Derm Syph 10: 371–375

15. Orton JJ (1896) Rectal gonorrhoea and gonorrhoeal endometritis. Med News (NY) 68: 408–409
16. Norris CC (1913) Op. cit. (13), p 395
17. von Bumm E (1884) Beitrag zur Kentniss der Gonorrhoe der weiblichen Genitalien. Arch Gynaecol 23: 327–348
18. Wertheim E (1932) Ascending gonorrhoea in the female. Bacteriologic and clinical studies. Med Life 39: 573–583
19. Stephenson S (1907) Ophthalmia neonatorum. George Pulman, London, pp 34–36
20. Pott R (1883) Die specifische Vulvo-Vaginitis in Kindesalter und ihre Behandling. Jahrb Kinderh 19: 71–78
21. Fraenkel E (1885) Bericht über eine bei Kindern beobachtete Endemie infectioser Colpitis. Virchows Arch Pathol Anat 99: 251
22. Holt LE (1905) Gonococcus infections in children with especial reference to their prevalence in institutions and means of prevention. NY Med J 81: 521–526, 589–592
23. Brown DK (1930) Vulvo-vaginitis in children. Br J Vener Dis 6: 285–300
24. Petrone LM (1883) Sulla natura parasitaria dell' artrite blennorrhagica. Riv Clin di Bologna 3: 94–113
25. Höck H (1893) Ein Betrag zur Arthritis blennorrhoica. Wien Klin Wochenschr 6: 736–738
26. Hewes HF (1894) Two cases of gonorrhoeal rheumatism with specific bacterial organisms in the blood. Boston Med Surg J 131: 515–516
27. Vidal E (1893) Éruption généralisée et symmétrique de croûtes cornées, avec chute des ongles, d'origin blennorrhagique coincident avec une polyarthrite de même nature. Ann Dermatol Syph (Paris) 4: 3–11
28. Buschke A (1899) Ueber exantheme bei Gonorrhoe. Arch Dermatol Syph (Wien) 48: 181–204
29. Thayer WS (1896) On the cardiac complications of gonorrhoea. Johns Hopkins Hosp Bull 7: 57
30. Thayer WS (1922) On the cardiac complications of gonorrhoea. Johns Hopkins Hosp Bull 33: 361–372
31. Valentine FC (1900) The irrigation treatment of gonorrhoea. William Wood, New York
32. Harrison LW (1949) Half a lifetime in the management of venereal diseases. Med Illust 3: 318–324
33. Valentine FC (1900) Op. cit. (31), p 159
34. Stecher RM, Solomon WM (1936) The treatment of gonorrhoeal arthritis with artificial fever. Am J Med Sci 192: 497–517
35. Neisser A (1900) Gonorrhoea: its dangers to society. Med News NY 76: 41–45, 85–89
36. Harrison LW (1931) The diagnosis and treatment of venereal diseases in general practice, 4th edn. Humphrey Milford, Oxford University Press, Oxford p 332
37. Kampmeier RH (1983) Introduction of suphonamide therapy for gonorrhoea. Sex Transm Dis 10: 81–84
38. Leading article (1944) Sulphonamide-resistant gonorrhoea. Lancet ii: 693–694
39. Wainwright M, Swan HT (1986) CG Paine and the earliest surviving clinical records of penicillin therapy. Med Hist 30: 42–56
40. Leading Article (1944) Penicillin in gonorrhoea. Lancet i: 345–346

Recommended Further Reading

Norris CC (1913) Gonorrhoea in women. Saunders Co, Philadelphia, pp 17–43
Harrison LW (1955) Neisser and neisserian principles in venereology. Br J Vener Dis 31: 65–73

Bloomfield AL (1958) A bibliography of internal medicine: communicable diseases section. 11: Gonorrhoea and gonococcal infection. University of Chicago, Chicago, pp 184–193

Chapter 11. Viruses and Chlamydiae

1. Beswick TSL (1962) The origin and use of the word herpes. Med Hist 6: 214–232
2. Turner DA (1714) Of the herpes: a treatise of diseases incident to the skin. Bonwicke, London, pp 48–49
3. Astruc J (1736) De morbis veneris, vol 1, translated by W. Barrowby London, p 420
4. Bateman T (1813) A practical synopsis of cutaneous diseases. Longman, London
5. Alibert JL (1832) Monographie des dermatoses. Daynac, Paris, p 89. Quoted Hutfield DC (1966) History of herpes genitalis. Br J Vener Dis 42: 263–267
6. Greenough FB (1881) Herpes progenitalis. Arch Dermatol 7: 1–29
7. Boret M de (1838) Considérations pratiques sur quelques maladies de la peau: herpès phlyctenoide, herpès preputialis. J Méd Chir Prat (Paris) 9: 347–348
8. Unna PG (1883) On herpes progenitalis, especially in women. J Cutan Vener Dis 1: 321–334
9. Du Castel (1901) Herpès: Le pratique dermatologique, tome II. Masson, Paris, pp 814–815
10. Bumstead FJ, Taylor RW (1883) The pathology and treatment of venereal diseases, 5th edn. Henry C Lea's Sons, Philadelphia, pp 271–274
11. Diday P, Doyon A (1886) Les herpès genitaux. Masson, Paris
12. Unna PG (1896) The histopathology of diseases of the skin, translated by N. Walker. McMillan, New York
13. Levaditi C (1922) Ectodermoses neurotropes. Masson, Paris, p 225
14. Lipschütz B (1921) Untersuchungen über die Aetiologie der Krankheiten der Herpesgruppe (Herpes zoster, Herpes genitalis, Herpes febrilis). Arch Dermatol Syph 136: 428–482
15. Goodpasture EW (1929) Herpetic infection with especial reference to involvement of the nervous system. Medicine 8: 223–243
16. Sharlit H (1940) Herpes progenitalis as a venereal contagion. Arch Dermatol 42: 933–936
17. Legendre F (1853) Mémoire sur l'herpès de la vulve. Arch Gén Méd 2: 171
18. Batignani A (1934) Congiuntivite da virus erpetico in neonato. Bull Ocul 13: 1217–1220
19. Hass M (1935) Hepatoadrenal necrosis with intranuclear inclusion bodies: report of a case. Am J Pathol 11: 127–142
20. Bäfverstedt B (1967) Condylomata acuminata – past and present. Acta Dermatol Vener (Stockh) 47: 376–381
21. Dionysius (sixth century AD) Quoted Hyde CD (1917) Condyloma acuminatum in the anal region in the male. NY Med J 106: 1125–1126
22. Lanfranc (of Milan) (1400) Quoted Hudson EH (1961) Historical approach to the terminology of syphilis. Arch Derm 84: 545–562
23. Hunter J (1786) A treatise on the venereal disease. London, p 250
24. Dease W (1776) Observations on venereal warts. Medical and Philosophical Commentaries 4: 335–347
25. Bell B (1793) A treatise on Gonorrhea Virulenta and Lues Venerea, vol 1, James Watson and Co, Edinburgh, pp 405–415
26. Jourdan A-J-L (1826) Traité complet des maladies vénériennes. Mecuignon-Marvis, Paris, pp 185–190
27. Lancereaux E (1868) A treatise on syphilis, vol 1, translated by G. Whitley. New Sydenham Society, London, pp 179–180

28. Wharton LR (1921) Rare tumours of the cervix of the uterus of inflammatory origin – condyloma and granuloma. Surg Gynecol Obst 33: 145–153
29. Cooper, A (1835) Lectures on the principles and practice of surgery, 8th edn, Cox and Portwine, London, pp 497–498
30. Gémy (1893) Quoted Frei E (1924) Zur Frage der aetiologischen Beziehung der Warzen und spitzen Kondylome. Schweiz Med Wochenschr 5: 215–219, 239–243
31. Frei E (1924) Op. cit. (30)
32. Bumstead FJ (1864) The pathology and treatment of venereal diseases. Blanchard and Lea, Philadelphia, p 230
33. Kranz (1867) Beitrag zur Kenntniss des Schleimhaut-papillomas. Dtsch Arch Klin Med 2: 79–88
34. Heller J (1921) Zur frage der Kontagiosität der spitzen Kondylome. Derm Zeit 34: 342–344
35. Harkness AH (1950) Non-gonococcal urethritis. Livingstone, Edinburgh, pp 166–170
36. Barrett TJ, Silbar JD, McGinley JF (1954) Genital warts – a venereal disease. JAMA 154: 333–334
37. Parnell JG (1929) Observations upon the venereal lesions of the rectum and anus. J Roy Nav Med Serv 15: 77–84
38. Smith RR (1903) A case of condyloma acuminatum in an infant. Am Gynecol 3: 515–517
39. Goldman L, Clarke GE (1940) Infectious papilloma (so-called condyloma acuminatum) with genital, perineal and lip lesions in a three-year-old child. Urol Cutan Rev 44: 677–678
40. Kaplan IW (1942) Condylomata acuminata. N Orleans Med Surg J 94: 388–390
41. Halberstaedter L, von Prowazek S (1907) Ueber Zelleinschlüsse parasitärer Natur beim Trachom. Arb K GesundhAmt 26: 44–47
42. Heymann B (1910) Uber die Fundorte der Powazekschen Koperchen. Berl Klin Wochenschr 47: 663–666
43. Lindner K (1910) Zur Atiologie der gonokokkenfreien Urethritis. Wien Klin Wochenschr 23: 283–284
44. Fritsch H, Hofstatter O, Lindner K (1910) Experimentelle Studien zur Trachomfrage. Albrecht von Graefe's Arch Ophthalmol 76: 547–558
45. Waelsch L (1904) Uber nicht-gonorrhoische urethritis. Arch Derm Syph Wien 70: 103–124
46. Thygeson P (1934) The etiology of inclusion blennorrhoea. Am J Ophthalmol 17: 1019–1034
47. Thygeson P, Stone W (1942) Epidemiology of inclusion conjunctivitis. Arch Ophthalmol 27: 91–122
48. Harrison LW, Worms W (1939) The relation between some forms of non-gonococcal urethritis, lymphogranuloma inguinale, trachoma and inclusion blennorrhoea: a critical review. Br J Vener Dis 15: 237–259
49. Moulder JW (1963) The psittacosis group as bacteria (CIBA lecture in microbial biochemistry). Wiley, New York
50. King AJ (1970) A. H. Harkness FRCS 1889–1970. Br J Vener Dis 46: 511
51. T'ang F-F, Chang H-L, Huang Y-T, Wang K-C (1957) Trachoma virus in chick embryo. Nat Med J China 43: 81–86
52. Jones BR, Collier LH, Smith CH (1959) Isolation of virus from inclusion blennorrhoea. Lancet i: 902–905
53. Dunlop EMC, Jones BR, Al-Hussaini MK (1964) Genital infection in association with TRIC virus infection of the eye. III. Clinical and other findings: preliminary report. Br J Vener Dis 40: 33–42
54. Dunlop EMC, Harper IA, Al-Hussaini MK et al. (1966) Relation of TRIC agent to "non-specific" genital infection. Br J Vener Dis 42: 77–87
55. Gordon FB, Quan Al (1965) Isolation of the trachoma agent in cell culture. Proc Soc Exp Biol Med 118: 354–359

56. Hunter J (1786) Op. cit. (23), p 265
57. Wallace WP (1833) Treatise on venereal disease and its varieties. Burgess and Hill, London, p 371
58. Ricord P (1838) Traité pratique des maladies vénériennes, Paris, p 149
59. Klotz HG (1890) Über die Entwicklung der sogennanten strumösen Bubonen und die frühzeitige Extirpation der selben. Berl Klin Wochenschr 27: 132, 153, 175
60. Durand M, Nicolas J, Favre M (1913) Lymphogranulomatose inguinale subaiguë d'origine génitale probable peut-être vénérienne. Bull Soc Méd Hôp 35: 274
61. Godding CC (1896) On non-venereal bubo. Br Med J ii: 842 (also 1897, i: 1475)
62. Frei W (1925) Eine neue Hautreaktion bei lymphogranuloma inguinale. Klin Wochenschr 4: 2148–2150
63. Desruelles H (1844) Observations dhypertrophie particulière de la vulve. Arch Gén de Méd series 4a, 4: 314
64. Huguier PC (1849) Mémoire sur l'esthiomène, ou dartre rongeante de la région vulvo-anale. Mém Acad Natl Méd 14: 501–596
65. Fournier A (1881) Leçons cliniques sur la syphilis, Paris, p 536 *et seq*
66. Stannus HS (1933) A sixth venereal disease. Baillière Tindall and Cox, London, pp 170–178
67. Koch F (1933) Experimentale untersuchungen über das Lymphogranuloma inguinale. Derm Ztschr 65: 207–227
68. Jones H, Rake G, Stearns B (1945) Studies on lymphogranuloma venereum. III. The action of sulfonamides on the agent of lymphogranuloma venereum. J Infect Dis 76: 55–69
69. Bell B (1797) A treatise on gonorrhoea virulenta and lues venera, vol 1. Watson Mudie and Murray, Edinburgh, p 416
70. Brodie BC (1818) Pathological and surgical observations on diseases of the joints. Longman, London, pp 51–63
71. Launois MP (1899) Arthropathies récidevantes: amyotrophie généralisée, troubles trophiques multiples (cornes cutanées, chute d'un ongle) d'origine blennorrhagique. Bull Mem Soc Méd Hôp Paris 16: 736–744
72. Reiter H (1916) Ueber eine bisher unerkannte Spirochäteninfektion (*Spirochaetosis arthritica*). Dtsch med Wochenschr 42: 1535–1536
73. Schachter J, Dawson CR (1978) Human chlamydial infections. PSG Publishing, Littleton, Mass., pp 141–152
74. Harkness AH (1949) Reiter's disease. Br J Vener Dis 25: 185–199
75. Keat A (1983) Reiter's syndrome and reactive arthritis in perspective. New Engl J Med 309: 1606–1615
76. Brewerton DA, Caffrey M, Nicholls A et al. (1973) Reiter's disease and HLA 27. Lancet ii: 996–998

Recommended Further Reading

Cumston CG (1926) The history of herpes from the earliest times to the 19th century. Ann Med Hist 8: 284–291
McNair Scott TF (1986) Historical aspects of *Herpes simplex* infections. Int J Derm 25: 63–70, 127–134
Oriel JD (1971) Natural history of genital warts. Br J Vener Dis 47: 1–13
Schachter J, Dawson CR (1978) Human chlamydial infections. PSG Publishing, Littleton, Mass

Chapter 12. Venereologists and Others

1. Roberts RS (1969) The first venereologists. Br J Vener Dis 45: 58–60
2. Waugh MA (1971) Attitudes of hospitals in London to venereal disease in the 18th and 19th centuries. Br J Vener Dis 47: 146–150

3. Lees R (1961) The "lock" wards of Edinburgh Royal Infirmary. Br J Vener Dis 37: 187–189

4. Waugh MA (1973) Venereal diseases in sixteenth century England. Med Hist 17: 192–199

5. Adler MW (1980) The terrible peril: a historical perspective on the venereal diseases. Br Med J ii: 206–211

6. Action W (1857) Prostitution considered in its moral, social and sanitary aspects in London and other large cities, with proposals for the mitigation and prevention of its attendant evils. Churchill, London, p 142

7. Fessler A (1951) Venereal disease and prostitution in the reports of the Poor Law Commissioners 1834–1850. Br J Vener Dis 28: 154–157

8. Fessler A (1949) Advertisements on the treatment of venereal disease and the social history of venereal disease. Br J Vener Dis 25: 84–87

9. Solly S (1868) In: Report of the Committee appointed to enquire into the pathology and treatment of the venereal disease with the view to diminish its injurious effects on the men of the Army and Navy. Her Majesty's Stationery Office, London (Cd 4031)

10. Power d'A (1934) Venereal disease in literature (discussion). Br J Vener Dis 10: 176

11. Wickham L (1889) The organisation of instruction in dermatology and syphilis in Great Britain. J Cutan Genito-Urin Dis 7: 225–228

12. Anon (1851) Review of W. Acton's "Practical treatise of the urinary and generative organs in both sexes." British and Foreign Medico-Chirurgical Review 8: 203

13. King A (1974) The life and times of Colonel Harrison. Br J Vener Dis 50: 391–403

14. Harrison LW (1949) Half a lifetime in the management of venereal diseases. Med Illust 3: 318–324, 376–385

15. Harrison LW (1934) The design of venereal diseases treatment centres. Br J Vener Dis 10: 223–232

16. Davenport-Hines R (1991) Sex, death and punishment. Collins, London, pp 251–254

17. Fluker JL (1990) Personal reminiscences of a venereologist before penicillin. Int J STD AIDS 1: 443–446

18. Cullis WC (1937) Mary Scharlieb. Dictionary of national biography 1922–1930, Oxford University Press, London, 749–751

19. Morton RS (1991) Did Catherine the Great of Russia have syphilis? Genitourin Med 67: 498–502

20. Perdrup A (1961) Gonorrhoea in Denmark. Br J Vener Dis 37: 115–118

21. Ackerknecht EH (1967) Medicine at the Paris Hospital 1794–1848. Johns Hopkins Press, Baltimore, pp 174–176

22. Acton W (1850) On the present condition and treatment of venereal diseases in Paris. Lancet ii: 51–53

23. Waugh MA (1977) The Viennese contribution to venereology. Br J Vener Dis 53: 247–251

24. Finger E (1913) Zur Geschlichte der Wiener Schule für Haut-und Geschlecht-krankheiten. Wien Med Wochenschr 63: 2309–2327

25. Clarke W (1936) Professor Ernest Finger today. Am J Syph 20: 562–565

26. Schonfeld W (1939) Friedrich Wilhelm Felix von Baerensprung (1822–1864). Urol Cutan Rev 43: 470–475

27. Neisser A (1890) Ueber den Nutzen und die Notwendigkeit von Spezialkliniken fur Haut- und Venerische Kranke. Klinisches Jahrbuch, vol II, Berlin, pp 194–211

28. Anon (1879) Obituary; Freeman Josiah Bumstead. Med Rec 16: 551–552

29. Fox GH (1920) Anniversary address: New York Dermatological Society. Arch Dermatol 1: 80–89

30. Anon (1934) Morrow, Prince Albert. Dictionary of american biography, Charles Scribner's Sons, New York, pp 236–237

31. Brandt AM (1987) No magic bullet: a social history of venereal disease in the United States since 1880. Oxford University Press, Oxford, p 43
32. Becket PC (1939) The City Hospital: a history of its dermatologic division. Arch Dermatol 39: 674–678
33. King AC, King AJ (1990) Strong medicine. Churchman Publishing, Worthing and Folkestone, p 208
34. Pottle FA (ed) (1950) Boswell's London journal 1762–1763. Heinemann, London, p 157
35. Rolleston JD (1934) Venereal disease in literature. Br J Vener Dis 10: 147–174
36. Bell B (1868) The life, character and writings of Benjamin Bell FRCSE, FRSE. Edmonston and Douglas, Edinburgh, p 112
37. Tilton EM (1947) Amiable autocrat: a biography of Oliver Wendell Holmes. Henry Shuman, New York, p 128
38. Beeson BB (1930) Philippe Ricord MD, 1800–1889. Arch Dermatol Syph 22: 1061–1068
39. Bayly HW (1932) Free treatment at venereal clinics. Lancet i: 1229
40. Anon (1926) Obituary: John Astley Bloxam. Lancet i: 261
41. Stokes JH (1930) The syphilology of today and tomorrow. Arch Dermatol Syph 22: 201–224
42. Anon (1908) Obituary: Sir Alfred Cooper. Br Med J i: 660–661

Recommended Further Reading

Goodman H (1944) Notable contributors to the knowledge of syphilis. Froben Press, New York

Crissey JT, Parish LC (1981) The dermatology and syphilology of the nineteenth century. Praeger, New York

Chapter 13. Public Health Matters

1. Hirsch EW (1930) A historical survey of gonorrhoea. Ann Med Hist 2: 416
2. Norris CC (1913) Gonorrhoea in women. Saunders, Philadelphia and London, pp 21–22
3. Morton RS (1962) Some aspects of the early history of syphilis in Scotland. Br J Vener Dis 38: 175–180
4. Acton W (1857) Prostitution. Considered in its moral, social and sanitary aspects. Churchill, London, pp 142–143
5. Mort F (1987) Dangerous sexualities. Medico-moral politics in England since 1830. Routledge and Kegan Paul, London, pp 75–76
6. Petrie G (1971) A singular iniquity. The campaigns of Josephine Butler. MacMillan, London
7. Osler W (1917) The campaign against venereal disease. Br Med J i: 694–696
8. Morrow PA (1901) Report of the committee of seven of the medical society of the county of New York on the prophylaxis of venereal disease in New York city. NY Med J 74: 1146
9. White D (1912) Discussion on syphilis. Proc Roy Soc Med 5: 143–150
10. Morris M (1913) A plea for the appointment of a Royal Commission on venereal disease. Lancet i: 1817–1819
11. MacCormac H (1947) "A vignette": Sir Malcolm Morris KCVO, FRCSE and John James Pringle MB, FRCP. Urol Cutan Rev 51: 609–612
12. Royal Commission on Venereal Diseases (1916) Final Report of the Commissioners. HMSO, London
13. Reid GA (1920) Prevention of venereal disease. Heinemann, London, p 337
14. Champneys F (1917) The fight against venereal infection. Nineteenth Century 82: 1052–1054

15. Beardsey EH (1976) Allied against sin: American and British responses to venereal diseases in World War I. Med Hist 20: 189–202
16. Harrison LW (1949) Half a lifetime in the management of venereal disease. Med Illust 3: 318–324, 376–385
17. Kitchener HH (1914) A message to the soldiers of the British Expeditionary Force, to be kept by each soldier in his Active Service Pay-book. In: Arthur G (1920) Life of Kitchener, vol 3. Macmillan, London, p 27
18. Leading Article (1916) Venereal disease in the army. Lancet i: 305–306
19. Brandt AM (1987) No magic bullet – a social history of venereal disease in the United States since 1880. Oxford University Press, Oxford, pp 96–121
20. Snow WF, Sawyer (1918) Venereal disease control in the army. JAMA 71: 456–462
21. Thibierge G (1918) Syphilis and the army. University of London Press, London p 170
22. Harrison LW (1931) The diagnosis and treatment of venereal diseases in general practice. Humphrey Milford, Oxford University Press, Oxford, pp 446–448
23. Leading Article (1944) Legislative control of venereal diseases. Lancet ii: 17–18
24. Wigfield AS (1972) 27 years of uninterrupted contact tracing. The "Tyneside scheme." Br J Vener Dis 48: 37–50
25. Special Committee on Venereal Disease (1921) Prevention of venereal disease. Williams and Norgate, London
26. Burke ET (1919) The venereal prevention committee (letter). Br Med J ii: 509–510
27. Brandt AM (1987) Op. cit. (19), p 125
28. Ibid., p 142
29. Leading Article (1943) Prevention of venereal disease in the army. J Army Med Corps 81: 35–37
30. Stokes J (1942) Civilian measures for the control of venereal disease in World War II: discussion. JAMA 120: 882
31. Leading Article (1945) The venereal disease contact. Br J Vener Dis 21: 1
32. Moore JE (1956) Venereology in transition. Br J Vener Dis 32: 217–224

Recommended Further Reading

Marcus S (1966) The other Victorians. Weidenfeld and Nicolson, London
Adler MW (1980) The terrible peril: a historical perspective on the venereal diseases. Br Med J ii: 206–211
Costello J (1985) Love, sex and war. Collins, London
Brandt AM (1987) No magic bullet – a social history of venereal disease in the United States since 1880. Oxford University Press, Oxford
Mort F (1987) Dangerous sexualities – medico-moral politics in England since 1830. Routledge and Kegan Paul, London and New York
Davenport-Hines D (1990) Sex, death and punishment. Collins, London

Chapter 14. No Happy Ending

1. King A (1958) "These dying diseases." Venereology in decline? Lancet i: 651–657
2. Morton RS (1977) Gonorrhoea. Saunders, Philadelphia and London, pp 204–234
3. Phillips I (1976) Beta-lactamase producing, penicillin-resistant gonococcus. Lancet ii: 656–657
4. Mårdh P-A, Ripa T, Svensson L, Weström L (1977) Chlamydia trachomatis infection in patients with acute salpingitis. N Engl J Med 296: 1377–1379
5. Beem MO, Saxon EM (1977) Respiratory tract colonisation and a distinctive pneumonia syndrome in infants infected with Chlamydia trachomatis. N Engl J Med 296: 306–310

6. Naib ZM, Nahmias AJ, Josey WE, Kramer JH (1969) Genital Herpetic infection. Association with cervical dysplasia and carcinoma. Cancer 23: 940–945
7. Solnik B (1926) Ueber syphilitische Primäraffekte am Anus bei Männern und Kindern. Dissertation, Leipzig. Quoted Hinrichson J (1944) op. cit. (9)
8. Taylor RW (1890) Some unusual modes of infection with syphilis. J Cutan Genitourin Dis 8: 201–216
9. Hinrichsen J (1944) The importance of a knowledge of sexual habits in the diagnosis and control of venereal disease, with special reference to homosexual behaviour. Urol Cutan Rev 48: 469–486
10. Jefferiss FJG (1956) Venereal disease and the homosexual. Br J Vener Dis 32: 17–20
11. Leading Article (1957) The Wolfenden report. Br J Vener Dis 33: 205
12. Leading Article (1957) Homosexual offences and prostitution. Lancet ii: 527–529
13. Gaupp R (1922) Das Problem der Homosexualität. Klin Wochenschr 1: 1033–1038
14. Centers for Disease Control (1981) Pneumocystis pneumonia – Los Angeles. Morb Mortal Weekly Rep 30: 250–252
15. Porter R (1986) History says no to the policeman's response to AIDS. Br Med J 293: 1589–1590
16. Hegel GWF (1830) Lectures on the philosophy of world history: introduction, translated by H.B. Nisbet. (1975) Cambridge University Press, Cambridge
17. Brandt AM (1988) AIDS in historical perspective: four lessons from the history of sexually transmitted diseases. Am J Publ Health 78: 367–371
18. Moore JE (1956) Venereology in transition. Br J Vener Dis 32: 217–224
19. Dunn RA, Rolfs RT (1991) The resurgence of syphilis in the United States. Curr Opin Infect Dis 4: 3–11

Recommended Further Reading

Catterall RD (1963) The advance of the venereal diseases. Lancet ii: 103–108
Austoker J (1988) AIDS and homosexuality in Britain: a historical perspective. In: Adler MW (ed) Diseases in the homosexual male. Springer, London, Berlin, Heidelberg, pp 185–197
Grmek MD (1990) History of AIDS, translated by R. C. Maulitz and J. Duffin Princeton University Press, New Jersey

Subject Index